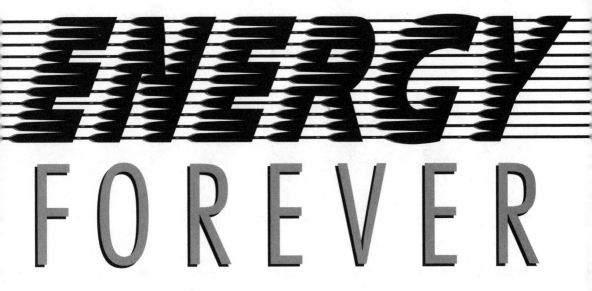

ENERGY FOREVER

MORE THAN 1,000 QUICK AND EASY TIPS AND TECHNIQUES TO BEAT FATIGUE AND *TURBOCHARGE* YOUR LIFE

BY SID KIRCHHEIMER, GALE MALESKEY
AND THE EDITORS OF *PREVENTION* MAGAZINE HEALTH BOOKS

Rodale Press, Inc.
Emmaus, Pennsylvania

Notice

This book is intended as a reference volume only, not as a medical manual. The information given here is designed to help you make informed decisions about your health. It is not intended as a substitute for any treatment that may have been prescribed by your doctor. If you suspect that you have a medical problem, we urge you to seek competent medical help.

 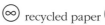
The "Know Your Glycemic Index" table on page 6 was adapted with permission from the *American Journal of Clinical Nutrition*, October 1985; volume 42: page 606.

Library of Congress Cataloging-in-Publication Data

Kirchheimer, Sid.
    Energy forever : more than 1,000 quick and easy tips and techniques to beat fatigue and turbocharge your life / by Sid Kirchheimer, Gale Maleskey and the editors of Prevention Magazine Health Books.
        p.   cm.
    Includes index.
    ISBN 0–87596–321–8 hardcover
    1. Fatigue—Prevention. 2. Medicine, Popular. I. Maleskey, Gale. II. Prevention Magazine Health Books.
RB150.F37K57   1997
613—dc20   96–9342

Distributed in the book trade by St. Martin's Press

2   4   6   8   10   9   7   5   3   1   hardcover

OUR PURPOSE

*"We inspire and enable people to improve
their lives and the world around them."*

Energy Forever *Editorial Staff*

EDITOR: **Alice Feinstein**

SENIOR MANAGING EDITOR: **Edward Claflin**

WRITERS: **Sid Kirchheimer, Gale Maleskey**

CONTRIBUTING WRITERS: **Kathleen N. Beans, Michelle Bisson, Jan Bresnick, Brian Chichester, Philip Goldberg, Ellen Michaud, Peggy Morgan, David Roth**

RECIPE DEVELOPMENT: **Sharon Sanders**

HEAD RESEARCHER: **Bernadette Sukley**

RESEARCHERS AND FACT-CHECKERS: **Elizabeth A. Brown, Carlotta Cuerdon, Christine Dreisbach, Kathryn Piff, Sally A. Reith, Margo Trott**

BOOK DESIGNER: **Vic Mazurkiewicz**

ASSOCIATE ART DIRECTOR: **Faith Hague**

STUDIO MANAGER: **Joe Golden**

TECHNICAL ARTIST: **Thomas P. Aczel**

LAYOUT ARTIST: **Mary Brundage**

COPY EDITOR: **Karen Neely**

PRODUCTION MANAGER: **Helen Clogston**

MANUFACTURING COORDINATOR: **Patrick T. Smith**

OFFICE STAFF: **Roberta Mulliner, Julie Kehs, Bernadette Sauerwine, Mary Lou Stephen**

Rodale Health and Fitness Books

VICE-PRESIDENT AND EDITORIAL DIRECTOR: **Debora T. Yost**

ART DIRECTOR: **Jane Colby Knutila**

RESEARCH MANAGER: **Ann Gossy Yermish**

COPY MANAGER: **Lisa D. Andruscavage**

Albert M. Kligman, M.D., Ph.D.
Professor of dermatology in the School of Medicine at the University of Pennsylvania in Philadelphia and an attending physician at the Hospital of the University of Pennsylvania

Jeffrey R. Lisse, M.D.
Associate professor of medicine and director of the Division of Rheumatology at the University of Texas Medical Branch at Galveston

Jack W. McAninch, M.D.
Chief of urology at San Francisco General Hospital and professor and vice-chairman of the Department of Urology at the University of California, San Francisco

Morris B. Mellion, M.D.
Clinical associate professor of family practice and orthopaedic surgery at the University of Nebraska Medical Center, and medical director of the Sports Medicine Center, both in Omaha

Thomas Platts-Mills, M.D., Ph.D.
Professor of medicine and head of the Division of Allergy and Immunology at the University of Virginia Medical Center in Charlottesville

David P. Rose, M.D., Ph.D., D.Sc.
Chief of the Division of Nutrition and Endocrinology at Naylor Dana Institute, part of the American Health Foundation, in Valhalla, New York, and an expert on nutrition and cancer for the National Cancer Institute and the American Cancer Society

William B. Ruderman, M.D.
Practicing physician, Gastroenterology Associates of Central Florida in Orlando

Yvonne S. Thornton, M.D.
Visiting associate physician at Rockefeller University Hospital in New York City and director of the Perinatal Diagnostic Testing Center at Morristown Memorial Hospital in Morristown, New Jersey

Lila A. Wallis, M.D.
Clinical professor of medicine and director of "Update Your Medicine," a series of continuing medical educational programs for physicians, at Cornell University Medical College in New York City

Andrew T. Weil, M.D.
Associate director of the Division of Social Perspectives in Medicine at the College of Medicine, University of Arizona in Tucson

Richard J. Wood, Ph.D.
Associate professor at the School of Nutrition at Tufts University in Medford, Massachusetts, and chief of the mineral bioavailability laboratory at the U.S. Department Agriculture Human Nutrition Research Center on Aging at Tufts University in Boston

Contents

Introduction ix

Part 1:
The Building Blocks of Energy

Eating for Energy 3

    Recipes for Energy .28

Environments for Energy 51

Exercising for Energy .66

Relationships for Energy 79

Relaxing for Energy 96

Scheduling and Organizing for Energy 107

Sleeping for Energy .116

Part 2:
Instant Energizers

Affirmations 131

Altruism and Volunteering 135

Aromatherapy 138

Bathing 142

Clear Thinking and Decision Making 145

Coffee 150

Daydreams and Fantasy 154

Deep Breathing 156

Forgiveness 158

Gratitude 162

Hugging 165

Journal Writing 168

Laughter 171

Looking out the Window 176

Meditation 180

Music 184

Naps 191

Pets 193

Prayer 197

Sex 202

Smiling 206

Snacks 208

Sunlight 211

Tai Chi 218

Touching 220

Toys 225

Vacations 228

Walking 235

Water 242

Part 3:
Beating the Energy Demons

Aging 247

Alcohol 254

Allergies 259

Boredom 263

Burnout 269

Child Rearing 276

Chronic Disease 283

Chronic Fatigue Syndrome 287

Colds and Flu 298

Commuting 305

Depression 308

Difficult People 312

Entertaining 317

Getting Up in the Morning .322

Grief 326

Headaches 331

Holidays 337

Housecleaning 343

Low Self-Esteem 348

Major Life Changes 353

Medication 357

Meetings 365

Mononucleosis 368

Moving 371

Overweight 374

Poor Posture 378

Pregnancy 385

Premenstrual Syndrome 390

Situational Insomnia 395

Smoking 402

Taxes 409

Teenagers 411

Television 416

Worry 422

Index 427

Introduction

When the editors of *Prevention* Magazine Health Books work many months on a single book, we're likely to get very involved with the subject—so much so that the advice in that book actually becomes a part of our lives and our day-to-day habits. Not surprisingly, that happened quickly when we started working on *Energy Forever*.

I think we're fairly typical of many people who have numerous demands, stresses and obligations. We have families, careers, community commitments, pets, houses, yards and hobbies. Like so many busy people, we often feel as though we don't have time to do everything that needs to be done—much less find fun-time to recharge our batteries.

Well, if you're in that overworked, under-relaxed group, you'll find plenty of help in the pages that follow.

I know this information really worked for me. For instance, it seemed as though I could never find time to try out some new recipes or take a bike ride through the countryside. But as I started doing the research for this book, I realized there might be some lifestyle habits that were whittling away my free time as well as undermining my enthusiasm.

I reconsidered those sugary muffins and the chocolate-laced coffee that I tossed down in the morning: Were the empty calories and shot of caffeine leaving me tired and starved by lunchtime? As for sleeping, what was the real energy cost of staying up 45 minutes past my bedtime to read or talk on the phone? And how about exercise: why was I avoiding it, and why did I often feel so stiff and muscle-bound after putting in time at the gym?

When I started interviewing the experts, I began to get some answers and started to apply some of their advice. Instead of having my usual breakfast, I started my days with some protein and complex carbohydrates and discovered that my energy was still going strong at noon. I cut off the phone and turned out the light at 11:00 P.M. and stopped hating the alarm clock the next morning. I started doing less weight lifting and more yoga and saw my endurance and flexibility—and energy—increase.

And something more. I found that anything that relieves stress and lifts self-doubt also boosts emotional, spiritual and physical energy. I began to look at some of the lifestyle elements that I had never associated with energy—things that the experts say are critically important. Along with nutrition, sleep and exercise, I started paying attention to sunlight, gratitude and affirmations.

I like to take a midday walk during the winter months—but in the past, I always wore dark sunglasses for my midday stroll. When I switched to a brimmed hat and a pair of yellow-tinted clip-ons, my energy took a leap upward. Why? See page 212. You'll learn that you get more of light's energizing effects this way, with less exposure to eye-damaging ultraviolet rays.

Gratitude? Experts say that being grateful allows you to live your life fully, no matter what comes your way. I started saying—and thinking—"thank you" a lot more often and realized how much I had to be thankful for. Sure enough, the release from negativity gave me a payoff—a lot more energy. That's why Gratitude is a full chapter in this book, beginning on page 162.

Affirmations? They're much more than wishful thinking. Affirmations are a way to focus on goals and assert your intentions. The words of affirmation deliver energy to your whole lifestyle. (On page 131, you'll find the affirmations that can have this kind of impact.)

These are the kinds of results you can get from all the energy boosters described in this book. It doesn't take any extra time to adopt these strategies. It only takes a slight bit of planning. And the rewards are enormous.

Certainly, if you're feeling extremely tired all the time, there may be some health problems that you need to discuss with your doctor. But keep in mind, this book offers more strategies than any single doctor ever could. That's because we've interviewed scores of experts in every area—including nutritionists, personal trainers, medical doctors and psychologists, as well as leading experts in industrial efficiency, music, color, sleep, massage, pet therapy, aromatherapy, hydrotherapy, play therapy, time management, sex and parenting. They have willingly shared their practical advice with us—and now with you.

Just read about these ideas, and I promise that you'll come away with dozens of little things that you can do to recharge your batteries. Discover the desk toys that enliven a workday. Try the music that can get your toes tapping. Use dialoguing techniques to renew a friendship. Negotiate more wisely to breathe new life into relationships. You can even discover what color to paint a room for the best overall energizing effect. (Clue: It's in the yellow band of the spectrum.) And along the way, you'll discover how to time your sex life to enhance energy, what lightbulbs to use to give your home an energizing glow and why dogs are more enlivening companions than other pets.

These and hundreds of other creative, practical ideas are in the pages ahead. So here's the best energy advice of all: Take the leap. Turn the pages to discover the experts' secrets. You'll find enough great ideas to keep your energy tuned up forever.

Gale Maleskey
Senior Writer
Prevention Magazine Health Books

1

The Building Blocks of ENERGY

Eating *for Energy*

There's a good reason for putting nutrition at the very front of this book. When it comes to having all the energy that you want, eating the right foods is as basic as getting enough sleep.

Poor nutrition all by itself can deplete energy. "Shortages of iron, vitamin B_{12}, folic acid, magnesium, protein and just about every other essential nutrient can all lead to fatigue," says Joanne Curran-Celentano, R.D., Ph.D., associate professor of nutritional sciences at the University of New Hampshire in Durham. So can eating the wrong foods at the wrong time or eating too much or too little. And what you don't eat is just as important as what you do eat.

Unless you have all the nutritional rules down pat and are following them religiously—which would make you a very rare individual, indeed—there are undoubtedly a number of dietary adjustments that you can make to boost your energy level throughout the day.

Here are the nutrition basics that experts say you need to know for maximum staying power.

Powering Up with Food

Most of us think of food as energy, and it is. Calories—units of energy from food—are burned in your body to provide energy, just as gasoline is combusted in an engine to make a car move, Dr. Curran-Celentano explains. You get calories from every single food you eat—carbohydrates (sugar and starch), fat, even protein.

But it takes more than just calories to produce energy. If calories were the only factor, you could live on sugar, which is almost pure energy, and overweight people would have the most energy of all. Each pound of fat they carry around is actually 3,500 calories' worth of stored energy.

To burn those calories—a process called energy metabolism—requires nutrients. These vital nutrients are the vitamins and minerals found in foods. "Certain nutrients such as some of the B-complex vitamins, magnesium and zinc act as catalysts for calorie burning," Dr. Curran-Celentano explains. "They help to move these chemical reactions along." Other nutrients—chromium, for example—help to transport glucose, or blood sugar, through cell membranes so that it can be burned for energy. You also need iron that delivers the oxygen inside the cells, "fanning the flames" to burn calories.

Many people in this country are overfed and undernourished, experts say. They get too many calories but, often, not enough of the nutrients that are needed to metabolize those calories. These people may be eating too much fat.

Others, following a strict heart-healthy diet, may get too much carbohydrate and too little protein for adequate energy production, says Mary Dan Eades, M.D., director of the Arkansas Center for Health and Weight Control in Little Rock and author of *The Doctor's Complete Guide to Vitamins and Minerals.* "They may even get too little cholesterol and essential fatty acids for optimum energy."

Nutritional experts say that perpetual dieters may be shortchanged on everything that they need to produce adequate amounts of energy—both calories and nutrients—and feel run-down as a result.

But how do you bypass these problems and ensure that your diet is not only healthful but also energizing? Nutrition experts have found a way, and here are some strategies.

Best Choice: Carbohydrates

These days, nutritionists recommend that complex carbohydrates, the stuff called starch and dietary fiber, take up the lion's share of people's plates. That means that you should be getting some 55 to 60 percent of your calories from things like bread, cereal, rice, grains and pasta. For an active woman eating about 2,200 calories a day, for instance, that comes to 8 servings. Servings could include bread (one slice per serving), cold cereal (one ounce per serving) and grains and pasta (one-half cup per serving). Active men need up to 11 servings a day.

Complex carbohydrates are considered the ideal choice as a basic fuel because they are easily converted into glucose, a type of sugar that is the body's main energy supply, explains Henry Hom, M.D., director of nutritional services at the Hoffman Center in New York City, which sees many patients with fatigue problems.

"Most complex carbohydrates take some time to be broken down to glucose, so they provide a steadier, slower burn than sugar," Dr. Hom explains. Some carbohydrates provide additional nutrients needed for energy production.

Here's the best way to pick and choose among the many carbohydrates.

Go for whole grains.

It's true that refined grains such as enriched white flour have added thiamin, niacin, riboflavin and iron. But many of the nutrients are missing from these foods, including some B-complex vitamins and minerals involved in carbohydrate metabolism. Refined grains, including white rice, are also missing fiber, the dietary component that makes sure that your body absorbs carbohydrates at a slow, steady pace.

"Stick mostly with brown rice, whole-wheat bread, oatmeal and whole-grain cereals to get the nutrients you need," recommends Nan Kathryn Fuchs, Ph.D., a nutritionist in Sebastopol, California, and nutrition editor of *Women's Health Letter.*

Turn up the pressure.

Pressed for time? Whole grains take a longer time to cook than refined grains, but you can prepare them faster by using a pressure cooker. Or buy an electric rice steamer that works like a Crock-Pot electric slow cooker. You can time it to start cooking the rice so that it's ready when you get home from work. Or you can cook grains the night before you'll need them.

Also, some health food stores carry faster-cooking versions of whole grains, so you can start meal preparations at the usual time.

Read the fine print on "whole-wheat" breads.

Some breads offer less healthy "wholeness" than their package labels would have you believe. Topping the label list are the main ingredients. So check to make sure that whole-wheat flour tops the list, says Dr. Fuchs. Also, don't trust the food color for assurance of "whole-graininess." Some manufacturers add coloring to their breads and other baked goods to make them look browner and more wholesome.

Go for a slow burn.

Unless you need a quick pick-me-up, you should choose carbohydrates that break down slowly in your body and provide a longer, steady flow of energy rather than a quick burst.

Why does oatmeal satisfy hunger for hours, while cornflakes ward it off for only an hour or two? The answer may be in what's known as their glycemic index; that's the speed at which a food converts to glucose in your body, says Dr. Fuchs. "Foods that convert quickly to glucose provide quick energy that fades fast. Foods that convert more slowly provide energy for longer periods of time."

To help you select the best steady-energy foods, you can check "Know Your Glycemic Index" on page 6. The higher the number, the faster the food converts to glucose. You may be surprised to see that carrots break down as fast as cornflakes, for example.

Know Your Glycemic Index

How fast does the food you eat reach you in the form of energy? It may be important for you to know.

The higher the number in this table, the faster a food converts to glucose—the form of sugar that your body burns to create energy. The numbers refer to the glycemic index—the relative rate at which blood sugar rises after various foods are eaten. A relatively high number translates into a quick energy boost. That may well be what you want. But, for some people, foods that offer quick bursts of energy ultimately cause fatigue by creating big peaks and drops in blood sugar and insulin levels, explains Ronald L. Hoffman, M.D., medical director of the Hoffman Center in New York City and author of *Tired All the Time*. "These people are considered to be sugar- or carbohydrate-sensitive," he says.

Some foods thought of as "good" carbohydrates may not be good for people who are sensitive to them, according to Dr. Hoffman. Baked potatoes, for instance, have a glycemic index that's higher than white bread's. So do carrots and cornflakes. Whole-wheat bread has a high glycemic index, as do millet and white rice. Shredded wheat and raisins have about the same glycemic index. Sucrose (refined sugar) has a lower index than corn-

Food	Glycemic Index (%)
BREADS	
White	100
Whole-wheat	100
Rye	83
CEREAL GRAINS	
Bulgur	65
Barley	31
Spaghetti	66
White rice	83
BREAKFAST CEREALS	
Cornflakes	119
Oatmeal, cooked	85
Shredded wheat	97

Food	Glycemic Index (%)
VEGETABLES	
Green peas	74
Carrots	133
Yams	74
Potatoes	
boiled	81
instant	116
baked	135
Corn	87
LEGUMES	
Red lentils	43
Kidney beans	51
Chick-peas	49
Baked beans	60
Lima beans	115
Peanuts	19

flakes or millet—and ice cream is even lower.

The trick for sugar-sensitive people is to eat carbohydrates like beans, lentils and whole grains such as brown rice, barley, bulgur, rolled oats, amaranth and quinoa, Dr. Hoffman says. These people may need to avoid flour, since it breaks down to glucose quicker than grains eaten as whole kernels. They may also need to eat frequently and consume more carbohydrate-free foods that have a glycemic index of zero: meat, fish, poultry, salad and eggs. (Oils and butter also have a glycemic index of zero, but you'll still want to eat these and other high-fat foods sparingly.)

To use the table, find a food on the left, then move to the right-hand column to find its glycemic index number. If you've found that you tend to be sensitive to sugar—you know, that "up" feeling followed later by a quick drop in energy—then you should choose energy foods with a lower number, says Dr. Hoffman.

The glycemic index measures the rise in blood sugar caused by a specific amount of a particular food compared to the rise caused by a reference food. In this case white bread has been chosen as the reference food and has been assigned a glycemic index of 100 percent.

Food	Glycemic Index (%)
FRUIT	
Apples	.53
Bananas	.79
Cherries	.32
Grapefruit	.36
Grapes	.66
Oranges	.67
Orange juice	.67
Peaches	.40
Pears	.47
Plums	.34
Raisins	.93

Food	Glycemic Index (%)
SUGAR	
Sucrose (table sugar)	.86
DAIRY	
Ice cream	.52
Milk	.49
Yogurt	.52

Choose fast foods with carbs in mind.

Let's face it, you won't always be "brown-ricing" it. So if you're grabbing fast food from the drive-through or sitting down for a quick lunch, steer toward high-carb alternatives, suggests Nancy Clark, R.D., director of nutrition services at SportsMedicine Brookline in Brookline, Massachusetts, and author of *Nancy Clark's Sports Nutrition Guidebook*. Even refined carbohydrates are better energy sources than fatty foods, so think bread and rice. "Order thick-crust instead of thin-crust pizza, submarine rolls rather than pita bread. And at Chinese restaurants have extra rice instead of egg rolls," she suggests.

Make the most of pasta.

Pasta—spaghetti, macaroni, noodles and the like—is low in fat. But since it's usually made from white flour, it doesn't have as many nutrients as you'd get from whole-wheat flour or whole grains.

To pack more nutritional punch into a pasta meal, load on the veggies, Dr. Fuchs suggests. To traditional red sauce add lightly steamed broccoli or escarole, red and green peppers, onions, garlic, mushrooms, zucchini or any other vegetables you like.

Don't carbo-load unless you plan to work it off.

Some professional athletes load up on all the carbohydrates that they can stomach in the days before a competition to boost stores of glycogen—a form of sugar—in their muscles. That lets them go longer before they poop out.

People who work out an hour or less at a stretch should eat adequate but not excessive carbohydrates, Clark says. "For people wanting to lose weight, extra calories from carbohydrates can prevent fat loss," she explains. "Plus, recreational exercisers are unlikely to run low on glycogen unless they exercise strenuously and continuously for more than an hour."

Beware of fat-laden carbs.

Croissants, biscuits, most crackers, potato and corn chips, french fries and processed macaroni and cheese can contain more calories from fat than from carbohydrates. And the same goes for packaged rice pilaf dishes, potatoes au gratin and some breakfast cereals, especially granola. Even pasta is fattening if it's layered with high-fat cheese. Make low-fat versions or eat these dishes only occasionally, if at all, Dr. Fuchs recommends.

Eat Just Enough—No More

We all know what it's like to plow our way through a Thanksgiving meal or an all-you-can-eat buffet. Afterward, we can barely roll home, and once there, a nap usually seems like an excellent idea. On the other hand, most of us also know what it's like to eat only as much food as our bodies require. The meal energizes us; it doesn't drag us down.

Overeating—constantly or occasionally—can cause sluggishness for several reasons. "To aid digestion, your body shunts blood to your intestines," explains Allan Magaziner, D.O., a doctor in private practice in Cherry Hill, New Jersey, who specializes in nutritional medicine and the treatment of chronic fatigue. "That diverts blood away from your muscles and brain, so they can't operate at their best."

Overeating fat sends fat molecules into your bloodstream, increasing the viscosity, or thickness, of blood, says researcher R. James Barnard, Ph.D., professor of physiological science at the University of California, Los Angeles, and consultant to the Pritikin Longevity Center in Santa Monica. The result is that oxygen-carrying red blood cells get sticky and clump up, which reduces your blood's oxygen-delivery capacity.

And if you have eaten an overload of starches and sugar, your brain chemistry changes, making you relaxed and more likely to become sleepy, Dr. Eades says.

"It makes sense that people who frequently overeat would feel sluggish," Dr. Barnard observes. "We see lots of people who overeat and then load up on coffee to try to keep themselves awake. Once people break out of this cycle, they often have more energy."

Here's how to retain control over your intake valve.

Have soup for starters.
Research has shown that people who have a bowl of soup at the beginning of a meal consume fewer calories than those who dive right into the main course. You'll want to pass on high-fat cream soups such as New England clam chowder or lobster bisque. But Manhattan clam chowder is fine, along with most vegetable-based soups. Bean soups are good, too, as long as they're not loaded with salt pork or sausage, says Dr. Fuchs. "And vegetable soups can be as tasty as those with meat, without the fat and salt."

Cinch yourself in.
Wear something that's snug around your waist when you go out to eat, suggests Sachiko T. St. Jeor, R.D., Ph.D., professor and director of the Nutrition Education and Research Program at the University of Nevada School of Medicine in Reno. Your expanding belly will signal when it's time to put your fork down.

Eat regularly throughout the day.
People who gorge at night often skimp on breakfast and lunch, Dr. Fuchs says. "They feel tired during the day, and they're more likely to gain weight eating this way." Being overweight is an energy drainer in itself.

Plan ahead to avoid temptation.

Most of us already know that we can't count on willpower to keep us out of trouble. Planning ahead, however, can help curb cravings that can lead to explosive eating. So plan real meals and healthy snacks, like whole-grain crackers and a slice of fat-free cheese or a piece of fruit. Eat something satisfying before you go mall prowling, where you'll be assailed by the odors of sticky buns and chocolate chip cookies, and take a snack such as almonds, pretzels or fruit juice–sweetened cookies with you. Keep food stashed away in cupboards, not visible on counters or in fully stocked bowls in front of the TV, suggests Dr. Fuchs.

Buy and serve in single portions.

That way, you'll have a built-in finish line. Measure out a half-cup or a one-cup serving to see what it looks like, suggests Clark.

Don't food-shop when you're hungry.

If cheese curls and butterscotch crumpets simply leap into your grocery cart, satisfy your cravings with some small concession before you head out to the supermarket, advises Clark. You'll do less impulse buying.

Cut back on fat at home.

Fat is the most concentrated source of calories, and if you're surrounded by high-fat foods, you're sure to overeat. Buy low-fat dairy products and salad dressings. Use no-stick pans instead of skillets and baking pans that require a lot of oil. And be sure to skim the fat from soups and stews, advises Dr. Fuchs.

Go low-fat—and eat slowly—when you eat fast food.

Your fast-food choices here aren't necessarily between a nice big, juicy burger or a measly, boring salad. They could be grilled chicken, a lean roast beef or turkey sandwich or a vegetarian sub, easy on the mayo. Ask for a pamphlet with nutritional information next time you're eating out. Then, check off the lower-fat food so that you'll be prepared to make choices.

The Ups and Downs of Sugar

Sugar can be a quick pick-me-up, that's for sure. It's broken down fast, so within minutes of eating, blood sugar is on its way to your brain and muscles, providing fuel for pencil pushing and foot stomping. That's why athletes who need a quick energy boost during competition may swill a sugary sports drink. "It's the next best thing to intravenous glucose," Dr. Hom says. It's also why people who do a lot of dreary desk work may call on sugar to perk them up when their brain cells are flagging.

Too much sugar, however, can be an energy drain for anyone. "That's because pure sugar has calories but none of the nutrients that help energy metabolism," says Dr. Magaziner.

Too much sugar can also wreak havoc on people's insulin and blood sugar levels. "This happens to everyone to some degree, but for some people it's a recognizable problem," says Dr. Eades.

These people develop a condition called reactive hypoglycemia. After they have eaten, their blood sugar first rises. Then their insulin levels rise, because their bodies need to secrete insulin in order to move sugar into the bodies' cells. Their insulin outputs last longer than their sugar bursts, and as excess insulin ushers more and more blood sugar into the cells, their glucose levels drop farther than they should. Two to five hours after they have eaten, people with this condition begin to feel spacey—unable to concentrate, weak, sleepy, and sometimes nervous, sweaty or dizzy.

"Sugary meals—and caffeine—make symptoms of reactive hypoglycemia worse," Dr. Eades says. Some sensitive people also have symptoms from a mostly complex-carbohydrate diet, she says. Those people may need to eat more protein and fewer carbs.

Getting Even: How to Smooth Spikes

Too much sugar and other carbohydrates can also set off spikes in insulin levels that leave people craving still more sweets and starches, Dr. Eades believes. "Falling blood sugar (from too much insulin) is a known appetite stimulant."

High blood levels of insulin also stimulate the storage of calories as fat in the body. Too much insulin also inhibits fat burning, Dr. Eades says. "When insulin levels are high, you actually have fewer calories immediately available to you for energy." So keeping blood sugar and insulin levels on an even keel can produce a more reliable energy supply.

Here's help to handle sugar.

Know your limits.
How much sugar is okay in terms of energy efficiency and healthy diet? For most people, about 10 percent of calories, Clark says. For a fairly active woman, for example, that would come to about 200 calories a day—slightly more than the 150 calories in one 12-ounce soft drink.

But most of us get much more than that. Research shows that the average American consumes 400 to 500 calories a day in sugar, corn syrup and other sweeteners, which is far more than we need. So for most people, limiting the amount of sugar to 200 calories a day means cutting back. For some, it means cutting way, way back.

Know that it will get easier.

People with a big sugar-monkey on their backs often go through withdrawal during the first few days or even weeks that they cut back or eliminate sugar, Dr. Eades says. They crave it and feel sluggish without it. "Over time, though, their sugar cravings diminish and their ability to taste the sweetness of fruits and even vegetables such as carrots is enhanced."

Make fruit your treat.

Fruit provides important nutrients, like potassium, fiber, beta-carotene and vitamin C. Pick fresh, ripe fruit in season. Keep a bowl of sliced fruit salad in the fridge for a quick, healthy snack. (Mix in some orange juice to keep the fruit fresh.) Pack a snack of a few dried apples or apricots with a few almonds or walnuts. But don't sugar-overload by eating more than a few pieces of dried fruit, Dr. Fuchs warns. Rule of thumb? Don't eat any more than what would equal a piece of fresh fruit. For apricots, that would be two pieces; for apples, about a third of a handful.

Plan healthy snacks for damage control.

"Don't let yourself get so hungry that you blow your good intentions on grease and goo," Clark says. If you know that you're going to be faced with a boxful of sugary doughnuts at 10:00 A.M., make sure that you have an acceptable substitute on hand such as whole-wheat banana bread from home. If you inhale cookies as soon as you get home from work, put some graham crackers or fruit salad in plain view.

Whip up some fast, healthy sweets.

Try a smoothie—a blenderized slush made with frozen bananas or any other kind of frozen fruit, citrus juice or skim milk. If you want, add a dollop of plain low-fat yogurt to the smoothie, suggests Dr. Curran-Celentano. With a banana and orange juice these drinks are loaded with potassium—a vital mineral that helps ward off fatigue and may not be found in sufficient amounts in your multivitamin supplement.

Or have a cup of plain low-fat yogurt topped with fresh fruit and a spoonful of granola or a crumbled-up oatmeal cookie. Have a whole-grain waffle or English muffin with a spoonful of fruit butter.

Save the best for last.

"There's nothing wrong with having a cookie after lunch," Clark says. "The problem is when you have cookies *for* lunch." Tagging a sweet onto the end of a meal means the fiber, protein and a bit of fat in your meal will slow the absorption of sugar, keeping blood sugar levels on a more even keel.

Be discriminating about juice.

Some fruit juices—filtered apple juice, for instance—aren't much more than sugar water. To get soluble fiber, potassium, vitamin C and other important nutrients, stick with citrus juices, like orange or grapefruit, and juices that have some "cloud" in them.

Or try vegetable juices. Carrot juice is an excellent source of potassium and beta-carotene, an anti-cancer nutrient. Low-sodium tomato juice or vegetable "cocktails" like V-8 also have lots of potassium, vitamin C and lycopenes, another set of compounds with anti-cancer potential, says Dr. Fuchs.

Suck on something sweet.
Some people are able to ration out bits of candy and can satisfy an occasional sugar craving without taking in a large sugar load. "Jolly Ranchers or Skittles are popular around here," Dr. Eades says. "Some people, however, are like an alcoholic with a drink. They need to avoid these sweets altogether, because they have a really hard time eating just one."

Don't get fooled.
It's easy to make the mistake of thinking that because a food is low in fat, it's low in sugar and calories, too. Some reduced-fat foods—cookies, cakes, ice creams and frozen yogurts, salad dressings, fruit yogurts—make up for their fat loss with extra sugar.

Know sugar by its many names.
It's everywhere, and often goes by an alias: dextrose, sucrose, glucose, honey, corn sweetener, brown sugar, fructose, high-fructose corn syrup, maltose, malt, fruit-juice concentrates, molasses, mannitol, maple syrup, turbinado sugar, sorghum, xylitol and sorbitol are all forms of sugar. "If you see any of these listed in the first three ingredients or see two or more in the top five, assume the food contains a hefty portion of sugar," Dr. Fuchs says.

Pro-Protein Proposals

Protein. It's what your body needs to build and repair tissue, to launch an immune defense, to make chemical messengers in your brain and to provide optimum energy.

"A diet that includes adequate amounts of protein helps to stabilize blood sugar and insulin levels," Dr. Eades says. "That in itself goes a long way toward alleviating fatigue." It may also help avert the sleepiness that some of us feel after a carbohydrate-rich repast.

Protein was once top dog in most diets, but nutrition educators don't stress it so much these days. They say that most Americans eat more than enough of the stuff. The protein that we get comes largely from saturated fat–laden red meat and dairy products, experts say. And there is no doubt whatsoever that a diet high in saturated fat can cause health problems. (Saturated fat, which is found mostly in meat and dairy products, is fat that is solid at room temperature.)

But some people, especially those trying their hardest to eat a healthy diet, may not be getting enough protein, Dr. Eades says. "Not everyone thrives on a high-carbohydrate diet. Some will do okay and some will do poorly. In my practice every week I see people who have tried those diets and gained weight and feel lousy." Those people may need more protein and fewer carbohydrates, she says.

"Some people may feel better if they get about one-third of their calories from protein," Dr. Eades maintains. Here's how to get the protein you need without going hog-wild.

Figure out your minimum.
How much protein you need depends on how much muscle (lean body mass) you're packing and how hard you work that muscle each day, Dr. Eades says. "You need a daily minimum of about a half a gram of complete protein from any source per pound of lean body mass just to repair the wear and tear on that lean mass." People working to build muscle with exercise may need almost twice that amount.

Best Food Sources for Protein

Complex carbohydrates—whole grains, fruits and vegetables—are all the rage these days. But that doesn't mean that you can afford to neglect your protein intake. Use this list to figure out how to get the protein you need every day.

Food	Protein Content (g.)	Food	Protein Content (g.)
Beef, select cuts (3 oz.)	22	Kidney beans (½ cup)	8
Clams (3 oz.)	22	Milk, 1% (1 cup)	8
Haddock (3 oz.)	21	Peanut butter (2 Tbsp.)	8
Tofu, firm (½ cup)	20	Cheese, Cheddar (1 oz.)	7
Cottage cheese, low-fat (½ cup)	15	Egg (1 large)	6.3
Oysters (3 oz.)	12	Sunflower seeds (1 oz.)	5.5
Soy burger (2.5 oz.)	12	Tahini (2 Tbsp.)	5
Yogurt (1 cup)	12	Almonds (1 oz.)	4.6
Chicken (3 oz.)	8	Egg white (from large egg)	3.5

So how does this translate into terms that make sense for your individual dietary needs?

A 125-pound woman with 22 percent fat (about average for women) would need 35 grams of protein a day. And a 170-pound bodybuilder with 10 percent fat may need as much as 55 grams of protein a day.

To determine whether you're getting enough protein, refer to "Best Food Sources for Protein."

Get friendly with fish.
Broiled, baked or poached, it's a great source of protein and is low in saturated fat. And fatty fish such as salmon, mackerel and tuna contain oils that may help prevent heart disease.

Try some "green protein."
A three-quarter-cup serving of lima beans offers seven grams of protein, while the same amount of peas contains more protein than a whole egg or a tablespoon of peanut butter.

Get an edge with eggs.
You probably won't want to eat more than three or four whole eggs a week, but "you can add some whites to a whole egg, scramble them up with a little oil and have a decent omelet," Dr. Eades says.

Have a bean blowout.
Besides being a good source of protein, beans bring a multitude of nutrients to the table. Try beans and rice, lentil soup or vegetarian chili. If gas keeps you from enjoying beans, try Beano, a digestive aid containing an enzyme that reduces flatulence. (The price for this little bottle, available at drugstores and supermarkets, may seem steep, but it goes a long way toward solving this problem, says Dr. Fuchs.)

Don't forget fowl.
There's more to poultry than baked chicken breasts. Try marinated chicken cubes in a stir-fry, ground-turkey meatballs or hearty, low-fat chicken vegetable stew (chill the stock and skim off the fat before adding vegetables).

Be creative with soy.
This nutritious, high-protein food is versatile enough to stand in for everything from cheesecake to meat loaf. In addition to tofu, try soy milk and soy cheese, available at health food stores. Experiment with dark or light miso, a fermented soy paste that makes a rich broth. Also try soy-based veggie burgers. "Some, such as Boca Burgers, taste so much like meat that I know vegetarians who won't eat them," says Dr. Fuchs. Veggie burgers can often be found in the supermarket's freezer or health food stores.

B Vitamins for Energy Burning

Think of them as little shuttle buses, helping to move carbohydrates along the chain of chemical reactions that ultimately result in energy production. That's what many of the B-complex vitamins do. In this role they're considered to be co-enzymes for carbohydrate metabolism.

Those playing this role include riboflavin, niacin, thiamin, vitamin B_6, pantothenic acid and biotin. Other vitamins and minerals play supporting roles in carbohydrate metabolism.

What happens when these nutrients are in short supply? These metabolic reactions may get sidetracked, leaving your body with a lot less energy than you should be getting from the food you eat.

Doctors argue whether B-vitamin deficiencies contribute to fatigue in this country. Those who believe it can play a role include Susan M. Lark, M.D., author of *Chronic Fatigue and Tiredness*. Dr. Lark points out that many weary women begin to perk up when they're getting enough B vitamins. Among the most important is vitamin B_6, which occurs naturally in whole-grain wheat. Vitamin B_6 gets removed during processing, and then it's not added back in to refined wheat flour.

B-ing There

Unless they are severe, experts say, many B-vitamin deficiencies are hard to detect. That's why "it's easier to simply make sure that you get plenty of all of them than to try to figure out if you don't have enough of one or the other," explains Dr. Curran-Celentano.

To make sure that you're getting the B vitamins that you need for energy, here's how to get good amounts in your food—and how to take supplements safely.

Eat some meat.
Most of the B vitamins—thiamin, vitamins B_6 and B_{12} and niacin—are concentrated in meat, especially in pork and beef. These foods also provide these vitamins in the form that allows them to be readily absorbed.

If your cholesterol levels are normal and you like meat, enjoy modest-size servings of lean cuts of beef or pork, Dr. Eades says. One savory way to do that is to add bits of marinated beef or pork to vegetables and rice.

Eat some whole eggs.
Eggs provide good amounts of folate (the natural form of folic acid), pantothenic acid, riboflavin, thiamin, vitamins B_{12} and B_6 and biotin. If your cholesterol lev-

els are normal, the American Heart Association recommends up to four whole eggs a week. If it's high, you'll be limited to fewer. Check with your doctor.

Get help from the deep blue.
Both finfish and shellfish are tasty and low in saturated fat, and they are a decent source of B vitamins and other vital nutrients. Enjoy broiled or baked salmon, swordfish, tuna, trout, cod, haddock, halibut, snapper, sea bass, mackerel, and herring as well as clams and oysters.

If you're a vegetarian, choose foods carefully.
The truth is that you're not going to get all the B vitamins you need from pizza and peanut butter. So include whole grains such as brown rice, oats, millet, peas and beans. Also try to include soybeans and foods made from soybeans such as tofu and miso, says Dr. Fuchs. Other foods that contribute B vitamins are sunflower, sesame and other seeds, nuts, orange juice and dark green, leafy vegetables such as spinach and broccoli.

Consider cereals.
Some packaged cereals are fortified with nutrients, making them an important source of B vitamins for some people. Check labels next time you're food shopping to see how much your favorite cereals contain. Among the top choices that are high in B vitamins but moderate or low in sweeteners include Whole-Grain Total, Grape-Nuts Flakes, King Vitaman, Wheaties and 100% Bran.

Take supplements if necessary.
Talk with your doctor or a nutritionist about your possible need for supplements, based on whatever dietary shortcomings you have. "Most people can take up to several times the Daily Value of B vitamins without any problems or need for medical supervision," Dr. Magaziner says. Look for a B-complex vitamin that includes all eight of the B vitamins: niacin, thiamin, riboflavin, B_6, B_{12}, biotin, pantothenic acid and folic acid.

It's best not to take more than 200 milligrams a day of vitamin B_6 without medical supervision, says Dr. Curran-Celentano. Amounts higher than this have been associated with neurological problems.

Magnify Energy with Magnesium

Magnesium is essential for more than 300 different chemical reactions in your body, including energy production at its most basic level. Every cell requires magnesium in its tiny generators, the mitochrondria, to crank out the energy needed to perform all its functions.

Are some people tired because they're not getting enough magnesium?

The Lunch That Won't Leave You in a Slump

If you find yourself longing for a nap come midafternoon, you're not alone—and you're perfectly normal. Changes in biochemistry that occur six to eight hours after you awaken, combined with the aftermath of a typical lunch, make a siesta seem mighty inviting.

So what's the best thing to eat for lunch if you need to remain your usual sharp self all afternoon? Nutritionists agree: Eat a light lunch based mainly on protein. It won't cause the sleepiness an hour or two later that a meal high in carbohydrates can cause. And unless you are digging ditches, it will provide enough energy to keep you going until suppertime.

What foods fit this bill? Fish, chicken, lean red meat, hard-boiled eggs, tofu or cottage cheese. But you'll want to avoid turkey, suggests Nan Kathryn Fuchs, Ph.D., a nutritionist in Sebastopol, California, and nutrition editor of *Women's Health Letter*. That's because turkey contains lots of tryptophan, an amino acid that converts to a brain-lulling neurotransmitter, serotonin.

If you're eating out, you may want to order grilled swordfish, salmon or chicken breast, along with a salad or other vegetables and a bit of complex carbohydrates—perhaps some rice. For maximum alertness it's best to start on the protein first, followed by the carbohydrates.

If a lunch-box menu is more your speed, try tuna, hard-boiled eggs or sliced chicken, along with sliced raw vegetables.

To avoid overeating at lunch, eat slowly, advises Liz Applegate, Ph.D., author of *Power Foods* and nutrition columnist for *Runner's World* magazine. It takes 20 minutes for your brain to get the message that your stomach is full.

Have fruit or a cup of instant soup midafternoon, when your brain may otherwise be scraping bottom. If you must have caffeine, stick with green tea, which offers a bit of an energy boost along with potential anti-cancer protection, Dr. Fuchs recommends.

"The people I see are usually tired for a number of reasons, and magnesium deficiency might be one of these," Dr. Magaziner says. In fact, British researchers found that 80 percent of the people with chronic fatigue syndrome and low blood levels of magnesium who received magnesium injections reported an improvement in symptoms.

It's possible to find out if you are low in magnesium by using a blood test that measures levels in red blood cells, Dr. Magaziner says. Unfortunately, most doctors, if they check magnesium levels at all, simply look at serum levels (serum is the clear liquid in blood). "That method can detect only a severe deficiency, not a milder type that might still cause tiredness," Dr. Magaziner says.

Dietary analyses show that many people don't get the Daily Value of magnesium—400 milligrams—in their diets. Women average about 200 milligrams per day, men a bit more than 300 milligrams.

Here's how to get what you need for maximum energy.

When it comes to grains, think whole.
Here's yet another reason for going for whole grains. Grains that have been refined—with the bran and germ removed—lose about 80 percent of their magnesium. One-half cup of cooked brown rice has 43 milligrams of magnesium. That's nearly four times the amount found in cooked white rice, which is just the processed form of brown. A half-cup of whole-wheat flour has 83 milligrams, six times as much magnesium as white flour.

Have bran.
Bran is the magnesium-packed outer layer that's been removed from grains during the refinement process. Rice bran is tops in magnesium, with 218 milligrams per one-third cup serving. Add it to cooked cereals, bread and other baked goods or sprinkle it on like a crumb topping. Also, a half-cup serving of 100% Bran cereal offers 80 milligrams of magnesium.

Seek seeds.
Pumpkin, sesame and sunflower seeds are all packed with magnesium. They are also high in calories, so you should use them sparingly as snacks or to garnish a salad. Look in your health food store for jars of tahini (sesame paste), which substitutes nicely for peanut butter and can be used to make creamy sauces and dressings. Check your favorite health food cookbook for ideas.

Get nutty.
Like seeds, just about any nut is a great source of magnesium. While nuts and seeds are high in fat, the fat is not saturated. That makes these foods good alternatives to butter and oil. Spread a little peanut butter on your toast instead of butter, and you'll be taking in extra nutrients, says Dr. Curran-Celentano. But remember that fat is still fat, so go easy. Unblanched almonds are tops in magnesium, with 86 milligrams per ounce, followed by filberts, cashews, pine nuts and Brazil nuts. Compared with other foods, peanuts are a decent source of magnesium, though they offer less than most other nuts.

Have halibut or haddock.
Here's another reason to have the catch of the day a couple of times a week. A 5½-ounce fillet of halibut, baked or broiled, provides 170 milligrams of magnesium. One 5½-ounce haddock fillet offers about 75 milligrams. Flounder, sole and oysters are also good choices.

Get friendly with beans.

Beans again? You bet. Some of the more exotic varieties of beans—moth beans, yard-long beans, cowpeas and hyacinth beans—are tops in magnesium, but their more pedestrian cousins, including soy, black, white, limas and kidney beans, also have much to offer.

If long cooking times discourage you from using fresh or dried beans, use canned instead. Add them to salads and soups or mash them for taco fillings or dips. Canned beans should be rinsed under cold running water to remove excess sodium and sugar, advises Dr. Fuchs.

Try tofu.

It's made from soybeans, a treasure trove of magnesium. Soy flour and soy meat extenders, also called texturized vegetable protein, have lots of magnesium, too.

Go on green.

A half-cup of boiled spinach or Swiss chard each has about 75 milligrams of magnesium. Two edible weeds, dock and purslane, are also good sources—so is seaweed. Look in a Japanese or macrobiotics cookbook for ways to use seaweeds like agar, spirulina, Irish moss and wakame.

Add avocados.

One average-size fruit offers 78 milligrams of magnesium. Substitute an avocado for the bacon in a bacon, lettuce and tomato sandwich, or use one to liven up a salad. Though it's true that avocados are fatty, they're high in monounsaturated fats that only seem to raise the level of high-density lipoprotein, the good cholesterol.

Add supplements as necessary.

No vitamin supplement can supply all the nutrients that you need. But if you want to get more magnesium fast or if you need more than your diet can supply, supplements are a safe addition. "Most of my patients safely take about 500 milligrams a day of magnesium," Dr. Magaziner says.

It's true that large amounts of magnesium can cause diarrhea. Two easily absorbed forms, magnesium gluconate and magnesium aspartate, are least likely to cause that problem.

Getting Action with Chromium

Chromium acts as the shovel that gets the fuel into the furnace. This trace mineral hooks up with insulin to help transport blood sugar across cell membranes and into cells where it can be burned for energy.

Those who are low or deficient in chromium can develop either hyperglycemia (diabetes) or hypoglycemia (low blood sugar). Chromium helps the

Should You Eat Like a Soldier?

How does a soldier get all the energy needed to dodge bullets, wriggle through ditches or peel a zillion potatoes?

Well, for one thing, he gets plenty of calories. If a soldier chows down all three of his ready-to-eat meals each day, he'll get 4,000 to 4,500 calories, explains Wayne Askew, Ph.D., professor and director in the Division of Foods and Nutrition at the University of Utah in Salt Lake City and formerly director of military nutrition research for the U.S. Army Research Institute of Environmental Medicine. That's about double the number of calories that a civilian would typically consume.

Those calories are 45 percent carbohydrates, 35 percent fat and 20 percent protein, Dr. Askew says. "These meals are not higher in carbohydrates because soldiers like and expect some fat," he explains. "Also, if the fat content were much lower, the volume of food the soldiers would have to carry and eat to get enough calories would be prohibitive."

If a soldier needs additional calories, he can consume the same sort of energy bars and sports drinks that athletes use, he says. Both of these foods contain a laboratory-concocted sweetener called glucose polymers. These are strings of glucose molecules, and glucose is the simple form of sugar that your body uses for energy. "Their advantage over single molecules of glucose or other simple sugars such as sucrose or fructose is that they cause less stomach cramping and diarrhea, since they don't draw as much water into the intestines for digestion," Dr. Askew explains.

While glucose polymers break down fairly quickly, they do so more slowly than the simple sugars found in most sweetened drinks and fruit juices. "That means that insulin secretion is less, so there is less danger of driving blood sugar too low, resulting in hypoglycemia," he says.

As for vitamins and minerals, soldiers get all they need without ever having to get near broccoli or chicken livers. Every food, from the chicken cacciatore to the apple brown Betty, is either naturally nutrient dense or fortified with extra vitamins and minerals. "For every 2,200 calories that a soldier eats, he or she gets the RDA of every vitamin and mineral," Dr. Askew explains. "Because of the way the rations are 'engineered,' we just don't see the kind of marginal vitamin deficiencies that occur in the general public."

What does all this mean for Joe Citizen who wants more energy? "*Our* situation closely parallels that of elite athletes," Dr. Askew says. For normal people, he recommends a diet of 30 percent fat or lower, heavy on the complex carbohydrates, with 20 percent of calories from protein.

body to utilize insulin, which is secreted by the pancreas, and makes blood sugar regulation more efficient.

People with adult-onset diabetes can experience fatigue, excessive thirst or hunger, difficulty losing weight and frequent yeast infections. On the other hand, hypoglycemia can result in headaches, feeling anxious or shaky, sweatiness, palpitations, sugar cravings or depression. Both of these conditions are worsened by eating too much refined sugar.

Since chromium helps insulin work better, it may also raise blood sugar levels in people with low blood sugar, studies by the U.S. Department of Agriculture (USDA) researchers show.

Most people don't get enough chromium in their diets, apparently. An analysis by Richard Anderson, Ph.D., a leading scientist in mineral nutrition at the USDA Human Nutrition Research Center in Beltsville, Maryland, found that even balanced diets designed by dietitians contain less than 50 micrograms of chromium. More often, these diets average about 15 micrograms. This is far less than the Daily Value of 120 micrograms.

Here's how to get more in your diet and how to safely take supplements.

Use brewer's yeast.
This malty-tasting stuff, found in health food stores, is used to brew beer. It's a top food source of a type of chromium called glucose tolerance factor (GTF)—a combination of chromium, nicotinic acid (a form of niacin) and amino acids. But since amounts of GTF in brewer's yeast vary from batch to batch, it's not as reliable a source as chromium supplements, Dr. Anderson says.

Brewer's yeast flakes or powder, available at health food stores, can be added to fruit shakes, milk shakes and baked goods, but not everyone can get used to the somewhat bitter taste.

Crank up the pepper mill.
Black pepper is loaded with chromium, although most of us don't use enough pepper for it to be a significant source. You can change that by generously sprinkling freshly ground spicy-hot black pepper on salads, soups, beans, meat, egg and cheese dishes, pasta and potatoes.

Add spice to your life.
Cinnamon, ginger and cloves all contain good amounts of chromium, Dr. Anderson says. As little as one-eighth teaspoon of cinnamon triples insulin efficiency, medical researchers report. Add cinnamon to oatmeal, applesauce and baked goods; ginger to stir-fries, cookies and cakes; and cloves to baked apples and ham. Or make a tasty tea using these spices.

Go bonkers for broccoli.
A one-cup serving offers 22 micrograms of chromium.

Have ham.
Turkey ham is tops here, with 10.4 micrograms per three-ounce serving. Regular ham has 3.6 micrograms per serving.

Stick with whole grains.
While they're not great sources of chromium, whole grains do offer more than refined grains. A whole-wheat English muffin, for instance, has 3.6 micrograms of chromium.

Consider supplements.
Taking up to 200 micrograms a day of supplemental chromium is safe without medical supervision, Dr. Magaziner says. Nutrition-oriented doctors tend to use chromium picolinate or polynicotinate, two easily absorbed forms. Most nutrients work together, though, says Dr. Magaziner, "so I usually give a multivitamin along with it and encourage a healthy diet."

Ironing Out Anemia

There's no doubt that iron-deficiency anemia is the best-known and most often diagnosed nutrition-related cause of fatigue. One out of every five women will have low iron levels sometime during her life. But that doesn't mean that you should automatically assume that if you're tired, you're low in iron, Dr. Fuchs says.

"A premenopausal woman can take up to 18 milligrams, the Daily Value, of supplemental iron a day," she says. "But she should not take more than this amount without blood tests to confirm that she needs it."

For men, women past menopause and anyone who's had cancer, the word is to proceed with caution. You should not take any amount of supplemental iron unless you have been advised to do so by a doctor who is knowledgeable in nutrition, Dr. Fuchs says. "Too much iron can cause immune system problems and may increase your risk of heart disease. And women who have had cancer or are at high risk for it should also avoid extra iron."

Iron is such an important factor because it's an essential part of hemoglobin, the protein in red blood cells that carries oxygen from the lungs to tissues. Oxygen is needed for energy metabolism in cells, just as it's needed to burn wood in a fireplace. When it's in short supply, you'll feel as though you're in slow motion.

And along with fatigue may come shortness of breath, faster heart rate, inability to concentrate and cold hands and feet. Some people with iron-deficiency anemia get a condition called restless legs: Odd sensations of movement in their legs keep them tossing and turning instead of sleeping at night.

Are Energy Bars for You?

Maybe you have seen them at health food stores, bike shops, sporting goods stores, even some supermarkets. With names like PowerBar, Thunder Bar and Performance Energy Bar, sports bars can be hard to resist, especially if you're feeling as though you could use a bit more pep. Are they a healthy food choice? Could be, depending on what you would eat otherwise.

Sports bars are designed as energy foods, no doubt about that. Most of them are packed with carbohydrates—both starch and sugar. But unlike typical candy bars, most sports bars provide additional goodies—protein, fiber, vitamins and minerals—usually without much fat.

"Sports bars offer much more in the way of nutrients than most snack foods," explains Liz Applegate, Ph.D., author of *Power Foods* and nutrition columnist for *Runner's World* magazine. Very digestible, these bars break down fast, providing quick energy. Plus, they're as convenient as food gets. "Sometimes you can't fuss with food," she says. "You just want to unwrap it and eat it."

So, if you have a sports bar instead of a candy bar, a handful of cookies or a chocolate brownie, you're doing yourself a nutritional favor. If you're having it instead of a healthy meal or a piece of fruit, you're not—although, on occasion, it may beat going hungry or running out of steam.

Compare labels between brands to make the best selection, Dr. Applegate recommends. The best bars offer 35 to 50 percent of the Daily Value of several vitamins and minerals, three to five grams of fiber, eight to ten grams of protein and, usually, 30 percent or less of calories from fat.

Same goes for sports drinks such as Gatorade. These drinks contain half the sugar found in sodas or sweetened teas or fruit drinks, along with small amounts of sodium and potassium, two minerals lost in sweat. So sports drinks are a good substitute for these soft drinks, says Dr. Applegate.

They're not such a good substitute for full-fruit juices like orange juice, which has eight times the potassium (more than 400 milligrams per eight-ounce serving, compared to about 50 milligrams for most sports drinks) along with good amounts of vitamin C, folate and other B vitamins.

But then again, orange juice usually isn't anyone's first choice for fluid replacement during exercise, Dr. Applegate says. "It's too acidy and too concentrated in sugar, so large amounts could cause stomach cramps." So save your juice for times when you're not guzzling to keep up with the pack.

Banishing the Blahs

You don't necessarily need to be anemic in order to benefit from additional iron, Dr. Fuchs says. "Ask your doctor to check your blood levels of ferritin, a storage form of iron. If that's low, studies show that extra iron may help restore your pep." Here's how to get what you need.

Feast on beast.
Unless you have a cholesterol problem, you can have reasonable-size servings of lean meat several times a week, Dr. Eades says. Meat supplies the most easily absorbed form of iron.

Add acid.
Acidic foods aid iron absorption. Add lemon juice to a spinach salad or, if you're taking iron supplements, take some vitamin C as well. Taking iron pills with orange juice will also aid absorption as the acidity of the juice helps the iron along.

Save tea and coffee for between meals.
Black tea and, to a lesser extent, coffee contain tannins, chemical compounds that can cut iron absorption in half, Dr. Fuchs says. So wait at least an hour after eating before you drink these beverages, she says, and never use them to wash down iron pills.

Avoid enteric-coated or delayed-release iron formulas.
Experts say that both the coating and the delayed-release ingredient can interfere with the body's ability to absorb the nutrient.

Nutrients to Bust Anemia

As mentioned, energy-depleting anemia can also be caused by shortages of vitamin B_{12} or folic acid. Both are needed to allow oxygen-carrying red blood cells to mature properly.

Strict vegetarians (vegans) are the only people who might not get enough vitamin B_{12} in their diets, since meat, eggs or dairy products easily provide the Daily Value of six micrograms. Older people and those with intestinal problems, however, may lose the ability to absorb vitamin B_{12} from foods. Over time, their vitamin B_{12} levels slowly drop. As they become more and more weary, they may have symptoms of tingling or numbness in their feet and hands and memory problems as well, Dr. Hom says.

Some studies show that B_{12} injections improve energy levels in some people who don't have anemia. "We often find that people who have low energy have improvement in their energy levels after B_{12} shots, and that's in spite of having normal B_{12} levels," Dr. Hom says.

People most likely to be short on folic acid have traditionally been elderly "tea and toasters" or other people eating a poor diet. More recent dietary studies show, however, that only 61 percent of Americans get half of the Daily Value of folic acid (200 micrograms). Folic acid deficiency is easily detected when it causes anemia, Dr. Hom says. "Sometimes, though, its only symptoms are fatigue and depression."

According to medical doctors, people seriously low in vitamin B_{12} or folic acid need injections of these nutrients, or supplements in some cases. But, otherwise, you can get enough of these nutrients from your diet. Here's how.

Beef up on B_{12}.
Your only sources of this important energy vitamin are dairy products, eggs or meat. Most folks need two micrograms a day of B_{12}, says Dr. Curran-Celentano. You can get this much in four eggs, two cups of milk or three ounces of chicken.

Feed on foliage.
Folic acid and folate get their names from their richest sources—dark, leafy greens. One-half cup of chopped spinach, turnip greens or mustard greens each provides about 54 micrograms of folate; a half-cup of romaine or cos lettuce, 38 micrograms. Broccoli, garden cress, cabbage, brussels sprouts and endive are also good sources.

Use parsley for more than pretty.
It offers 5.7 micrograms per tablespoon, so a parsley-based dish such as tabbouleh can really deliver folate.

Get some A-letter veggies.
With 113 micrograms of folate, one avocado will put you well on your way to meeting your daily needs. But be sure that you can handle the calories as avocados are high in fat. Also, a mere four spears of asparagus offers 90 micrograms.

For fruit, target oranges and papaya.
One cup of cubed papaya has 53 micrograms of folate and one navel orange has 47 micrograms. Make yourself a fruit smoothie with this tangy duo, and you'll end up with a hefty 100 micrograms of folate. Boysenberries are also an excellent source.

Reach for the beans.
Here's yet another reason to eat beans. Mung and adzuki beans, both used in oriental cooking, are among the top bean choices for folate. Following closely are chick-peas, lentils, and pinto, Great Northern, pink and black beans.

Get Your Timing Straight

When it comes to optimum energy, when you eat can be just as important as what you eat. The trick is to avoid feast or famine situations: You don't want to go too long without food, only to stuff yourself silly when you finally do pull up to the table. That leads to lows and highs in blood sugar and insulin levels that can make you as tired and crabby as a worn-out three-year-old, Dr. Eades says.

Here's how to schedule your fuel deliveries so that you don't run out of steam.

Begin with breakfast.
Unless you have been raiding the refrigerator at 2:00 A.M., chances are that you wake up without having eaten for at least seven or eight hours. That means that you're operating on empty.

You can fill your tank in any number of imaginative ways. Heat up leftover brown rice or couscous, then top it with fruit and milk. Make old-fashioned oatmeal—chewy, not mushy—by simmering steel-cut (Scotch or Irish) oats, uncovered, without stirring. For a tasty treat, add a little vanilla or cinnamon to the cooking water or mix in honey or maple syrup before eating.

On weekends make extra whole-grain pancakes to freeze. Pop them into the toaster oven on mornings when you're in a rush. Make a pancake-and-fruit-butter "sandwich" to eat in the car. When you're using your oven at night, bake a few sweet potatoes. They'll be quick, hearty fare for the next day's lunch or dinner.

Schedule mini-meals.
Some people have more energy, more of the time, if they eat a little something every few hours. If you're one of them, keep healthy snacks on hand for mid-morning and afternoon noshing. Some suggestions: bagels, rice cakes, fruit, plain popcorn, sunflower seeds, almonds and yogurt.

Make up missed meals.
If you do have to skip a meal, don't try to wait until the next meal comes along. Grab a nutritious snack as soon as you can. That may mean some low-fat cheese and an apple, yogurt and fruit, pretzels and skim milk, carrot sticks, even a bowl of cereal and a banana. Eating sugary snacks instead of meals may perk you up at first, but such eating ultimately leads to poorer health, Clark says.

Eat before exercise.
If you work out three or more hours after your last meal and, especially, if you find yourself feeling shaky or weak before you're done, have a high-carb snack an hour or so before you start sweating, Clark advises. It will give your muscles more to go on.

Recipes for Energy

What's your idea of energy food? A plateful of pasta? A doughnut and a cup of coffee? A candy bar?

It's true that carbohydrates—found in things like bread, pasta and sugary foods—can provide a quick burst of energy. But nutrition experts have found that we need more than these foods for enduring energy and good health.

Energy metabolism, the process that converts food into fuel, calls for a wide array of nutrients. These include most of the B vitamins—niacin, thiamin, riboflavin and the like. You also need adequate amounts of iron, magnesium and other minerals. Even protein and a bit of fat are needed for optimum energy.

You can get these nutrients by eating a variety of nutritious foods, including fruits and vegetables, whole grains, beans, fish and shellfish, low-fat dairy products and lean meats.

Once you start cooking with these basic foods, all needed by your body to create energy, your kitchen becomes a kind of alchemical laboratory. Just select the nutritious ingredients and combine them in ways that are temptingly tasty, and you'll have meals that boost your energy level in the days to come.

Following are 20 recipes that will get you started in combining these key energy-producing, nutrient-packed foods in countless delicious ways. Adding dishes like these to your menu will fuel your day-to-day energy challenges.

Tropical Fruit Smoothie

Energy-enhancing potassium gets more than a fair shake in this smoothie.

> 1   **ripe papaya, peeled, seeded and cut into chunks**
>
> 1   **medium frozen banana, peeled and cut into chunks**
>
> 1   **cup nonfat plain yogurt**
>
> ½   **teaspoon ground cinnamon**
>
> ⅛   **teaspoon ground ginger**
>
> ½   **cup skim milk**

In a blender jar, place the papaya, banana, yogurt, cinnamon, ginger and milk. Blend for 30 to 40 seconds, or until smooth. Pour into 2 tall glasses.

Makes 2½ cups; 2 servings.

Per serving: 263 calories, 0.9 g. total fat, 0.3 g. saturated fat, 5.1 g. fiber, 3 mg. cholesterol, 134 mg. sodium

Garden Patch Pasta

This quick pasta dish with a chunky vitamin-rich vegetable sauce provides energizing iron, copper, magnesium and B vitamins, along with carbohydrates. What's more, it takes less than 30 minutes to cook. Smart cooks can maximize the effort by making a double recipe of the sauce and freezing half for another meal.

1	**tablespoon olive oil**
1½	**cups sliced mushrooms**
1	**small green pepper, cut into ½" chunks**
1	**medium onion, coarsely chopped**
1	**clove garlic, minced**
⅓	**cup raisins**
1	**can (14½ ounces) diced tomatoes (with juice)**
10	**ounces (3 cups) uncooked penne or rotini pasta**
2	**cups broccoli florets and peeled stalks, cut into ¼"-thick slices**
3	**tablespoons grated Romano cheese**
	Red-pepper flakes (optional)

In a large no-stick frying pan, heat the oil. Add the mushrooms, peppers, onions and garlic. Cook, stirring occasionally, for 10 minutes, or until the vegetables are soft and golden. Add the raisins and tomatoes (with juice). Bring to a boil. Reduce the heat and simmer for 10 minutes.

Meanwhile, bring a large covered pot of water to a boil. Add the pasta, stir and return the water to a boil. Boil, uncovered, for 5 minutes, stirring occasionally. Add the broccoli and continue cooking for about 3 minutes, or until the pasta and broccoli are tender but still firm. Ladle out ¼ cup of the pasta cooking water and reserve.

Drain the pasta and broccoli, then return it to the cooking pot. Add the vegetable sauce, Romano and reserved cooking water; toss gently to coat. Set aside for 3 minutes so that the pasta absorbs some of the sauce. Serve sprinkled with the red-pepper flakes (if using).

Makes 4 servings.

Per serving: 426 calories, 6.8 g. total fat, 1.7 g. saturated fat, 4.5 g. fiber, 5 mg. cholesterol, 249 mg. sodium

Northern Italian Tuna-Bean Salad

This robust main-dish salad serves up dietary fiber, energy-producing B vitamins and heart-healthy fish oils, along with rich, hearty flavor. Accompany the salad with a slice of the toasted Wheat and Walnut Bread (see page 48) and a wedge of chilled cantaloupe.

- 1 **tablespoon extra-virgin olive oil**
- 1 **tablespoon red-wine vinegar**
- 2 **tablespoons nonfat plain yogurt**
- ¼ **teaspoon ground black pepper**
- 1 **can (15½ ounces) red kidney beans, rinsed and drained**
- 1 **can (12 ounces) water-packed tuna, drained and flaked**
- ¼ **cup minced red onions**
- 4 **cups packed, torn romaine lettuce or escarole leaves**

In a large bowl, whisk the oil, vinegar, yogurt and pepper until smooth. Add the beans, tuna and onions. Toss gently to coat with the yogurt dressing. Line 4 dinner plates with the romaine or escarole leaves. Spoon the tuna-bean salad on top.

Makes 4 servings.

Per serving: 244 calories, 5 g. total fat, 0.7 g. saturated fat, 8 g. fiber, 25 mg. cholesterol, 503 mg. sodium

Vegetable Miso Soup with Ramen Noodles

Get to know miso—a fermented soybean paste that's high in protein—in this hearty vegetable noodle soup. Miso paste is sold in Asian and health food stores and keeps beautifully in the refrigerator for months.

This dish boosts energy with copper, iron, half your daily requirement of vitamin C and decent amounts of B vitamins—including folate, riboflavin and thiamin.

2   **medium carrots, thinly sliced**

1   **medium leek, white and light green stem, thinly sliced**

2   **cups packed chiffonade-cut kale leaves (see hint)**

2   **cloves garlic, minced**

4   **cups water**

1½ **teaspoons grated fresh ginger**

2   **packages (0.3 ounce each) instant ramen noodles, without seasoning packets**

1½ **tablespoons light miso paste**

1   **cup frozen baby peas**

1½ **teaspoons sesame oil**

¼   **cup chiffonade-cut fresh mint or basil (see hint)**

Coat a no-stick Dutch oven with no-stick spray. Combine the carrots, leeks, kale and garlic in the pan. Cover and cook over medium-low heat, stirring occasionally, for 8 minutes, or until the vegetables are partially cooked.

Add the water and ginger to the pan. Cook over medium heat for 8 to 10 minutes, or until the vegetables are tender but still firm. Add the noodles and cook at a brisk simmer for 3 to 4 minutes, or until the noodles are almost tender.

In a small bowl, whisk the miso with ¼ cup of the cooking liquid. Add the miso water, peas, oil and mint or basil to the pan. Remove from the heat and allow to sit for 1 to 2 minutes before serving.

Cook's Hint: To quickly cut the kale and mint or basil (or any other salad or herb leaves) into thin strips called chiffonade, stack the leaves on top of one another and then roll them into a tight tube. Holding the tube with one hand, use a sharp knife to slice the tube crosswise into thin strips.

Makes 4 servings.

Per serving: 122 calories, 3.6 g. total fat, 0.4 g. saturated fat, 4.4 g. fiber, 3 mg. cholesterol, 393 mg. sodium

Turkey-Vegetable Wedges

This protein-rich (and practically fat-free) skillet dinner provides significant amounts of magnesium, zinc and B vitamins, which rev up energy levels by acting as calorie-burning catalysts.

 1 **pound ground turkey breast**

$1\frac{1}{2}$ **pounds small red potatoes, scrubbed, dried and quartered**

 1 **bunch scallions, white and light green stems, sliced**

 1 **medium yellow pepper or sweet red pepper, seeded and diced**

 1 **tablespoon crushed dried sage**

$\frac{1}{8}$ **teaspoon salt**

$\frac{1}{8}$ **teaspoon ground red pepper**

 1 **cup defatted reduced-sodium chicken broth**

Coat a large no-stick frying pan with olive no-stick spray. Place over medium-high heat until the pan is hot. Crumble the turkey into the pan. Cook, stirring frequently, for 5 minutes, or until the turkey is no longer pink. Transfer to a plate and set aside.

Remove the pan from the heat. Coat with the olive no-stick spray. Add the potatoes and sauté over medium-high heat, tossing occasionally, for 10 to 12 minutes, or until golden on all sides. If necessary, add a tablespoon of water at a time to reduce sticking. Add the scallions and yellow or sweet red peppers. Cook over medium-high heat, stirring occasionally, for 3 to 4 minutes, or until the scallions and peppers start to soften.

Return the turkey to the pan and mix to combine with the vegetables. Season with the sage, salt and ground red pepper. Add the broth. Cook over high heat for about 8 minutes, or until the liquid is absorbed and the bottom is crisp. Cut into quarters. Remove the wedges with a spatula.

Makes 4 servings.

Per serving: 277 calories, 1 g. total fat, 0.3 g. saturated fat, 0.3 g. fiber, 76 mg. cholesterol, 208 mg. sodium

Southwestern Pumpkin and White Bean Chili

This unique chili is an outstanding source of beta-carotene from the pumpkin. It also provides good amounts of energy-boosting nutrients—magnesium, iron and folate. Last but not least, this is a low-fat version of a popular dish that is notoriously high in fat.

3   **strips turkey bacon, chopped**

1   **large clove garlic, minced**

1   **teaspoon ground cumin**

1   **can (15 ounces) pumpkin puree**

3   **cups defatted reduced-sodium chicken broth**

2   **cans (15 ounces each) Great Northern or navy beans, rinsed and drained**

⅛   **teaspoon salt (optional)**

1   **jalapeño pepper or serrano pepper, seeded and minced (wear plastic gloves when handling)**

½   **cup nonfat plain yogurt**

¼   **cup minced fresh cilantro leaves**

Place the bacon in a no-stick Dutch oven. Cook over medium-high heat, stirring frequently, for 3 to 4 minutes, or until crisp.

Add the garlic and cumin. Cook for 30 seconds, or until fragrant. Add the pumpkin, then whisk in the broth. Add the beans and salt (if using). Cook, partially covered, over medium-low heat for 15 minutes.

Add the peppers. If the chili is too thick, stir in about ¼ cup water.

To serve, spoon the chili into 4 large bowls. Top each serving with 2 tablespoons yogurt and 1 tablespoon cilantro.

Makes 4 servings.

Per serving: 343 calories, 3.6 g. total fat, 1.2 g. saturated fat, 3.2 g. fiber, 7 mg. cholesterol, 461 mg. sodium

Tuscan Beans and Pork with Rice

Rosemary, tomato and succulent pork tenderloin give this dish true Italian gusto. Both the brown rice and the cannellini beans are appetizing sources of essential B vitamins, which help your body burn calories from food. Using quick-cooking brown rice cuts the preparation time considerably.

8 **ounces pork tenderloin, trimmed of all visible fat, cut into ½"-thick slices**

1 **can (19 ounces) cannellini beans, rinsed and drained**

1 **can (14½ ounces) diced tomatoes (with juice)**

1 **large clove garlic, minced**

2 **teaspoons crushed dried rosemary**

¼ **teaspoon ground black pepper**

2 **tablespoons grated Parmesan cheese**

3 **cups hot cooked brown rice**

Coat a large no-stick frying pan with olive no-stick spray. Place the pan over medium heat.

With the flat side of a large knife or with the palm of your hand, flatten the pork slices to ¼" thickness. Place the pork in the pan and cook for 2 minutes each side until golden. Remove to a plate and set aside.

To the pan, add the beans, tomatoes (with juice), garlic, rosemary and pepper. Cover and simmer over medium-low heat for 10 minutes, or until the tomatoes soften.

Meanwhile, cut the reserved pork slices into thin strips. Add the pork strips and any juices on the pork plate to the bean mixture and simmer for 5 minutes.

Just before serving, stir the Parmesan into the cooked rice. Divide the rice onto 4 dinner plates and spoon the stew on top.

Makes 4 servings.

Per serving: 365 calories, 5.6 g. total fat, 1.6 g. saturated fat, 11 g. fiber, 35 mg. cholesterol, 521 mg. sodium

Dilled Halibut Skillet Dinner

Dinner doesn't get more appetizing, quick or nutritious than this single-pan recipe. Each serving provides good amounts of energy-promoting protein, magnesium and B vitamins, including B_{12}, B_6, niacin, thiamin and riboflavin.

2   cups vegetable broth or water

1   cup quick-cooking barley

½   cup coarsely shredded carrots

1   cup coarsely shredded green cabbage

1   small onion, thinly sliced

1   tablespoon lemon juice

2   teaspoons coarse mustard

2   tablespoons nonfat sour cream

1   pound halibut fillets, ½" thick, cut into 4 equal portions

2   tablespoons minced fresh dill

In a large frying pan, combine the broth or water, barley, carrots, cabbage, onions and lemon juice. Cover and bring to a boil over high heat. Reduce the heat and simmer for 8 minutes.

Meanwhile, in small dish, combine the mustard and sour cream. With the back of a spoon, spread the mixture over the tops of the fillets.

Place the prepared halibut over the barley-vegetable mixture. Cover the pan and simmer for 10 to 12 minutes, or until the halibut is opaque all the way through. (Check by inserting a sharp knife into center of a fillet.)

To serve, place the halibut fillets on 4 dinner plates and surround with the barley-vegetable mixture. Sprinkle with dill.

Variations: You can also use fish broth in this recipe. If you don't have any homemade broth, substitute 1 cup bottled clam juice mixed with 1 cup of water.

Regular pearl barley can also be used for this dish. Add ½ cup more broth and cook the barley and vegetables in the first step for about 12 to 15 minutes.

Makes 4 servings.

Per serving: 329 calories, 3.9 g. total fat, 0.6 g. saturated fat, 7.9 g. fiber, 36 mg. cholesterol, 155 mg. sodium

Lentil Tacos with the Trimmings

This irresistible dish offers up a smorgasbord of energy boosters—copper, iron, magnesium, folate and vitamin B₆. It's also a good source of carbohydrates.

Make a double batch of filling for freezing. For an effortless weeknight meal, thaw the cooked lentils overnight in the refrigerator or in the microwave. Reheat in the microwave on medium power (50%), stirring the lentils once, for about 3 minutes, or until hot.

   1   **cup brown lentils, sorted and rinsed**

   1   **small onion, minced**

   3   **cups vegetable broth or water**

   2   **cloves garlic, minced**

   ½   **teaspoon ground cumin**

   1   **teaspoon dried oregano**

   2   **teaspoons reduced-sodium Worcestershire sauce**

   1   **small ripe avocado**

   1   **tablespoon lime juice**

   8   **corn tortillas, heated**

   1   **cup torn romaine lettuce leaves**

   ¼   **cup salsa**

   ½   **cup nonfat plain yogurt**

   ¼   **cup fresh cilantro leaves**

In a Dutch oven, combine the lentils, onions, broth or water, garlic, cumin, oregano and Worcestershire sauce. Bring to a boil over high heat, then reduce to medium low. Simmer, stirring occasionally, for 30 to 40 minutes, or until the lentils are tender.

Meanwhile, halve the avocado and remove the pit and skin. Cut lengthwise into ¼"-thick slices. Place it in a small bowl, add the lime juice and toss gently.

If the mixture is soupy after the lentils are cooked, turn the heat to high and cook, stirring constantly, for 4 to 5 minutes, or until the lentils are dry. Remove from the heat. With the back of a large spoon, smash some of the lentils against the side of the pan until the mixture resembles refried beans.

To serve, spoon the lentil puree down the center of the tortillas. Garnish with the avocado, romaine, salsa, yogurt and cilantro.

Makes 4 servings.

Per serving: 395 calories, 9.4 g. total fat, 1.4 g. saturated fat, 2.5 g. fiber, 1 mg. cholesterol, 304 mg. sodium

Bistro Pepper Steak with Herbed Oven Fries

This satisfying pepper steak pumps essential protein into your diet. This sometimes underrated nutrient alleviates fatigue by stabilizing blood sugar and insulin levels. An extra plus: This dish also provides B vitamins, along with copper and zinc—all important energy enhancers.

1¾	**pounds baking potatoes, scrubbed and dried**
½	**teaspoon crushed dried rosemary**
½	**teaspoon crushed dried thyme**
	Pinch of salt
1	**pound boneless top loin beef steaks, cut 1" thick and trimmed of all visible fat**
2	**teaspoons coarsely ground black pepper**
¼	**cup dry red wine or defatted reduced-sodium beef broth (see hint)**

Preheat the oven to 375°. Coat a large baking sheet with olive no-stick spray.

Cut the potatoes lengthwise into eighths. Pat dry with paper towels. Place in a single layer on the prepared baking sheet. Coat the potatoes lightly with olive no-stick spray. Sprinkle the rosemary, thyme and salt evenly over the potatoes. Toss with your hands to coat evenly with the herbs. Position the potatoes, skin side down, so that they don't touch. Bake for 35 to 40 minutes, or until puffed and golden.

About 10 minutes before the potatoes are cooked, pat the steaks dry and coat both sides evenly with the pepper.

Coat a medium cast-iron or aluminum frying pan with olive no-stick spray. Heat the pan over medium-high heat. Place the steaks in the pan and cook for about 3 minutes, or until seared on the bottom. Turn the steaks and cook for 3 to 5 minutes longer (for rare), or until cooked to desired doneness. Raise the heat to high. Add the wine or broth and bring to a boil, swirling pan gently so that the juices coat the steaks.

Remove the steaks and cut lengthwise in ¼"-thick slices. Arrange the steak slices on 4 dinner plates. Pour the pan juices over the steaks. Serve the oven fries on the side.

Cook's Hint: If using beef broth, adding 1 to 2 teaspoons red-wine vinegar will add a pleasant acidity to the pan juices.

Makes 4 servings.

Per serving: 529 calories, 9.9 g. total fat, 3.7 g. saturated fat, 0.3 g. fiber, 87 mg. cholesterol, 109 mg. sodium

Couscous Vegetable Medley

A bushelful of vitamins, minerals and dietary fiber comes with this delightfully spicy vegetable-grain main dish. Each serving delivers healthy amounts of energy-enhancing vitamin C, copper, iron, folate, magnesium and potassium.

1 **green pepper, cut into 8 wedges**

1 **large onion, cut into 8 wedges**

2 **medium sweet potatoes, peeled and cut into ½" rounds**

1 **can (15½ ounces) chick-peas, rinsed and drained**

2 **cloves garlic, minced**

¾ **teaspoon ground cumin**

½ **teaspoon ground coriander**

¼ **teaspoon ground cinnamon**

1 **can (11½ ounces) reduced-sodium vegetable juice cocktail**

1 **cup water**

1 **cup couscous**

2 **tablespoons chopped fresh cilantro leaves**

Hot-pepper sauce (optional)

In a Dutch oven, place the peppers, onions, sweet potatoes and chick-peas. Season with the garlic, cumin, coriander and cinnamon. Pour the vegetable juice cocktail and water over the vegetables. Cover and cook over medium-low heat, occasionally moving vegetables gently for even cooking, for about 25 minutes, or until the vegetables are tender when pierced with a sharp knife.

Sprinkle the couscous over the vegetables, tilting the pan, if necessary, to moisten all the couscous. Sprinkle the cilantro over the couscous-vegetable mixture. Cover the pan, remove from the heat and set aside for 5 minutes, or until the couscous absorbs most of the liquid.

Serve the vegetables and couscous with the hot-pepper sauce (if using).

Makes 4 servings.

Per serving: 381 calories, 2.5 g. total fat, 0.4 g. saturated fat, 16.2 g. fiber, 0 mg. cholesterol, 470 mg. sodium

Tabbouleh

A refreshing partner for grilled lean meat, baked fish or a bean salad, this cracked-wheat classic contains plenty of energy-boosting B vitamins. The key ingredient is bulgur, which is cracked, partially cooked wheat. You'll find that it's sold in most supermarkets, as well as health food stores.

¾ cup medium-grind bulgur

1 tablespoon extra-virgin olive oil

¼ cup nonfat plain yogurt

2 tablespoons lemon juice

1 small cucumber, peeled, seeded and diced

1 bunch scallions, white and light green stem, sliced

1 medium tomato, diced

1 cup minced fresh parsley leaves

¼ cup minced fresh mint leaves

½ teaspoon ground black pepper

Place the bulgur in a medium mixing bowl. Cover with plenty of cold water and set aside for about 1 hour, or until the grains are tender but still firm.

Meanwhile, in another medium mixing bowl, whisk the oil with the yogurt and lemon juice.

Drain the bulgur through a fine sieve. Place the bulgur in the bowl with the yogurt dressing. Add the cucumbers, scallions, tomatoes, parsley, mint and pepper. Toss to combine. Cover and chill in the refrigerator for at least 1 hour before serving.

Makes 4 servings.

Per serving: 157 calories, 4.1 g. total fat, 0.6 g. saturated fat, 6.8 g. fiber, 0 mg. cholesterol, 29 mg. sodium

Spinach-Orange Salad with Sesame

Sunny lemon juice and orange slices boost the body's ability to absorb the iron from the fresh spinach leaves. And more iron means more energy. This delightful salad pairs beautifully with Turkey-Vegetable Wedges (see page 32) for supper or brunch.

- **2 tablespoons lemon juice**
- **1 tablespoon honey**
- **2 tablespoons nonfat plain yogurt**
- **4 cups tightly packed, washed, dried and torn spinach leaves**
- **¼ medium red onion, thinly sliced**
- **1 navel orange, peeled, quartered, thinly sliced**
- **1 tablespoon toasted sesame seeds (see hint)**

In a large bowl, whisk together the lemon juice, honey and yogurt. Add the spinach, onions, oranges and sesame seeds. Toss to coat with the dressing.

Cook's Hint: To toast sesame seeds, place them in a small, heavy frying pan over medium heat. Cook, stirring frequently, for 5 minutes, or until golden and fragrant. Remove from the heat to cool. The seeds can also be toasted in a larger batch and stored in the freezer.

Makes 4 servings.

Per serving: 64 calories, 1.4 g. total fat, 0.2 g. saturated fat, 2.6 g. fiber, 0 mg. cholesterol, 51 mg. sodium

Top Secret Chocolate Pudding

This secret is worth sharing—a luscious chocolate dessert that's really rich in protein from reduced-fat silken tofu. The extra protein may help keep your blood levels of insulin on an even keel. And that's an important benefit, because big swings in blood sugar and insulin levels can play havoc with your energy supply.

3 ounces unsweetened baking chocolate

1 cup light corn syrup

2 packages (10½ ounces each) reduced-fat, firm or extra-firm silken tofu, drained

1 teaspoon vanilla

8 ripe strawberries (optional)

In a microwaveable small bowl or glass measuring cup, combine the chocolate and corn syrup. Microwave on high power for 2½ to 3 minutes, stirring occasionally, or until the chocolate melts. (The mixture can also be heated in a small saucepan over low heat on the stove top.) Remove from the heat and set aside.

Place the tofu in the bowl of a food processor. Process, scraping the sides of the bowl, as necessary, for about 2 minutes, or until very smooth and fluffy. With the machine running, add the chocolate mixture and vanilla through the feed tube. Process to combine, scraping the sides of the bowl with a spatula so that no white remains.

Spoon the pudding into a medium glass serving bowl or 8 dessert dishes. Cover and refrigerate to chill for several hours or overnight.

Top each serving with a strawberry (if using).

Makes 8 servings.

Per serving: 207 calories, 6.5 g. total fat, 3.3 g. saturated fat, 1.6 g. fiber, 0 mg. cholesterol, 101 mg. sodium

Whole-Wheat Buttermilk Pancakes with Blueberry Cinnamon Sauce

The whole-grain wheat flour in these pancakes provides magnesium, an important component of energy production. Each pancake also offers good amounts of blood-building copper and iron along with vitamins B_6, thiamin and riboflavin—all involved in energy metabolism.

You can make these moist and tender carbohydrate-packed griddle cakes with blueberry sauce for Sunday brunch. Or make only the pancakes, cool them on a baking rack, and then freeze them in a plastic bag, separated by pieces of wax paper. For a weekday breakfast, just pop a pancake into the toaster or toaster oven to thaw and heat. Cover with fruit spread and roll it up for a portable breakfast.

SAUCE

- 2 tablespoons sugar
- 1 tablespoon cornstarch
- ¾ teaspoon ground cinnamon
- 1 pint fresh blueberries or 1 pound loose-packed frozen blueberries, unthawed
- 1½ tablespoons lime juice

PANCAKES

- 1 cup whole-wheat pastry flour (see hint)
- ½ cup unbleached all-purpose flour
- 1 tablespoon sugar
- ¾ teaspoon baking powder
- ¼ teaspoon baking soda
- ½ teaspoon ground ginger
- 1¼ cups buttermilk

  About ½ cup skim milk

- ¼ cup fat-free egg substitute
- 1 tablespoon canola oil

To make the sauce: In a medium saucepan, combine the sugar, cornstarch and cinnamon. Add the blueberries and lime juice. Stir to combine. Cook over medium-low heat, stirring frequently, for 4 to 5 minutes, or until the blueberries are hot and a sauce forms. Remove from the heat and set aside.

To make the pancakes: In a medium mixing bowl, combine the whole-wheat pastry flour, all-purpose flour, sugar, baking powder, baking soda and ginger. Set aside.

In a large glass measuring cup or bowl, combine the buttermilk, ½ cup skim milk, egg substitute and oil.

Pour the liquid ingredients into the dry ingredients, stirring with a whisk or fork, just until combined. Add 1 to 2 tablespoons more skim milk, if needed, to thin the batter.

Heat a heavy aluminum or cast-iron griddle over medium-high heat. Coat lightly with oil. Ladle or pour pancake batter, in ¼-cup portions, onto the griddle. Cook for about 2 minutes each side, or until the pancakes are golden. Continue cooking until all the batter is used. Serve pancakes with warm blueberry sauce.

Cook's Hint: Whole-wheat pastry flour is sold in some health food stores and supermarkets. If unavailable, substitute regular whole-wheat flour combined with 1 tablespoon cornstarch.

Makes 12; 6 servings.

Per serving: 217 calories, 3.4 g. total fat, 0.6 g. saturated fat, 4.1 g. fiber, 2 mg. cholesterol, 179 mg. sodium

Gingery Date-Nut Bars

These cookies are a decent source of magnesium, an energy-enhancing nutrient that is responsible for more than 300 chemical reactions in the body.

1 **package (8 ounces) pitted dates, chopped**

1 **tablespoon finely chopped candied ginger**

2 **tablespoons granulated sugar**

½ **cup water**

½ **teaspoon vanilla**

1 **cup whole-wheat pastry flour (see hint)**

½ **cup rice bran**

¼ **cup packed brown sugar**

½ **teaspoon baking soda**

¼ **cup finely chopped walnuts**

2 **egg whites, lightly beaten**

2 **tablespoons canola oil**

Preheat the oven to 350°. Coat an 8″ × 8″ baking pan with no-stick spray. Set aside.

In a medium saucepan, combine the dates, ginger, granulated sugar and water. Cook the mixture over medium heat, stirring frequently, for 5 minutes, or until it thickens. Remove and set aside to cool slightly. Stir in the vanilla.

In a medium mixing bowl, combine the flour, bran, brown sugar, baking soda and walnuts. In a small bowl, combine the egg whites with the oil. Add to the dry mixture and toss with a fork or your hands to combine. The mixture will resemble streusel topping.

Press about two-thirds of the crust mixture into the prepared pan. Pat gently. Spread the reserved date filling over the bottom crust, then top with the remaining crust mixture. Pat gently.

Bake for about 30 minutes, or until the top crust is golden. Remove from the oven to cool. Cut into bars.

Cook's Hint: Whole-wheat pastry flour is sold in some health food stores and supermarkets. If unavailable, substitute regular whole-wheat flour combined with 1 tablespoon cornstarch.

Makes 16.

Per bar: 123 calories, 3.5 g. total fat, 0.3 g. saturated fat, 1.7 g. fiber, 0 mg. cholesterol, 49 mg. sodium

Apricot Cinna-Muffins

These delicious whole-grain muffins have the B-complex vitamins and minerals needed to metabolize the carbohydrates that fuel your body.

1¼   **cups whole-wheat pastry flour**

¾   **cup unbleached all-purpose flour**

2   **tablespoons granulated sugar**

2   **teaspoons baking powder**

1   **teaspoon baking soda**

¾   **cup chopped dried apricots**

2   **tablespoons packed brown sugar**

1½   **teaspoons ground cinnamon**

1   **cup buttermilk**

1   **egg, lightly beaten**

1   **egg white, lightly beaten**

3   **tablespoons canola oil**

Preheat the oven to 375°. Coat 12 regular-size muffin cups with no-stick spray. Set aside.

In a large bowl, combine the whole-wheat pastry flour, all-purpose flour, granulated sugar, baking powder, baking soda and apricots. Stir to mix.

In a small bowl, combine the brown sugar and cinnamon. Set aside.

In another small bowl, combine the buttermilk, egg, egg white and oil. Pour into the bowl with the flour mixture. Stir just until combined (do not beat).

Spoon half of the batter into the prepared muffin cups. Sprinkle half of the reserved cinnamon-sugar mixture over the batter in the cups. Top with the remaining batter and remaining cinnamon sugar.

Bake for 14 to 16 minutes, or until the muffins are golden and a toothpick inserted into the center of a muffin comes out clean. Remove from the oven to cool for 5 minutes.

Remove the muffins from the baking cups. Serve right away or freeze as soon as the muffins are cool.

Makes 12.

Per muffin: 154 calories, 4.4 g. total fat, 0.5 g. saturated fat, 2.4 g. fiber, 18 mg. cholesterol, 194 mg. sodium

Fruit-Bowl Cake with Orange–Cream Cheese Frosting

This exceptionally moist snack cake is a hit with children and adults. It contains an amazingly low 2 grams of fat per serving. A low-fat diet is the mainstay of healthy eating for energy, and tasty desserts that fit the bill can help you stick to your resolve to eat right.

CAKE

¾ **cup whole-wheat pastry flour (see hint)**

½ **cup unbleached all-purpose flour**

¾ **teaspoon ground cinnamon**

¼ **teaspoon ground cloves**

2 **teaspoons baking soda**

6 **tablespoons fat-free egg substitute**

½ **cup granulated sugar**

⅓ **cup unsweetened applesauce**

¼ **cup buttermilk**

1 **teaspoon vanilla**

⅔ **cup mashed ripe banana**

⅓ **cup canned crushed pineapple (with juice)**

FROSTING

1 **package (3 ounces) reduced-fat cream cheese, softened**

¼ **cup nonfat sour cream**

3 **tablespoons powdered sugar**

⅛ **teaspoon orange extract**

To make the cake: Preheat the oven to 350°. Coat an 8″ × 8″ cake pan with no-stick spray. Set aside.

In a small bowl, combine the whole-wheat flour, all-purpose flour, cinnamon, cloves and baking soda. Set aside.

In a medium mixing bowl, beat the egg substitute with the sugar. Stir in the applesauce, buttermilk, vanilla, banana and pineapple (with juice).

Add the dry ingredients to the wet ingredients, stirring just until combined. Pour mixture into the prepared pan.

Bake for approximately 30 minutes, or until a toothpick inserted in the center of the cake comes out clean. Remove from oven to a wire rack to cool.

To make the frosting: In a small mixing bowl, beat the cream cheese and sour cream until smooth. Add the sugar and orange extract. Beat until smooth. Spread the frosting on the cooled cake.

Cook's Hint: Whole-wheat pastry flour is sold in some health food stores and supermarkets. If unavailable, substitute whole-wheat flour combined with 1 tablespoon cornstarch.

Makes 9 servings.

Per serving: 171 calories, 2.1 g. total fat, 1.1 g. saturated fat, 1.9 g. fiber, 4 mg. cholesterol, 363 mg. sodium

Wheat and Walnut Bread

This whole-grain bread, enriched with extra wheat germ, has a moist crumb that makes it taste great when it's toasted. Each slice provides a bit of magnesium, copper, iron, thiamin, niacin and riboflavin. All these nutrients play a role in energy metabolism.

Try slicing the loaves before freezing so that you can conveniently thaw a slice at a time in the toaster.

    1   **package active dry yeast**

    2   **teaspoons sugar**

    3   **cups warm (110°) water**

    ½   **cup instant nonfat dry milk**

    2   **tablespoons canola oil**

    ½   **teaspoon salt**

    4   **cups whole-wheat flour**

    ½   **cup wheat germ**

    ½   **cup finely ground walnuts**

 2½–3 **cups unbleached all-purpose flour**

In a glass measuring cup, dissolve the yeast and sugar in ½ cup of the water. Set aside for 5 minutes until the mixture bubbles.

In the bowl of a heavy-duty mixer fitted with beaters or a dough hook, combine the milk, oil, salt and the remaining 2½ cups water. Mix on low speed to combine. Add the yeast mixture and the whole-wheat flour, 1 cup at a time. Mix until blended. Add the wheat germ and walnuts. Mix until blended. Add the all-purpose flour, 1 cup at a time, until the dough can no longer be mixed by machine.

Turn the dough onto a lightly floured board. Scrape the bowl and beaters or dough hook to remove all the dough. Knead for 10 minutes, working in as much of the remaining all-purpose flour as the dough will absorb. The dough should be smooth and elastic, moist but not sticky.

Coat a large bowl with no-stick spray. Place the dough in the bowl and coat lightly with no-stick spray. Cover with plastic wrap and set in a warm spot for 1½ hours, or until doubled in bulk.

Coat two 9″ × 5″ loaf pans with no-stick spray.

Punch down the dough and place on a lightly floured surface. Divide into two equal portions. Shape into two loaves. Place the loaves in the prepared pans. Spray lightly with no-stick spray. Cover with plastic wrap and set in a warm spot for 45 minutes to 1 hour, or until the loaves rise to the tops of the pans.

Preheat the oven to 400°. Bake for 15 minutes, then reduce the temperature to 350°. Bake for 20 to 25 minutes more, or until the loaves sound hollow when tapped. Or check with an instant-read thermometer for an internal temperature of 190°. Remove from the oven and turn the loaves onto a wire rack to cool.

Makes 2 loaves; 36 slices.

Per slice: 101 calories, 1.9 g. total fat, 0.2 g. saturated fat, 2.2 g. fiber, 0 mg. cholesterol, 36 mg. sodium

Sweet and Spicy Snack Mix

Splurge on good-for-you, low-fat, low-sugar snacks—eaten throughout the day—to keep your body up and running.

In addition to providing low-fat carbohydrates, this snack is a source of nutrients that play a role in carbohydrate metabolism—magnesium, copper, iron and thiamin.

1	**egg white**
2	**tablespoons cold water**
2	**cups Life cereal**
1	**cup raw, shelled, mixed nuts such as walnuts, unblanched almonds or pecans**
2	**tablespoons sugar**
½	**teaspoon ground cinnamon**
¼	**teaspoon ground ginger**
¼	**teaspoon ground cloves**
⅛	**teaspoon ground red pepper (optional)**

In a large mixing bowl, lightly beat the egg white and water with a fork. Add the cereal and nuts. Toss with a fork to coat the dry ingredients completely.

In a small bowl, combine the sugar, cinnamon, ginger, cloves and pepper (if using). Sprinkle over the cereal mixture. Toss with a fork until the cereal and nuts are coated with the spicy sugar.

Preheat the oven to 350°. Coat a large baking sheet with no-stick spray. Scatter the cereal mixture in a single layer on the baking sheet. Bake, stirring occasionally, for 18 to 20 minutes, or until the mixture is golden and crisp.

Remove from the oven to cool. Store in a cookie tin in a cool spot.

Makes 3¼ cups.

Per ¼ cup: 93 calories, 6 g. total fat, 0.5 g. saturated fat, 1.2 g. fiber, 0 mg. cholesterol, 42 mg. sodium

Environments
for Energy

No doubt about it, where we are has a lot to do with how energized we feel and what we can do. Michelangelo's talent really hit the roof at the Sistine Chapel. Thoreau's writings from Walden Pond were anything but all wet. And Lady Godiva seemed most energized on top of her proud steed . . . well, at least the crowd was energized.

Unfortunately, the everyday surroundings for the rest of us can be anything but energetic. Unlike the vaulted expanse of the Sistine Chapel, a suburban tract house or cramped office isn't exactly an environment for divine inspiration—or is it?

Look to the Unexpected

"There seems little doubt that your environment affects your energy level," says Maria Simonson, Sc.D., Ph.D., professor emeritus at Johns Hopkins University Medical Institutions in Baltimore and director of its Health, Weight and Stress Clinic. "But it's not as though you need to be someplace special to get more energy. No matter where you are, any surrounding can help you become more energized if you know what to do."

Some of the environmental tinkering you can do to turn up your energy level is obvious: You seek silence from barking dogs and noisy lawn mowers (both of which seem to be highly energized on sleep-deprived Sunday mornings). You open the curtains and windows to let sunlight and fresh air into your home or workplace. You play your favorite music when you're feeling down or want to stay up—or readily hand over the car keys to your heavy metal–loving offspring when he insists on playing his.

Less obvious, but perhaps more important, are these lesser-known ways of manipulating and masquerading your surroundings to give you optimum energy.

Color: Power from the Palette

When you say you're "in the pink" or "feeling blue," you're not just talking slang. You're talking science.

That's because colors actually give off electromagnetic wave "bands" of energy—with each shade having its own wavelength. It doesn't matter if it's paint on a wall or a picture, a bright flower or a piece of clothing, scientists say these color waves send impulses to the pituitary and pineal glands in the brain, which control mood, energy levels and heart rate.

"I was the first one in the mid-1950s to prove that color has a predictable and measurable effect on the autonomic nervous system—pulse rate, blood rate and blood pressure. Some colors raise them, others lower them," says Harry Wohlfarth, Ph.D., president of the International Academy of Color Sciences at the University of Alberta in Edmonton, Canada. "Color also has an impact on psychological factors as well, so something as simple as painting your walls or wearing a certain color of clothing can have an energizing effect."

These color waves occur even if you can't see the colors. Dr. Wohlfarth found that severely handicapped blind children reacted to the wavelengths of colors in the same way that seeing children did—both physiologically and psychologically.

Repainting for Vigor

In his studies, which some experts believe are the cornerstone of "color therapy," Dr. Wohlfarth found that yellow shades tend to have the most energizing effect on people; next come the other warm colors of orange and red. And, generally, cooler shades of blues, greens and grays have a more relaxing effect. Other researchers have made similar findings.

"We had some nursing homes, which typically have walls painted in browns, grays and dull greens, repainted with bright colors and done in graphics—lots of splashes of reds, yellows and oranges as well as coral shades, emerald greens and colors like that," says Dr. Simonson. "Once this was done, we found the activity level of the patients there soared. Old ladies who did nothing all day were getting out of bed and having people come in to do their hair. Men got up to shave. They got more involved in social activities. And now a lot of nursing homes and hospitals are getting away from the dull greens and grays and going with brighter and warmer colors."

Both experts say that colors can have the same impact on your environment. Here's what they recommend.

Find your own color profile.

While studies show yellow is the best energizing color for most people, there is no one color that has exactly the same effect on everyone. "A lot of it depends on your personality—whether you're an introvert or an extrovert," says Dr. Wohlfarth.

Introverts benefit most from colors that excite—warm hues of yellows, oranges and reds. But these colors can overstimulate extroverts, who usually run on full throttle. Cooler colors like blues and greens may be better to help extroverted people relax and recharge their batteries for more energy, according to Dr. Wohlfarth.

Pick the right shade.

It's not enough to just pick a color; you also have to give some thought to picking the right shade. "Not all yellows will energize and not all blues will relax you," says Dr. Wohlfarth. "For instance, if you come home from a stressed day at work and you're all wound up, you need to calm down, but with a *warm* shade of blue—one with red and yellow tints. A cool blue with green tints may be too depressive."

No matter what your personality type, for maximum energy Dr. Wohlfarth advises sticking with colors that have yellow tints. His recommendations for painting your walls: Glidden color 73–85, a light warm yellow, is best for an overall energizing effect.

For those high-strung type A people who need to relax for better energy, Dr. Wohlfarth advises Glidden color 77–30, a light blue with subtle yellow tints. You will find both colors—or similar shades—at most paint stores or home-improvement centers.

Get smart with art.

If you find the idea of repainting your walls anything but energizing, take an easier route—which might be even better for boosting energy: hang paintings, posters and other pieces of artwork. "The more colors there are, the better," says Dr. Simonson. "In fact, pictures and paintings are a great way to get splashes of energizing colors like red and orange that might be too much for an entire wall."

The key is to choose something you like—and will continue to like for months on end, says Linda Gantt, Ph.D., a registered art therapist and former president of the American Art Therapy Association in Mundelein, Illinois. "You'll be much more satisfied if you choose a piece that you can look at for a very long time, like a Monet, as opposed to the kind of artwork you buy at a gas station parking lot on Saturday afternoons," she says. "It doesn't really matter if it's abstract or a scenic setting. The key, other than color, is to just get something that you won't tire of."

Hue and You

If you're true to blue—or any other color—your raves for that shade may have more to do with personality traits than just personal choice. Researchers believe that we favor certain colors, particularly our "favorites," because of our internal makeup, disposition and other factors that can influence our energy levels.

"These are merely observations," notes Maria Simonson, Sc.D., Ph.D., professor emeritus at Johns Hopkins University Medical Institutions in Baltimore and director of its Health, Weight and Stress Clinic. "But they are observations we found to be consistent among several hundred people studied."

Red tends to be the choice of people who are decisive go-getters. "It indicates a somewhat impulsive, emotional person who likes to stay on top of things," says Dr. Simonson. "These are people who are aggressive and make lasting impressions."

Still, it's a color that shouldn't be used for the long term. It's best as an accent color, used on a short-term basis, like wearing a red scarf when you want to generate ideas or having accent pillows as opposed to four walls painted red. Too much red can be counterproductive since it stimulates the flow of adrenaline, raising pulse, blood pressure and energy levels. Such reactions probably date back to prehistoric times, when hunters got excited by the sight of blood from their day's kill.

Yellow is favored by those who are cheery, optimistic and fun-loving. "They have plenty of personality and like novelty in their lives," says Dr. Simonson. But when yellow is in your environment, it can contribute to anxiety and short tempers in excitable people. Studies show, for example, that babies cry more frequently in yellow rooms.

When you need long-term energy, yellow is a good choice for rooms or clothing, and it's popular on assembly lines because it energizes employees. The color is also popular with industries that deal with "temporary" services—real estate, rental car agencies and fast-food restaurants.

Orange is best liked by those with gregarious personalities. "These people thrive on fun, have unique ideas and are very determined and creative," says Dr. Simonson. It's a bad choice for the kitchen because it stimulates the appetite (which is the reason why the color is popular in many fast-food restaurants). But it is a good overall energy booster.

Blue, the most popular color, tends to be the favorite of Everyman. "These are no-nonsense individuals, perhaps even conservative," says Dr. Simonson. "They tend to be even-tempered and may even appear cool, but underneath are very sensitive." It's a good color for relaxing and daydreaming because it stimulates the brain to secrete tranquilizing hormones. Blue is an excellent choice for the bedroom or den, rooms where you want to wind down.

Green is the choice of those who are creative, outspoken and treasure their freedom. "People who prefer green tend to be 'joiners' who are very loyal friends and persevere in what they do," says Dr. Simonson. Green is a comforting color to many people and helps them relax, which is why it's often used in training rooms, personnel offices, hospitals and schools. Exposure to green helps lower the heart rate and reduce stress.

Purple is the color preferred by artistic types, says Dr. Simonson. "They tend to be highly creative, emotional and generally have an ambitious and philosophic streak. They are witty and observant, but tend to also be moody." But the color has its drawbacks: Purple decreases the appetite and slows muscular response, so it's not a good choice for those seeking energy.

Black is liked mostly by those who see themselves as strong and sophisticated. Since it's seen as depressing by many, black's a poor choice for energy.

White is liked by those who are serene and cool—nonemotional types. "But they tend to be very neat and fussy," says Dr. Simonson. It's the most popular color for work and home environments—but a bad choice for energizing because it causes the eye to shut down, resulting in unconscious squinting, increased fatigue and a general wearing down. In terms of energy, experts advise going with off-white, eggshell and other colors more in the beige family instead of a snowy white.

Gray is favored by those who put their noses to the grindstone. "They are careful people who are hard workers and have cool, nonemotional personalities," says Dr. Simonson. Although the color has no direct effect on energy, research shows that office workers are most productive in light gray environments.

Floor 'em.

Don't assume that the walls are the only place where colors play a role in boosting energy. "I have Persian rugs all over my apartment because there is plenty of color to keep me energized," says Dr. Wohlfarth. "In my bedroom I have a red rug because it's very sexy—and, like a lot of people, my bedroom isn't used only for sleeping."

Don't snicker. Dr. Wohlfarth and other experts say that men in particular often associate their overall energy level with their sex drive. In other words, when guys are "energized" below the waist, they tend to think of themselves as energized all over.

Dress for success.

Even if you can't redecorate your environment—at the workplace, for instance—you can still energize your surroundings.

"You just need to be around or exposed to that color—and that can come from dressing in a particular shade, having an object like a flower on your desk or even just looking at a piece of paper in that color," maintains Dr. Simonson. "That's one reason why children get more excited when playing with yellow toys as opposed to toys of other colors—no matter where they are playing."

Her advice: Dress in energizing colors like yellow, red and orange—or at least include splashes of those colors in scarves or other accessories. At work you can place roses or black-eyed Susans on your desk—or at least keep a sheet of paper in an energizing color handy.

Lighting: Brighten the Mood

Of course, the cause of those doldrums could be over your head—quite literally. So if you know the right kind of lighting to choose, say researchers, you may be able to short-circuit fatigue and boost energy levels.

"We've long known that the type of lighting you have in your home or workplace can influence mood and productivity," says Robert Baron, Ph.D., an industrial psychologist at Rensselaer Polytechnic Institute's Lighting Research Center in Troy, New York, and chairman of its psychology department. Dr. Baron is also one of the nation's foremost authorities on the effects that lighting has on personality. "Whether mood relates to energy may be a point of debate, but many people argue that a positive mood includes exhilaration and feelings that you're able to do stuff, which is very much related to a high energy level," he says.

His studies also indicate that the proper lighting helps improve creative problem-solving and conflict-solving abilities—other factors associated with high energy. "You also tend to work harder because you don't want to spoil that good feeling," he says.

Best of all, achieving these benefits can be as easy as changing a lightbulb, according to Dr. Baron. "There's no doubt that certain lightbulbs—as well as certain types of lighting—put people in better moods and increase their productivity," he says.

Warm up to "warm" fluorescent bulbs.

Every major manufacturer makes two types of bulbs—the widely used cool-white bulbs that give off a brighter, bluish hue and the less popular warm-white bulbs that have a reddish yellow hint to make the skin look rosier. Which ones should you choose?

"The warm bulbs seem to produce a more positive mood and better productivity in people," says Dr. Baron. "It's not that the cool-white bulbs make you depressed, but that most people find the lighting too harsh and not as pleasing, and as a result, it fatigues them."

Warm-white fluorescent bulbs are available at most places where lighting fixtures and bulbs are sold and cost only pennies more than cool-white bulbs. "At work, I recommend that you specifically ask for warm-white bulbs," says Dr. Baron. "They are readily available."

Get into incandescents.

There's no doubt that fluorescent lights are the choice of most workplaces and even some homes—because they're cheaper to buy and operate. But even if you work under these long tubes, still try to have a table lamp nearby.

The reason is that although they appear to be on all the time, many fluorescent lights actually flicker about 60 times per second. This flickering may not seem noticeable, but it tends to fatigue the brain, causing headaches and fatigue. (Although some fluorescent lights have been improved in recent years to avoid this, others still flicker, Dr. Baron says.) Besides, fluorescent bulbs tend to produce a lot of glare.

"At home many people tend to stay away from fluorescents because they are associated with a work setting or hospitals," says Dr. Baron. "The best thing is to try to shut off the fluorescents if you can. But even if you can't, having a lamp with an incandescent bulb will help."

Switch to dimmers.

Those on-off switches may be turning off your energy more than you might think. "People tell us they tend to be in a better mood when the illumination is relatively low, but that's not always practical," says Dr. Baron. "Besides, people want to be able to control the lighting in their environment—whether it's their homes or workplaces."

His answer: Install dimmer switches wherever possible. That way, you can not only reduce the amount of light for less glare but also flex some control—a "mental" energizer in itself.

"With fluorescent lights you may not be able to control the amount of light from the individual bulbs, but you can still control the overall lighting with dimmers for the specific activity," says Dr. Baron. "For instance, if you have fluorescent lights in your kitchen like I do, you keep all the lights on when you're baking. But if you're having coffee, you can use less light."

Fragrances: The Nose Knows

Another way to sniff out more energy from your environment is to do just that—sniff.

"The quickest way to induce a change in emotions or mood is through smell, because the sense of smell reacts more quickly on the brain than other senses," says Alan R. Hirsch, M.D., neurological director of the Smell and Taste Treatment and Research Foundation, a leading facility in fragrance and smell research in Chicago. "And in many cases, feeling energized—or fatigued—is due to the kind of mood we're in."

Because of this, Dr. Hirsch and others believe that adding fragrances can be among the most effective ways to add energy to your surroundings—as well as the fastest.

"When we talk about energy, we're really talking about two things: the activation of the systems in the brain that make us awake and alert as well as the ability to deal with fatigue," he says. "We studied both and found that fragrances play a role in both."

Scents That Make Sense

There's a lot of evidence that certain odors can impact wakefulness, says Dr. Hirsch. "It's the same principle as using smelling salts or cutting into an onion and crying. You stimulate the irritant nerve, and that triggers wakefulness."

In Japan always-on-the-go executives start each morning with alarm clocks that, ten minutes before sounding, actually spray a scented mist to make the mind and body more alert. (They're not available in the United States.)

Dr. Hirsch has also discovered that certain fragrances can distract people enough to make them "forget" they're fatigued, and even improve mood. "And when you're in a better mood," he adds, "there's at least the perception that you have more energy."

While smelling any aromas that you particularly enjoy is beneficial, studies at his research center indicate that some odors are better than others. So here's how to use those sweet smells for success.

Get jazzed with jasmine.

Different odors actually have an effect on brain waves, and altering brain waves can change your energy level, says Dr. Hirsch.

"Smelling jasmine tends to induce beta waves in the front of the head, which are associated with a more alert stage. Meanwhile, if you want a more relaxed stage or have trouble sleeping (a problem frequently associated with fatigue), try lavender because it increases the alpha waves in the back of the head, which help put you to sleep." If you have no jasmine plants, you can buy jasmine-scented incense or oils at some health food shops and other stores to reap these benefits.

Desert stress with dessert scents.

Dr. Hirsch has found that certain smells are best for distracting you from those everyday stresses that zap your energy.

"We looked at exercise strength when people were exposed to certain odors and found that certain smells helped them exercise longer—probably because of a distraction factor." This is similar to what happens when people watch TV or have the company of another person while exercising—they exercise longer, according to Dr. Hirsch. "And we found that the best smell for this was strawberries and buttered popcorn." Although his tests used a combination of both scents, he adds that either smell alone would probably be beneficial.

Induce "the mood" with food.

No red rugs in the bedroom? Then check out the kitchen cabinets.

"There is little doubt that the more sexually excited a man is, the more energized he feels," says Dr. Hirsch. "And we found that certain smells can help increase penile blood flow and excite a man sexually." Incredibly, these aren't odors that would automatically pop into mind.

The top odor for putting men in the mood was a combination of pumpkin pie and lavender, followed by black licorice and freshly baked doughnuts. For older men, the smell of vanilla was the most sexually stimulating, he adds.

Take a whiff of the old days.

Scientists believe that the more positive your mental or emotional state, the more energized you feel. "When you're in a more positive mood, things seem to bother you less, and feeling fatigued can be the result of letting these things get to you," says Dr. Hirsch.

So how do you get into a better mood? Take a whiff of a childhood memory. Since most people tend to have fond memories of childhood, odors associated with those memories can improve mood—although those evocative odors vary from person to person.

"Those born before 1930 are most likely to describe natural scents as their favorites—pine trees, flowers and the like—while those born after 1930 are more likely to favor artificial smells such as Pez candy, baby powder and VapoRub," says Dr. Hirsch.

Where you lived when you were growing up has a lot to do with it, too. The childhood odors found most pleasing were baked goods (especially to residents of the East Coast), fresh air (favored by Southerners), barbecued meat (for Westerners) and farm animals (by those from the Midwest).

Slice a lemon.
"Actually, just about any pleasing odor is beneficial," says Dr. Baron. "If you like the smell of chocolate chip cookies, then bake some, and it will probably improve your mood." But there is one smell, he says, that is pleasing to just about everyone: citrus.

Since many commercial air fresheners and potpourris are so strong that they can actually turn you off, Dr. Baron recommends slicing an orange or lemon and inhaling deeply. "You don't need anything fancy to benefit from fragrances," he says. "In fact, the more natural, the better."

Airing Problems Out

Tarzan, you'll notice, is one heck of an energized guy—swinging from tree to tree and yelling at the top of his lungs, while many men his age would get fatigued jogging once around the block. Maybe genes have something to do with it. But check out his environment and you may get another explanation.

"Being in an environment where there are plenty of plants absolutely helps a number of psychological and physiological factors—possibly even including boosting energy levels," says Bill Wolverton, Ph.D., a former research scientist with NASA's John C. Stennis Space Center, who now runs his own environmental research firm in Picayune, Mississippi. "It makes you feel alive!"

That's because whether they're in your home, office or the Amazon rain forest, plants give off low levels of hundreds of different chemicals, says Dr. Wolverton. "Some of these chemicals protect the plants against insects," he notes. But there are other plant-released chemicals whose purpose is unknown.

Scientists do know, however, that many of these chemicals purify the air and battle "sick building syndrome," two factors that play a key role in fighting fatigue and keeping energy high. "We took an indoor room that had no plants and

Plants for Pep

How does a spider plant get rid of formaldehyde fumes from your new carpeting? Microorganisms living in potting soil use airborne toxins as a source of food. Plant roots absorb the waste produced by those microorganisms and then release cleaner air in your home.

"Some plants work better because their root systems prefer pollutants and use them as food faster than others," says Bill Wolverton, Ph.D., a former research scientist with NASA's John C. Stennis Space Center, who now runs his own environmental research firm in Picayune, Mississippi. Figuring the number of plants to best do the job isn't easy, and he advises that you overestimate that number rather than underestimate it.

But it's easy to figure out the types of plants to use. Here are 11 of the best—and easiest to maintain—household plants to hold down pollution levels in your home for better breathing and energy.

- Bamboo or Areca palm
- Boston fern (or any fern)
- Chrysanthemum
- Corn plant (or any dracaena)
- English ivy (or any ivy)
- Gerbera daisy
- Golden pothos
- Peace lily
- Philodendron
- Snake plant
- Spider plant

placed a common variety of readily available houseplants in it," says Dr. Wolverton. "There were 50 percent fewer dangerous airborne particles than before."

Among the chemicals absorbed by plants are carbon dioxide, acetone, methyl alcohol and ethyl acetate—chemicals given off when humans exhale. Plants also absorb some dangerous toxins like formaldehyde, benzene and other contaminants found in building supplies, furniture and carpeting. "These building contaminants can cause flulike symptoms, general fatigue and are even suspected of triggering some cases of cancer," says Dr. Wolverton. After absorbing these contaminants, the plants then return clean air.

Houseplants also help control the humidity of your environment, which is important in hot weather: When high heat combines with humidity, both can rob you of energy. "Certainly, when it gets too warm, you don't do as well and get tired faster," says Jack Loeppky, Ph.D., an environmental physiologist in Albuquerque, New Mexico. What plants do is absorb excess humidity into their

(continued on page 64)

How the Chinese Energize

The newest trend in designing environments for energy is a method that's been around for more than 2,000 years on the other side of the world. Masters of this method claim that subtle influences all around could be contributing to your fatigue in things that create a problem with your chi or a failure of your yin to balance properly with your yang.

Feng shui (pronounced fung shway) is the Chinese art of arranging your home and working environment to produce maximum positive energy—or *chi*. Feng shui makes use of architecture and design concepts such as location of doors and windows, interior decorating and even furniture placement. When chi is flowing appropriately, the theory goes, you feel energized, positive and productive. And when it's not, you are ineffectual and anxious.

Besides chi, feng shui's other foundation is based on the Taoist philosophy of *yin/yang*. Yin and yang represent opposing energetic forces: yin being the dark and passive qualities like sleep and yang being the active qualities. The theory holds that the two are complementary and must be in good balance for you to have maximum energy. One purpose of feng shui, say experts, is to help you achieve that perfect balance.

"Feng shui is based on superstition, geometry and even horoscope and is very important in Chinese culture," says George J. Grover, Jr., an Asian-American feng shui expert who owns Intergraph Environmental Planning and Design, an architectural firm in San Francisco. "Doing feng shui helps you be more energetic and productive and, as a result, more prosperous."

Feng shui is beginning to gain popularity among Westerners—especially along the West Coast. "It can be very complex, since it takes individual factors into account like your birthday, where you were born, even the direction the building faces," says Grover, who incorporates feng shui principles into the buildings he designs. "But it can also be as simple as placing your furniture a certain way in order to achieve maximum chi."

Although Western scientists are not about to put their stamp of approval on feng shui, billions of Chinese have maintained for centuries that this art energizes them. If something like this makes them—or you—feel better, who's to say it doesn't work? Here are a few energizing tips from Grover.

Head to your bed.

Some of feng shui's most important—and all-purpose—principles revolve around where you spend one-third of your time: in the bedroom. "You should never place a bed so that your feet directly face the door," says Grover. "That's bad because the belief is that your spirit leaves your body at night and if the room is too open, the spirit might go away and not come back. You want something to block it, like a wall."

That means it's okay to have the foot of the bed facing toward the door, as long as it's not a straight shot. In other words, when lying in bed, you shouldn't be able to see directly out the bedroom door, he says.

Check your exits.

If you have a shotgun style of home—where the front and back doors are in a straight line with nothing in between—then you could be depleting your chi. "The belief is that a good element can come in the house and just leave. You need something to block a straight line between the front and back doors, like a wall, a partition or even some furniture," says Grover.

Play the numbers.

"The first thing Chinese people do when buying property is look at the address, because numbers mean something—and the same goes for a telephone number," he says. "The numbers eight and two are good, a sign of wealth and good chi." While you can't change your address, you can do what many believers in feng shui do: When getting a new phone number, request that it contain these numbers, he advises.

Look overhead.

Beamed and sloped ceilings may be the rage in design, but they add up to bad chi in feng shui. "You don't want to sleep or sit directly under a beam, because it sits on your chi all the time," says Grover. "A higher ceiling is better because it gives your energy more of a lift."

Let there be light.

Windows play a big part in feng shui, because sunlight helps boost chi and, as a result, energy levels. While you may not be able to add more windows to an existing structure, Grover recommends allowing as much light in as possible with the right type of window treatments.

Cut a rug.

Tile is hard on your feet, the bottom of your chi, according to Grover. "You want something soft and friendly underneath, such as a rug," he says. "So if you have hard floors, put down an area rug or carpeting."

Plan those plantings.

One of the worst things you can do in feng shui is to plant a tree directly facing the entrance of your home. "If you can walk outside your home without something blocking your chi, that's good," says Grover. "But if a tree or other landscaping is blocking your chi, that's bad."

root systems and release it when the environment is drier, thus keeping surroundings more comfortable.

Seeing Is Believing

Just *seeing* plants can put people in a better frame of mind, a cornerstone of increased energy. "Studies show that hospital patients whose rooms overlook trees or a garden have a better recovery rate than those who don't," says Dr. Wolverton. "Maybe it's just psychological, but it seems to be consistent in all the studies." He adds that while he worked at NASA, he noted that the first request from dog-tired Russian cosmonauts returning from space was for "a picture of trees."

So here's how to use Mother Nature's greatest gift for maximum energy.

Do your math.
Dr. Wolverton suggests a minimum of one plant for every 100 square feet of living space—the typical 10- by 10-foot room. "Of course, the more you have, the better," he adds. "You can't have too many plants if your environment has central heat and air conditioning."

Buy quality.
The quality of plants you bring into your environment has a lot to do with their effectiveness. "You want to buy the plants where you know they've been well-cared-for and not have a lot of insects," says Dr. Wolverton. It's no energizer to have plants around that look as if they're dying of mite or aphid infestations. "I'm not saying that discount-store plants are full of bugs or of inferior quality, but the chances are they will have more bugs than a plant you get from a quality nursery."

Reason with the seasons.
Keeping your plants well-watered—but not drowned—is the best way to keep them healthy and able to control room humidity. If plants are brown-leaved and drought-afflicted, they're not going to be good energy companions. Ideally, water should be given in a slow and steady flow, rather than a massive gushing once or twice a week.

"Many people don't know this, but most houseplants need two to three times more water in the winter," says Dr. Wolverton. That's when heating systems tend to dry indoor air so its relative humidity is around 15 percent—drier than Death Valley. A room should have at least 35 percent relative humidity, but properly watered houseplants can keep cold-weather air over 40 percent, making it more comfortable.

Keep an eye on the thermostat.

Even with a comfortable humidity level, be sure to keep an eye on the temperature itself. Most people feel more energized in cooler temperatures than in warmer ones, but there is no ideal range.

Don't keep your house too cold, though, warns Thomas Adams, Ph.D., professor of physiology at Michigan State University in East Lansing. "You need to watch out especially for small children; because of their smaller body mass, children tend to heat up and cool down faster than adults."

If you have an elderly member of your household, you might want to provide an especially warm room for their comfort—so other members of the household don't have to live in an overheated house. Since metabolism slows with age, the elderly tend to like their surroundings warmer, which can rob energy from other household members. "The key," says Dr. Adams, "is to take everyone's needs into account—and everyone has different needs."

Exercising
for Energy

You know how to tell when a juggler is tired. Instead of keeping all those balls in the air, he starts dropping them. Well, you may identify with that pooped performer when you're juggling life's varied responsibilities. Funny thing is, any kind of exercise—even as low-key as juggling—can help you keep all your balls in the air and even charge up your juggling style.

It's true that exercise requires you to expend energy. But it's equally true that regular exercise, in any form, frequently gives people an energy boost—physically and mentally.

In fact, exercise offers regenerating benefits to every part of your body, from your brain to your bones—and that equals more energy. People who exercise regularly become more resistant to stress, an insidious energy drainer. They have better-quality sleep, and so, may function better on fewer hours than sedentary people do.

Iron-Pumping Payoffs

Instead of losing muscle as they age, exercisers can maintain or rebuild muscles. They slash their chances of developing such energy-draining illnesses as heart disease and diabetes. And because their immunity gets a boost from activity, exercisers may have fewer bothersome colds and flus, which can leave people wiped out for days.

If you're trying to lose weight, exercise automatically shores up your resolution by increasing your hunger for carbohydrates, says William McCarthy, Ph.D., director of science at the Pritikin Longevity Center in Santa Monica, California. Dr. McCarthy calls regular exercise "the best 'marker' that people will stay on the wagon when it comes to such energy-enhancing lifestyle habits as maintaining proper weight, eating healthfully and not smoking."

With exercise such an important component of any energy-restoring program, it deserves to be near the top of your daily "to do" list. If you haven't exercised regularly for a while, here are ways to safely ease into it. And even if you do get a regular workout, there are some ways to make your exercise easier, more effective and fun.

Getting Started

People who are just starting out have different needs than longtime exercisers, whose main concern may be the battle against boredom, says Tedd Mitchell, M.D., medical director of the Cooper Wellness Program in Dallas. Here's what beginners need to know.

Sneak in exercise.
You don't have to run two miles a day, or even go to a gym, to be more fit. You'll benefit if you get a total of 30 minutes a day in short bursts of moderate activity around your house, Dr. McCarthy says. Activities can include such things as walking up stairs, walking short distances quickly, gardening, doing housework, raking leaves, dancing and playing with children or pets.

"The most health benefits from this sort of activity are for people who otherwise would be completely sedentary," he adds. "All these daily choices will make a difference."

Get help before you get hurt.
Consider professional help in designing your exercise program right from the start, says Dr. Mitchell. A professional trainer can assess your current fitness level and come up with a plan that lets you exercise safely and with maximum improvement. "Even people who are simply planning to walk can avoid injury by getting tips on correct posture and shoes." The personal fitness assessment doesn't substitute for a doctor's evaluation, so you should let the trainer know about any health problems your doctor has identified.

The best places to find help? Try a good health club or the local Y. Local chapters of the Arthritis Foundation or the American Heart Association can also point you in the right direction. Or you can call the American Council on Exercise (ACE) at 1-800-529-8227. They may be able to recommend ACE-certified trainers in your area.

Establish the habit.
"Initially, consistency, not intensity, is the most important thing people need to develop in an exercise program," Dr. Mitchell says. "That's especially important for some who say, 'I don't have enough energy to get through the day. I don't see how I can exercise.' "

Getting Your Doc's Go-Ahead

If you're out of shape, but still want to reap the many energy-enhancing benefits of exercise, you just need to exercise a little caution first. If exercise is new to you, it's wise to see a doctor before you get started, says Tedd Mitchell, M.D., medical director of the Cooper Wellness Program in Dallas. Just about everyone can exercise, even those with heart disease, as long as they follow a program designed to be safe for them, he says.

Dr. Mitchell recommends that men age 40 or older and women age 50 or older get a medical evaluation before they begin exercising. The evaluation should include a treadmill stress test, which can detect serious coronary blockage, and blood pressure and cholesterol measurements.

He also recommends a treadmill stress test for older men who have been exercising for years—especially if they plan to gear up for a special event such as a marathon. "It's possible to be very fit without being healthy," Dr. Mitchell says. A case in point is world-class runner Jim Fixx, who died of a massive heart attack—and who refused to be tested for heart disease, despite a family history of the problem.

It's true that many older people begin walking for exercise without ever getting a stress test. "We don't want to discourage these people from walking, and probably most can safely do this," says Dr. Mitchell. Still, it's best to get your doctor's permission for your own peace of mind. Some people may need to begin exercise under medical supervision.

To get such people started, Dr. Mitchell has them exercise three days a week for as little as 5 to 10 minutes a day for a month. If a person thinks he can't exercise on a given day, he is told to reschedule meetings or appointments or substitute some other physical activity. Dr. Mitchell stresses the importance of establishing a time designated for exercising only.

"We're not worrying about heart rate or distances, we're not worrying about anything except getting it done for those 5 to 10 minutes," Dr. Mitchell says. After a month, he'll boost people to five days a week of 5 to 10 minutes a day for another month. "Then, and only then, will we start working on increasing the time." After people have started walking five days a week for 20 to 30 minutes a day for a month, he starts working on the intensity of the exercise.

Be a tortoise, not a hare.
People who catch exercise fever tend to do too much too soon, says Diane McDevitt, a personal trainer at the Bethlehem Racquetball Club in Bethlehem,

Pennsylvania. "They say, 'This is it. I'm going to exercise every day.' And, usually, they're dieting as well," she says. "They tear right into it, and three to four days later they are completely out of steam."

That sets the stage for injury, exhaustion and, ultimately, defeat. The trick is to start out with an exercise regimen that is suitable for your level of fitness, McDevitt explains, "and for people who haven't exercised for a long time, that's S-L-O-W."

Stop before you run out of gas.

One way to make sure that you don't initially overdo it is to stop your activity before you get too tired to go on. "Even at the start, your new exercise program should not make you more tired," Dr. Mitchell says.

"You may have a little muscle soreness and feel a little tired in a relaxed sort of way, but if you're exhausted or you have less energy during the rest of the day, you are doing too much," explains McDevitt.

Don't expect to perk up right away.

If you're easing into your exercise program gradually, it could take up to six months to notice an improvement in endurance and strength, Dr. Mitchell says. People who start out more fit, however, may get returns on their energy investment within a few weeks. Improved mood, better sleep and more staying power are among the first things people notice, McDevitt says.

Take advantage of energy peaks.

Exercise during the time of day when your body naturally has the most energy. For some people, that's first thing in the morning. For others, it's later in the day.

"Everyone has a different cycle, and it's hard to break that cycle. So the best thing may be to work with it," says Richard Bullough, Ph.D., adjunct professor of nutrition at the University of Utah in Salt Lake City. "If I exercise in the morning, for instance, by midday I am starting to wear down. I don't feel invigorated anymore. I have to wait until at least 4:00 P.M. to exercise, and then, for me, it's like a second breath. If I go out and do a workout, my evening's great. It makes a big difference."

If you're having a hard time getting going or feel tired after you exercise, experiment with switching your workout to different times of the day, Dr. Bullough suggests.

Pump Air with Aerobics

Aerobic, which simply means "with oxygen," describes exercises that force you to breathe a lot. As the result of aerobic exercise, you get a greater concentration of oxygen in your blood, and that means more oxygen-rich blood flowing to your muscles.

Aerobic exercise is a proven mood elevator and stress reducer. "It's just purging adrenaline, an anxiety-producing biochemical," Dr. Mitchell explains. "With stress, adrenaline rises. Aerobic exercise simply gets rid of adrenaline."

Aerobic exercise also increases your heart's pumping capacity, which means you're less likely to seriously jack up your heart rate during normal daily activities. "With aerobic exercise your heart actually increases in size, so it ejects more blood with each squeeze," Dr. Mitchell explains. "The result is a lower heart rate."

And that's a good sign. The average heart beats 70 to 75 times a minute. A heart conditioned through exercise can beat 45 to 50 times a minute but delivers the same amount of blood as the average person's heart. A conditioned heart gets to rest more, which results in less wear and tear on your cardiovascular system.

Aerobic exercise also makes muscles more efficient at extracting oxygen and nutrients from blood. So as you get your muscles conditioned, you're less likely to experience muscle cramps or heaviness in your legs, Dr. Mitchell observes.

Another plus: Aerobic exercise increases your lungs' ability to expand and take in oxygen and to expel air fully so that stale air doesn't linger. That lets you use oxygen better, so you're less likely to feel out of breath when you exert yourself in everyday activities—when you're dragging a vacuum cleaner up the stairs, for instance.

Air-Raising Experiences

Since aerobic exercise is the base of an energy-expanding program, you need some ways to get comfortable with it. Here are some approaches that experts recommend.

Walk into energy.
You don't need an aerobics instructor and rock music to get an aerobic charge. In fact, one of the best aerobic exercises, experts say, is the first thing we learn after crawling.

"Walking is wonderful—it's practical, it's inexpensive and it works," says athletic trainer Marjorie J. Albohm, of the Center for Hip and Knee Surgery in Mooresville, Indiana.

Count on a warm-up.
Even a good warm-up is a nice pick-me-up when your eyelids are lowering. But warming up has practical benefits, too. "You need to warm up first to prevent injuries such as muscle strains and tears," says Dr. Bullough. "It's especially

important for people with desk jobs, people who aren't exercising regularly and for everyone as they get older."

A good warm-up gets your heart rate and breathing up a bit and produces a light sweat. It gets blood into the muscles that you plan to exercise. In most cases simply starting slowly is enough to warm you up. Lifting very light weights, walking or easy jogging, light pedaling on an exercise bike or a few minutes on a rowing machine can all constitute a warm-up, he says. After you've warmed up, stretch a bit before you start the more vigorous part of your exercise routine, suggests Dr. Bullough.

Take a talk test.
A personal trainer can help you determine your target heart rate, the range into which you want to get your heart rate while you're exercising. But you can also do a simple "talk test" to determine whether you're working too hard or not hard enough during aerobic exercise, says Jeffrey Tanji, M.D., associate professor in the Department of Family Practice at the University of California, Davis, School of Medicine.

"If you're maintaining a good aerobic level, you should be breathing too hard to sing, but not too hard to talk," Dr. Tanji says. Keeping this in mind will help you take your aerobics in stride—and prevent you from overdoing it.

Try stair climbing.
It's one of very few high-intensity, low-impact workouts around, and it allows you to get a good cardiovascular workout in record time.

Just make sure that you can stand up straight on this machine, McDevitt warns. "Some people don't have the muscle strength to hold themselves in an upright position while climbing at higher intensities. If you're hunched over the stair-climber, you need to reduce your intensity to the point where you can stand up straight. For the best results, it's important that you keep your weight on your feet and be sure not to lean on the handlebars," she says. "When clients are seriously deconditioned, I prefer to start them out on a stationary bike or walking."

Be a biker.
Cycling outdoors—in addition to riding a stationary bike—is another fine low-impact, high-intensity activity. And it can provide year-round enjoyment. "If you get a road bike or mountain bike, you can enjoy biking outdoors during good weather," Dr. Bullough says. Once you have the outdoor bike, it doesn't take much to turn it into an indoor exerciser as well. "For less than $130, you can get a training stand to pedal away happily when rain or snow keeps you indoors."

Alternate.
If you do a weight-bearing activity such as running or aerobics one day, do a non-weight-bearing activity such as swimming or biking the next day, McDevitt

recommends. "This is how you avoid injury." As you become more conditioned, you may also want to alternate hard workout days with take-it-easy days.

Include rest days.
Three days a week, 20 to 30 minutes a day, is the minimum amount of aerobic exercise you need to improve cardiovascular fitness, Dr. Mitchell says. "And I prefer people doing five days a week." Everyone should allow at least one day of rest, he notes.

If you need more than two days of rest, you're probably overtraining and need to pull back on the intensity of your sessions, McDevitt says.

Go Steady with Strength Training

While aerobic exercise can build some muscle—witness the thighs on serious bikers—it's strength training, or weight lifting, that's specifically meant to add muscle mass.

"Muscles are important for energy because it's our muscles that do any kind of physical work," Dr. Bullough says. Regularly exercised muscles do the job with less effort and don't poop out so fast. That means you're less likely to develop muscle fatigue—weakness, heaviness or shaking—when you're doing routine or even not-so-routine things around the house.

For instance, if you've been building your shoulders with strength training, you'll find it's easier to hold up that board while your partner hammers it in place. If you've been doing squats, it will be easier to endure the bending and lifting of garden work for a long time before your quadriceps call it quits.

Strength training also counters the effects of inactivity. If you don't exercise at all, you lose muscle as you age—an estimated half-pound a year, beginning in your mid-twenties. That amounts to five pounds of lost muscle each decade. And as you're losing that muscle, it's usually replaced with fat. "With muscles, it really is use it or lose it," Dr. Mitchell says.

But don't think you need to spend endless hours in some smelly gym to see results. Thirty minutes of resistance training, two or three times a week, is all that's required to start seeing new muscle. In one study approximately 30 minutes of weight lifting, three times a week, produced an average gain of three pounds of muscle—and a loss of four pounds of fat—in just 12 weeks. "As incredible as it may seem, people in their eighties and nineties have been able to build muscle using weight training," Dr. Mitchell says. One caution, however: Weight lifting can cause spikes in blood pressure. "You may need to avoid this activity if your blood pressure is already high," he says.

Stronger and Stronger

Want to reap the energizing rewards of strength training? It's not hard to get started. Here's how.

Join the club.
There are definite advantages to heading off to a health club, especially for beginners. Many clubs have an array of exercise machines, which allows you variety in your workout. Professional advice is also at hand. And you're never alone. The enthusiasm and energy others bring to their workouts can be contagious.

Get some lift tips.
If you've never lifted before, get instruction, McDevitt advises. An instructor at the club or a personal trainer will be able to help you with proper form and technique. If you get the guidance up front, you're much less likely to get hurt, and you'll progress faster, she says.

Warm up first.
Walk pumping your arms, ride a stationary bike or use a rowing machine to get those muscles loosened up and warmed up before you work them, McDevitt says. Again, a health club instructor or personal trainer can be very helpful in showing you the right way to use the equipment.

Start big.
For maximum muscle building, work the big muscles—your chest and back, for example—before your biceps.

Go for challenge, not pain.
During your workout, don't think you need to lift a ton to build muscle. In fact, when you're starting out, one of the greatest risks of injury comes from lifting too much too soon and using improper technique. "Lift only as much weight as allows you to do eight to ten repetitions of the movement in a slow, controlled manner," advises Miriam Nelson, Ph.D., a physiologist with the Human Physiology Laboratory at Tufts University in Boston.

Exercise every muscle group efficiently.
"Six to ten different exercises are all you'll need to get a thorough, whole-body workout," assures Dr. Nelson. And, for best results, each exercise should be repeated twice within each 30-minute workout session. If a set is 8 to 10 repetitions of a particular lift, for instance, you want to do 16 to 20 repetitions during the workout.

Focus on your muscles.
You're lifting weights to stimulate your muscles, so it often helps to actually feel a muscle with your free hand while you're lifting, says McDevitt. You can feel

your muscles contracting as they push, pull and tug against resistance. Doing so may keep you from being distracted, and it assures you that you're really exercising the muscles that you want to.

Try counting during a lift.
Count silently and slowly to yourself—one, two, three, four—each time you lift and lower a weight, McDevitt advises. "Don't rush the negative or lowering phase. It is just as important as the lifting phase. Counting can help you slow that movement," she says. Slow lifting through the full range of motion helps maximize strength gains.

Balance your building.
Work opposing muscles during each workout, Dr. Bullough recommends. You should build your back as well as your chest muscles, and both the fronts and backs of your legs. "This helps prevent muscle imbalances, which can lead to injuries," he says.

Build in recovery time.
Between lifting sessions, when your muscles are recovering, new muscle tissue develops. To give that process time to occur, most experts recommend lifting every other day—no more. Some actually prefer every third day.

Make Any Time Flex Time

Does stretching, by itself, give you more energy, the same way aerobic exercise or strength training can? Experts say no. Rather, they recommend stretching to keep muscles flexible, so they won't get sprained or torn while you're using them.

That's not to downplay the need for stretching, however. "The power of stretching is underestimated," Dr. Bullough says. "Those who get the most out of their bodies aren't just strong, they're flexible."

If you ask the most dedicated stretchers—yoga instructors—you'll hear even stronger affirmation of stretching's power. Stretching does generate energy, they say. "Certain yoga postures help to open up and expand your chest area, which allows you to take deeper, calming, rejuvenating breaths," explains Lilias Folan, a widely recognized yoga teacher whose hour-long yoga program, *Lilias!*, has aired on the Public Broadcasting Service (PBS) for many years. "Replacing stale air with fresh, oxygen-rich air has an immediate energizing effect," she observes.

Yoga—and other forms of stretching—can also relieve muscle and emotional tension, increase blood circulation, relieve pain and neutralize the most common physical responses to stress, Folan says.

Yoga includes meditative aspects that help you release emotional energy blocks as well, adds Michael Lee, founder of Phoenix Rising Yoga Therapy, whose national training office is located in Housatonic, Massachusetts.

The Next Move

Whether you're trying yoga-style stretching or just reaching for tension relief, here's how to make every move count.

Find a good yoga class.
Ask your friends if they know of a good yoga teacher, look for a teacher who individualizes instruction and take a trial class if you can before you invest for the long term, Folan recommends. For suggestions about what to look for in a yoga teacher, write to the American Yoga Association, 513 South Orange Avenue, Sarasota, FL 34236. And check out some yoga videos at your local library, including Folan's own "Energize with Yoga." For more information on where to find a yoga teacher near you, write to Yoga Journal Teachers Directory, 2054 University Avenue #600, Berkeley, CA 94704.

Warm up beforehand.
Even people doing yoga warm up first with some very easy movements or a few minutes of walking and swinging their arms. When you need stretching the most—that is, when you're really stiff—is the time to warm up first, Folan says.

Target the muscles that need it most.
Not all muscles are equally tight, McDevitt says. "You want to stretch the short ones and be careful not to overstretch the ones that are already too long." A personal trainer can do some tests to determine which of your muscles are tight.

"Most people have short hamstrings (the muscles on the backs of your upper thighs), and their lower backs are usually tight, so those are areas you want to focus on," Folan says. Most people are also tight in the neck and shoulders, she adds.

Relax into the stretch.
Move slowly and never, ever force your body or push it until it hurts, Folan says. "Feel yourself release into a stretch. Imagine yourself breathing warmth into the muscles and see the muscles let go of tension as they relax and lengthen."

Never bounce.
Reaching down and "bouncing" as you try to touch the floor can trigger a reflex mechanism that will actually tighten the muscles you're trying to stretch. The bouncing motion can tear rather than stretch muscles, Folan says.

Still, within a stretch there can be some very gentle controlled movements as you "play with the edge" of a posture, Folan says. "As you exhale, you can ease into the stretch, and as you inhale, you can relax back a bit," she says. You'll want to hold a pose for two or three breaths.

Exorcise That Afternoon Slump

It's 3:00 P.M. Do you know where your brain is?

Lots of people have an afternoon slump, the kind of boy-do-I-need-a-nap fatigue that can leave you staring mindlessly out the window, if you're lucky enough to have one, or reaching for a cup of coffee you really don't want.

If you just can't sneak in a nap, you may be able to re-energize with some mindful moves, says Lilias Folan, creator of the videotape "Energize with Yoga" and star of a long-running Public Broadcasting Service (PBS) show, *Lilias!* Here's what she recommends.

Get those shoulders moving.

Stand up and roll your shoulders slowly in one direction, 6 to 12 times. Repeat, rolling the shoulders in the opposite direction.

Try a chest expander.

Clasp a belt, scarf or hand towel behind you with the palms of your hands facing your buttocks and your hands about six inches apart. Slowly straighten one arm, then the other. Inhale, slowly raising both arms behind you as high as you can, lifting your face toward the ceiling. Then exhale slowly as you release the tension, lowering both your hands and your face. Repeat the action three to six more times. Never force or strain. Keep it steady and comfortable.

Move your spine in six different directions.

Bend forward, back, left and right. Twist left, then right. Keep all motions slow, steady and comfortable.

Reach for the sky.

Stretch by reaching your hands high over your head, leading with first one, then the other. See if you can coax a yawn as well, Folan suggests.

Focus on your effort.

If you venture out, make the most of your foray. Swing your hips and arms and take deep, energizing breaths. "Think about what you're doing," Folan says. "Say, 'I am energizing myself. I am releasing tiredness.' "

Smile when you stretch.

"It's hard to be tense when you're grinning," says McDevitt.

And Folan agrees. "A genuine smiles helps your body relax in subtle ways. Enhance your smile with a positive thought," she says. "Turn the corners of your mouth up so you can feel your cheeks rise slightly and add to that a genuine feeling of gratitude, so there's a good feeling connected to the smile."

Consider an aquatic setting.

Exercising in water lets you stretch and strengthen in a warm, gravity-free environment, which is perfect for people with arthritis or weight problems, says Dr. Mitchell. Call a nearby Y for details on aquarobics or contact your local branch of the Arthritis Foundation, which sponsors a nationwide Aquatic Program in conjunction with the YWCA.

Staying at It

What counts most in any exercise program? You have to actually *do* it, McDevitt says. "Even a professionally designed program is worthless if the person never gets around to doing it."

What compels you to keep going depends on personal motivation. But here are some pointers from experts on tactics that may help keep you exercising.

Take lessons.

Improve your backhand, learn the butterfly stroke or spend a week learning how to use a sea kayak. "Mastering an athletic skill provides people with the kind of enjoyment that makes them stick with it," Dr. Bullough says.

Chart your progress.

An exercise diary, or even a simple chart or log that marks each workout, lets you see just how far you've come and reinforces feelings of accomplishment, McDevitt says.

Feel the sun on your face.

One way to break a boring routine is to get outdoors to exercise, Dr. Bullough says. "I love to hike or bike in the woods or meadows, even to walk in the rain. The scenery and the elements can provide distraction and pleasure."

Love it.

Explore the wide range of healthful physical activities available to you. Dr. Bullough believes that the key to beginning a regular exercise program is getting out there and finding a physical activity that you really love to do. "Once you find that activity, or those activities, consistency becomes automatic," he says.

Schedule exercise when interference is least likely.

"For most people, that's first thing in the morning," Dr. McCarthy says. "You can control morning schedules better than evening schedules, and anyone who has kids, typically, will find out that if they wait until the evening to work out, it doesn't happen."

Plan on change.

People who keep doing the same sort of exercise year after year usually get bored eventually. They may keep doing it, but it's no fun.

The way to get around that? "Anticipate that you will need change in your exercise routine to keep it enjoyable," Dr. McCarthy says. "Build in some kind of regular exploration of alternatives so you have something handy if you get bored, injured or are traveling." Those alternatives need not be as exotic as snowshoeing or mountain biking. They could include dancing, hiking or swimming.

Monitor your contentment level.

"Ultimately, it is contentment, or a sense of being fulfilled, that you are looking for," Dr. McCarthy says. "I suggest people worry less about a particular way to do something, but explore the ways that make them feel good about doing it."

Add a safety net.

Health behaviors reinforce each other, Dr. McCarthy says. You might have to stop smoking or start eating right if you haven't already. These lifestyle improvements help to energize your exercise program, in his view. "I call it a kind of lifestyle conspiracy that prevents you from going back to your old ways."

Keep it convenient.

Join a gym close to home or work, buy equipment that you can use at home, keep a bag of workout clothes and sneakers in your car, even try going to sleep in your morning workout clothes. In other words, do whatever you need to make exercise relatively hassle-free.

Buddy up.

Especially on those days when excuses scream louder than reason, it's helpful to know that someone, somewhere, is expecting you to show up. That could be a walking partner or the participants in an exercise class. "People who begin exercising for health reasons will find there are social reasons as well for continuing with a group," Dr. McCarthy says. "On those days when they feel tired, they might nevertheless feel compelled to go because friends are expecting them."

Just do it, and do it and do it.

Even if you intend never to enjoy exercise, you can always reap its benefits—more energy and increased alertness and calmness. "How you feel afterward may be motivation enough," Dr. Mitchell says.

Relationships
for Energy

*I*t is the best of experiences. It is the worst of experiences. If Charles Dickens were a modern author-psychologist, his best-selling title might be *A Tale of Two Relationships* instead of *A Tale of Two Cities*.

"Our relationships are among the most positive and potentially the most negative life experiences we have," says Barry Lubetkin, Ph.D., clinical director of the Institute for Behavior Therapy in Manhattan and author of *Why Do I Need You to Love Me in Order to Like Myself?* "When people are in stable relationships—where they're understood, their needs are met, they feel trust and they give the goodies of love back and forth—it's an energizing experience. People constantly report that when their relationships are going well, they feel better, eat better and sleep better. And their work environments are more tolerable.

"And, of course, the opposite is true—divorce or a breakup of a relationship is a major event on the stress charts." According to statistics kept by insurance companies, "married people seem to be healthier and live longer than unmarried people," Dr. Lubetkin observes.

Love Equals Energy

The simple fact is that "if a relationship is healthy, you feel energized," says Linda De Villers, Ph.D., a psychologist in El Segundo, California, and author of *Love Skills.* "If it's dysfunctional, you feel sapped."

Spouses, friends and family members are the star players in your cavalcade of relationships. But there are other kinds of partnerships, too. A dynamic exercise class can rev you up and give you the energy to stick with a demanding workout. Coping with a difficult boss or colleague, on the other hand, can drain all the vital juice that you need to complete a work project or help the kids with their homework when you get home.

"There's growing evidence that our relationships are extremely powerful," says Dr. Lubetkin. A University of New Mexico study of more than 250 elderly people in Albuquerque, for example, found that those with the strongest relationships had the lowest risk of disease. And a Duke University study of 1,368 people with heart disease found that the folks with even one good friend were three times less likely to die after a heart attack. After surveying a group of studies linking friendships to longevity, the California Department of Health advises state residents to "make a friend" because "friends are good medicine."

When it comes to energy enhancement, the quality of the relationship—whether it is positive or negative—is everything.

The Folks to Know

You usually don't need to be a palm reader or have a psychology degree to figure out whether a friend or relative is an energy booster or an energy sapper. But sometimes you're not really sure. In these cases answering a few simple questions will provide the answer, says Ellen McGrath, Ph.D., executive director of the Psychology Center, which has offices in Laguna Beach, California, and New York City, and author of *When Feeling Bad Is Good*.

"What do you do after an encounter with a particular person?" she asks. "Are you so tired that you want a nap? Do you eat because you're stressed or depressed? Or do you go back and do some productive work with renewed energy?"

If you want to assure yourself that any new acquaintance will become an energy provider rather than an energy sapper, here are a few guidelines to follow.

Be yourself.
A true friend or lover is a person who lets you feel like you can just be yourself. "You feel that the other person really sees who you are. So you feel like you're known and understood," says Ervin Staub, Ph.D., professor of psychology at the University of Massachusetts at Amherst.

If you're comfortable around someone, you don't have to censor your opinions or put on a fake happy face. But if you find yourself walking on eggshells around a potential friend or lover, if you're afraid to say this or that, if your smile feels like it's cracking your face, or if, conversely, you have to tame your humor, then that person isn't likely marriage or friendship material, says Dr. Staub.

Go heart-to-heart.
Another defining element in a great friendship is the ability to confide your deepest secrets or concerns, says Dr. Staub. Even if you don't want to burden

your buddy with the hard stuff, you feel that you could if you had to. But that's not all. Your most serious thoughts, your highest dreams and most yearning desires—your dumbest jokes, too—can be put on the table. You'd never think, "Oh, I couldn't tell him that."

Check the edge.

Beyond comfort and companionship, Dr. Lubetkin looks for a certain edge in a successful relationship. "You don't want to feel anxious or inadequate, but you need a slight challenge—intellectually or sensually or emotionally."

If you're a very neat person, for instance, it won't do you any harm to hang out with someone who's a bit of a slob.

"The thing is that you should enjoy the other person's personality," observes Dr. Lubetkin. "That doesn't mean it has to be like yours; it can be quite different from yours. That difference sometimes provides that edge, that challenge."

The Art of Communication

Friends, and especially spouses, are often both energy boosters and energy sappers, changing roles depending upon the interaction between the two of you. But in any marriage, the fear of communication that sometimes builds up between couples can become a major energy drain.

"Over a period of time, some couples learn what not to say to each other," says Louise Merves-Okin, Ph.D., a marriage and family counselor in private practice in Philadelphia. "They can't talk about her mother or religion or what happened at work without a fight. So their communication becomes very stilted. Before they talk to each other, they go through a mental dialogue of all the things they can't say. And that's very draining."

There are techniques to prune the prickly thorns of communication. Many of these apply to close friendships as well as to marriage.

Nip it in the bud.

"When a person in love just goes along with whatever the other does or says because she's afraid of endangering the relationship, it can become destructive. If something bothers her, she has to take action and say something before his behavior solidifies," says Dr. Staub. "You have to talk about issues early in the relationship rather than later, because then they've become a way of life. At that point you'll meet a lot of resistance because the other person sees the behavior as normal. If you air issues earlier, you'll be less angry and you can talk about them more gently and sensitively."

If it irritates you that your spouse doesn't put shoes back in the closet, talk

The Loving Touch

Psychologists who practice couples therapy often recommend a sensual exercise called pleasuring to the folks who come to them for help. "It's an opening exercise for couples to begin to reconnect," says Louise Merves-Okin, Ph.D., a marriage and family counselor in private practice in Philadelphia. Massage, as anyone knows who has experienced it, is a wonderfully relaxing and energizing experience.

Essentially, the exercise is a massage that each partner gives the other. And it's sensual, not sexual. "It doesn't lead to the next thing. It is what it is. In a way, it's more intimate than having sex for a lot of people because it makes them vulnerable; they have to take the pleasure of receiving someone's touch," she says.

Here's how to do it.

Plan ahead.

Schedule a 40-minute appointment in your calendar with your mate—"a rendezvous," says Dr. Merves-Okin. "That tells your partner, 'Now you're my first priority.' " If you need to hire a babysitter, line one up.

Set the scene.

Together, decide how you'd like your love bower to look and smell and sound. Pick out a favorite compact disc to enjoy together, stock up on scented candles or even summer roses—let your romantic imagination roam. Then buy massage oil at a bed-and-bath shop, a department store or a drugstore. Each of you should have your own massage oil, however, so that she doesn't have to smell like his pine oil and he doesn't have to smell like her lilac scent.

Picking out candles or oils or compact discs can be done together, or

about it as soon as you notice that it bothers you. If you wait too long, your partner might greet your concern with surprise and resentment: "Well, it never used to bother you."

Listen up.

Psychologists call this communication technique active listening. "It's a way of listening without judgment or reaction," says Dr. Merves-Okin. "You just hear the other person and make sure that you understand him."

To listen actively, "focus on what the other person says. Then tell him, 'I think you're saying this . . .' or 'I think you're saying that . . .' Tell him what you thought you heard him say. He can then agree with your interpretation or say, you can divvy up duties. Sharing the preparation is important. "One of you shouldn't wind up doing all the preparation," Dr. Merves-Okin says.

Agree to be alone.

Make a pact not to answer the door or the telephone. Turn on the answering machine.

Turn up the heat.

Adjust the thermostat if the room needs to be warmer. Let the oils heat up in a container placed in a bowl of hot water for about five minutes. Before you start to massage your partner, dab some oil onto your palm and rub your hands together to warm the oil.

Take turns.

Decide who's going first. You can trade off going first each time you do the exercise.

Touch and tell.

"Massage the entire body," says Dr. Merves-Okin. "Don't worry about being a massage therapist. Just make sure you give each other feedback on what feels good, what you like, what's too hard, what's too soft. Ask questions: 'Do you like this? Is this better? Or is that better?' I call it going to the eye doctor—'Is this lens better . . . or is that lens better?' We might not even know—we wind up learning about our bodies.

"This really opens the door to begin communication," says Dr. Merves-Okin. "Maybe he hates to have his ears kissed. Or he's been touching you too hard. And you've been doing that for 30 years. You can correct that. After that exercise you can go on from there and face each other and learn to be verbal again. It puts a lot of energy back into the relationship."

'No, not exactly. It's more like this . . . ' And you can go over it again," she says.

"It sounds simple, but it's actually one of the hardest things to do, because we're not trained this way," she adds. "Active listening is energizing because you can talk about anything and be listened to and understood."

Use the I-word, not the Y-word.

"Don't communicate in the form of blaming the other person," says Dr. Staub. "Don't say, 'Look, you haven't been doing this . . . ' Say what you need and what you don't feel you've been getting. That mode is very important."

Here's an example from Dr. McGrath: "You state what behavior bothers you, how it makes you feel and why. In a close relationship with a friend, relative or partner, you might say, 'When you raise your voice like that, I feel so upset that I can't remember what you're saying.' "

"When you actively communicate, it creates energy," adds Dr. McGrath.

Cut it short.

Dr. Merves-Okin has another listening tip: "One of the keys is talking less, in shorter amounts. People often talk too long, and the other person only hears what's said at the end. Talk for five minutes at the most and then let the other person talk."

Making Your Marriage Work

What exactly does a great, mutually energizing marriage relationship look like? "Each partner draws out the best in each other. They support each other's dreams and goals. They're facilitators and cheerleaders for each other. They're full of energy," says Dr. De Villers.

But even the happiest couples can occasionally get on each other's nerves and sap each other's precious energy reserves. Here's a little energy-boosting behavior brushup for couples.

Play fair.

Probably the most important area to spruce up is the division of housework, says Dr. De Villers. "If you feel you have to do the bulk of the domestic navigation, that isn't good," she says. "There has to be shared responsibility for tasks, because a sense of inequality concerning domestic chores is a major predictor of divorce. Chores don't have to be divided down the middle, but there has to be the sense that the division is fair in order for the relationship to be energized. This isn't petty stuff. It's the foundation of whether the relationship is equitable or not."

Collaborate.

Collaboration, instead of compromise, is the current word of choice, says Judy McQueen, educational program coordinator for the Women's Resource Center at Michigan State University in East Lansing and also a longtime lecturer on conflict resolution, assertiveness training, friendship and family life.

This is how it works, she says: "Say you want Italian food and he wants Chinese. Instead of compromising on something like Thai food and having neither of your top choices, figure out how you can have both. Go out for Italian food one night. He can eat the one Italian thing he likes—like minestrone. Then the next time you go out to eat, get Chinese food. And you can eat the one thing you like—an egg roll or something."

Be reliable.

"Failing to keep commitments is a big drain on a relationship," says Dr. De Villers. "Tardiness may be the main problem, especially when it's unpredictable.

"Or maybe you have to be the marital CEO all the time—you always have to ask, 'Did you pick up the plumber's helper?' or 'Did you get the milk?' or 'Did you pick Mary up at school?' because he often says, 'I forgot.' That's a big burden on the person who has to pick up the pieces. It goes back to the issue of equity in the relationship."

Respect those feelings.

"Probably the greatest single problem I see in my work with couples is their inability to validate and respect each other's feelings," says Dr. De Villers.

That can easily happen when couples don't practice active listening. "Nobody says, 'Let me see if I understand exactly what you're feeling.' Instead, they devalue those feelings and try to talk the other one out of having them," says Dr. De Villers.

Take ten.

Life sweeps us in and out on the tide of its daily sea. To make sure that you and your partner aren't boats sailing past each other, hook up for ten minutes every night to swap news, suggests Dr. Merves-Okin. "Set aside those ten minutes to talk to each other. Tell the other person how you're doing in your life, and then after five minutes listen to your partner talk for five minutes. Make sure you ask each other how you think you're doing together."

Dr. De Villers agrees, "If you have a regular time set aside to talk, it reduces the scare of 'Uh-oh, we're gonna have a talk' or 'Uh-oh, what's wrong?' "

Romancing the Relationship

Remember the last time you fell in love—the sheer energy high that it gave you?

We all know that marriage doesn't always feel that vibrant and compelling. On the other hand, something is wrong when it has the opposite effect—when being with your partner makes you feel like someone pulled the vitality drain.

Dr. Merves-Okin describes a typical couple who comes to her for counseling: "They love their children, their home, their furniture, their friends. They might even like their jobs. They like everything in their life . . . except the other person. The other person looks unattractive to them all of a sudden. They don't really think of divorce, though, because they really like their life together. And they don't want to be single. Yet everything they do together is no fun. There's no energy there. And there's nothing safe to talk about except the weather."

Can this marriage be saved? "Yes, you can often do a lot with that relationship," she says. "You can re-romanticize it." Here's how.

Relive your honeymoon.
"In marriage therapy we often bring people back to the time when they first met—where they met, what they wore, what they said, what their dates were like," says Dr. Merves-Okin. "They re-experience the positive time they had so that they can look at the other person and see what made them feel that way." A couple can feel energized just by that experience of reliving the honeymoon, according to Dr. Merves-Okin. "Sometimes you see them smile at each other, grab each other's hands and talk about the time they were so happy together."

You may experience a similar re-enactment by going back to the scene of your honeymoon, physically, not just emotionally. "It's a nice thing to do for a special anniversary. You can go back to that place and plan it as much like before as you can," she says. Or you could opt for something quicker and cheaper like a visit to your favorite courting restaurant.

Leave mash notes.
"You don't have to go away for a week or spend lots of money. You can do simple things for each other, like leave love notes—maybe a surprise note in the car about something special that you like about your partner," Dr. Merves-Okin suggests. You could write "I love you" on the grocery list. Or tuck a note in a briefcase.

Do two-a-day.
Love letters are one nice spice to add to your marriage. But don't stop there. "Try to do two things a day for the other person," Dr. Merves-Okin suggests. "Get them coffee or tea when they sit down. Or take the snow off their car when it snows. Get them a gift you know they like. For me it would be something like herbal tea or flavored water. It could even be an item for their workouts.

"Couples forget how well they know each other, what each other likes, what pleases them. In a draining relationship they often tend to use that knowledge against each other."

Spring a surprise.
"Planning surprises is an old couples-therapy assignment. But it almost always works," says Dr. Merves-Okin. "The surprise should be something that the planner wants to do, too, not just something that pleases the partner. It can cost nothing. Or you can go to Disneyland. Be creative. Just tell your partner whether to eat beforehand or not. And tell him what to wear. It's amazing how effective this is. It creates such a sense of goodwill and fun."

Dating Your Spouse

Sometimes time is scarcer than love or goodwill. Too often, in even the most solid marriage, this is the scene: Your spouse reaches for you late at night. You rest your head against that comforting shoulder; then the Sandman hits you over the head. "Honey, I'm exhausted," you manage to murmur before sleep descends. Even when you cherish your marriage, how do you get the time for romancing it?

One thing you can do is to treat your marriage like your other A+ priorities. Block out regular date time in your weekly schedule, says Harold H. Bloomfield, M.D., a psychiatrist in Del Mar, California, and co-author of *The Power of 5: Hundreds of 5-Second to 5-Minute Scientific Shortcuts to Ignite Your Energy, Burn Fat, Stop Aging and Revitalize Your Love Life*. That may sound bloodless but, in practice, it's romantic.

Here's how to date your husband . . . or wife.

Hire a sitter.
"At least one night or afternoon a week, get a babysitter for the kids. Then you'll really be able to relax with one another and connect in a nonfrantic way," says Dr. Bloomfield.

"You can barter time with another couple—watch their kids in exchange for them watching yours," says Dr. Merves-Okin. "You need time to talk and enjoy yourselves together without having to be parents. So you have to find ways to have quality time not as parents or a family but as a couple."

Have an AFFAIR.
"AFFAIR is an acronym that stands for adventure, fun, fantasy, affection, intimacy and romance," says Dr. Bloomfield. "You can use all week to anticipate it."

Some couples plan a Saturday-night dinner out. Other people get very creative with their scheduled time, he says. Some cover their beds with rose petals, cool a bottle of champagne or light incense and candles. But sex isn't the only point of the planning.

"The main thing is to have those heart-to-heart talks, to find out what's been important to your partner," he adds. "You need to know what's going on emotionally with your partner and to let your partner know what you appreciate."

Bailing Out

Communication techniques can turn around a tired marriage or a stale friendship. "You can convert negative relationships into positive ones. But you need to be able to decide whether it's worth it to try," says Dr. McGrath.

Your Relationship Inventory

If you're confused about which people are good for you and which are bad, in terms of being energizing or de-energizing, you can take steps to find out. "Taking inventory, writing it down, helps you get control over your relationships," according to Ellen McGrath, Ph.D., executive director of the Psychology Center, which has offices in Laguna Beach, California, and New York City, and author of *When Feeling Bad Is Good*. Here are her suggestions for creating a Relationship Inventory.

1. Write down the names of all the key people and close friends in your life—family members, spouse or significant other, colleagues from work.

2. Make a list by putting three headings across the top of a sheet of paper: "Positive," "Negative" and "Toxic."

3. Look at the names of the key people on your list and determine how each one makes you feel. "If encounters with that person make you feel energized and enhanced—good about yourself—by appreciating who you are and by being there for you when you need them, put him or her under the 'Positive' heading," says Dr. McGrath.

   Under "Negative," list anyone who makes you feel depleted and depressed, she says. "Those are people who are unreliable or self-centered. Or they take a great deal and don't offer much in return. Or they're simply not available enough."

   Under the "Toxic" heading, "include any of those people who consistently leave you feeling bad instead of good, who poison your self-esteem through criticism, exploitation, competitiveness or attacks," Dr. McGrath says.

4. Next to each name, "jot down a word or two to remind you why that person falls into that particular category," she says.

Many people can't be divided into categories so neatly. Some of your friends and family may cruise through two or even all three categories. In those cases, suggests Dr. McGrath, "list their names in each category and draw arrows connecting them to remind you how fluid these people can be in stimulating the best and worst in you."

When you have finished taking stock and have thought about the people in your life and how they make you feel, you can decide to spend more time with the Positives, she says. And you can protect yourself against the Negatives and the Toxics.

"Some relationships are toxic—destructive to self-esteem or even danger-ous, as in cases of abuse," she says. Other relationships are merely so draining that they're simply not worth pursuing.

"Sometimes we simply outgrow a relationship and have to release it," says McQueen.

"We have to come face-to-face with the fact that the relationship takes away from who we are and the kind of life we want to live and our happiness," adds Dr. McGrath.

Here are a couple of ways to help you cut the ties that hurt.

Let it go.
It's not always necessary to announce the dissolution of a friendship or love af-fair, says Dr. Lubetkin. "The actual act of breaking off can be as direct or indi-rect as you need it to be," he says. "A lot of people are assertive enough to speak up about what they feel. That's ideal. But many of us are unable to do that because it's too painful. It's perfectly okay to just let the relationship drift apart. You can do things like not call the person back. Or don't show interest in the things you used to show an interest in."

Keep a miserable-memory list.
Even the rockiest relationship can prompt post-separation regrets. So you want to have something on hand to remind you of why you broke up. "For at least a few weeks before you break off, keep a journal of all the things about your en-counters that really turn you off," suggests Dr. Lubetkin. Write down everything that is unsatisfying, he advises. "Then, when you have those inevitable second thoughts, the list will remind you that you really did make the right decision about breaking up."

Protecting Yourself

You can't shoo away every energy vampire who swoops down in your di-rection. Sometimes, you just have to grin and bear it. Maybe it's command ap-pearances at family functions that leave you totally pooped and aggravated. Maybe you have bitter colleagues or a boss with bite.

"When you have the choice, you never put yourself in the company of peo-ple who take it all out of you," advises McQueen. "Try to eliminate the energy drainers from your life. But most people have to work and they have families—and those two groups are full of energy sappers. So you have to plan events that involve them very carefully."

Here's how.

Choose the battleground.

When you have to deal with a drainer, try to initiate the meeting so that you have control over when it starts and ends and where it takes place, advises McQueen. That way, you can choose to meet with that person either by phone or in your office, in public or at home—whichever way you're most comfortable and wherever you'll be most at ease. That way, you're not trapped by the other person at a time and place not of your choosing. You also have time to prepare what you're going to say and do.

Fill up the schedule.

"Especially with family things, it helps to plan lots of activities," says McQueen. You don't want to wind up on a couch in a living room, either bored witless and thoroughly depleted or seething with anger. "Go out to dinner," she suggests. "Go to a movie—but pick uplifting ones so that there's less to be negative about. Try to change the negatives to positives, but realize that there will always be negative downers who like to rain on your parade.

"Then, after the movie, if you still have to spend more time with your relative, go have coffee and dessert."

Take along a buffer.

If you can take a good friend along to awful Aunt Ida's or nasty Uncle Ned's, you can make the dreaded visit much nicer, at least for you. That way, you get to talk to someone you like. And friends are both energizing and calming.

In one of the many studies of friends and friendship, researchers at Carnegie–Mellon University in Pittsburgh measured the blood pressure of 90 students as they each gave a speech in front of a group—a high-stress situation for almost anybody. Not surprisingly, the blood pressure of every student rose. But the blood pressure of the students who were accompanied by friends rose significantly less than that of the students who spoke alone.

Buffers are sometimes helpful in work situations, too. For instance, if you and one or more of your colleagues are concerned about your department head's inaccessibility, two or three of you together could ask him to schedule a meeting to discuss it. Then you won't have to delegate one lone person to carry the meeting by herself.

Stay public.

Aunt Ida or Uncle Ned may rail at you in private about your un-Ida- or un-Ned-like life. But they probably won't make a scene in a restaurant or at a movie theater. Many of the scariest relatives believe in putting on a good face in public, so public spaces are often good meeting places for problem people. "A restaurant can be the safest place for a visit or meeting," says McQueen.

Not always, though. If your relative has any spark of volatility, he can blow up anywhere. "I do remember one altercation where I was yelled at in a restaurant. So I just got up and left," McQueen adds.

Working It Out: Managing Your Work Relationships

You may love your job, but if your supervisor gets your goat, your job can also be a major-league energy drainer. "Working with an intimidating person can make you hate your job," says Leonard Felder, Ph.D., a psychologist in private practice in Los Angeles and author of *Does Someone at Work Treat You Badly?* If you have to work for a boss who screams with anger, you're more likely to make mistakes, observes Dr. Felder. "You can alter the way you experience abusive behavior, though, and dramatically improve the way you interact with people."

Hear the valuable stuff.
"Don't go deaf when your boss yells at you," says Dr. Felder. "He's giving you valuable information about your performance even if his behavior is inappropriate. Stay alert and managerial."

He suggests repeating this silent mantra to calm yourself during a tirade, "Hear the valuable stuff. Ignore the anger. It's not mine." Dr. Felder notes that "you'll be surprised at how much it can help you deflect the anger and allow you to separate out any valuable information you need to hear."

Give a little positive back talk.
Mantras aren't the only way of handling a bellicose boss. A good comeback line may be more in your nature. Here are three useful ones.

• *Stop! I don't appreciate being talked to like this.* "This straightforward sentence doesn't waste a lot of time criticizing the other person or being apologetic," says Dr. Felder. "It's simple and direct and lets the volatile person know that you won't permit him or her to walk all over you."

• *Time out! I want to hear what you're saying, but I have to ask you to slow down a bit.* "This statement is a little gentler and much more specific," says Dr. Felder. "It's more like an invitation—'I want to hear what you're saying.' It can lighten up the mood a little and make the screamer stop shouting for a few minutes."

• *Let's talk about this. You go first, and I won't interrupt. Then when you're done, I'll see if I have any questions.* "This sounds very managerial and even more professional," says Dr. Felder. "You become the facilitator/director of the conversation. And you let the screamer know that you won't interrupt him or her. Their fear is that they won't be heard unless they yell and hurry."

Turn Boring into Energizing

Talking to boring people can be more tedious than watching grass grow on a summer day. Trying to make small talk with a lackluster conversationalist can dull your mental edge. But with a few well-timed queries and conversational strategies, you can learn to turn an energy sapper into a booster.

Even the dullest people can be interesting. But often, you have to play verbal detective with them to find that conversational gold mine.

"Part of the problem with boring people is that we tune them out because they're boring. But if you really listen to people, you'll get enough out of them to make the conversation a two-way street," says corporate trainer Stephan Schiffman, president of the New York–based sales training firm D.E.I. Management Group and author of *Cold Calling Techniques (That Really Work)*.

Here are some recommendations from the experts.

Apply the Five Ws.

An interviewing method popular with journalists is to ask who, what, where, when and why. With a little finesse you can apply the five Ws tactfully and without sounding like an interrogator. If you're talking to someone who mutters that he'd rather be collecting stamps than making small talk, pipe up, "Really? What kind of stamps do you collect?" Then casually follow up with, "When did you start? Where do you keep them? Why do you do it?"

Questioning like this (if you're sincere) is a good way to turn small talk into scintillating conversation.

Don't talk about yourself.

If you fill conversational voids by talking about yourself, you'll learn nothing about the other person and you'll probably bore them as much as they're boring you. You'll not only learn more by listening and questioning, you'll be more likely to stay alert.

Ask about their first job—it's a sure bet.

"I remember seeing this interview of Barbara Walters and she said that question worked best for her over the years. It really works," says time-management and etiquette expert Elizabeth L. Craig, author of *Don't Slurp Your Soup*, a book on office etiquette.

Most people have strong feelings about their first jobs, not to mention a few good stories. So tapping this topic can be a verbal gold mine, Craig says.

Ask questions.

If your boss is a perfectionist who picks apart or trashes all your projects, go the question route. First, question yourself. "Ask what part is accurate and what part is just negative complaints," suggests Dr. Felder. "If you're unsure or beaten down, get a second opinion from someone who would know.

"Then ask your boss for specific, useful, constructive ideas about your work. Ask, 'Exactly what part of the project do you think could be improved?' Then, 'What would you like this part to be like?' and 'What are you looking for that you didn't receive?' "

Keep a warm fuzzy file.

If you walk into your office, still reeling after being raked over the coals by your supervisor, you'll feel better if you keep a collection of kudos and compliments and congratulatory letters that you can turn to, says McQueen. "I have a bright yellow private file. And I put into it thank-you notes and everything nice I get," she says. "With something like that, you can retreat into your safe office after an altercation and get some reaffirmation of your worth."

People Wattage

Dealing effectively with negative people is, of course, an important part of holding on to your precious energy reserves. The flip side is also important— taking full advantage of people power in helping to build those energy reserves in the first place.

Ask the people who attend exercise classes why they pour themselves into spandex and drive to a gym instead of sweating unseen at home. They'll say something like, "But I wouldn't work out at home. I need the energy of a class."

A group generates energy. That's why people form groups to tackle problems. And the same people-power principle applies to support groups and to group therapy. "I've learned over the years that you can have more success and create more in a group than you can individually," says Dr. McGrath, who leads group as well as individual therapy sessions.

In this era of frequent moves and high divorce rates, "we need a feeling of family more than ever before," Dr. McGrath says. "We need to connect. We need support." Here are a few suggestions on how to do just that.

Form a group.

You can start your own high-energy, stress-busting support group. That's what McQueen did when she found herself dealing with the pangs of divorce at the age of 40.

Here's how she did it: First, she called up 12 of her best girlfriends and

Taming Temper Tantrums

Why is it that every time Junior throws a tantrum, you're the one who winds up feeling exhausted?

"Temper tantrums actually wear parents down," says Philip C. Kendall, Ph.D., professor of psychology and head of the Division of Clinical Psychology at Temple University in Philadelphia. Such tantrums are sure to be tiring both mentally and emotionally, he points out.

"The good news is that if you start when a child is young and don't give in to temper tantrums, you'll be fine," Dr. Kendall adds. "The bad news is that if you give in, it's going to take a lot longer to teach the child to behave properly."

You can oust the outburst—or at least keep it from ousting your energy—by following this sage advice.

Ignore and praise.

Ignore temper tantrums, no matter how difficult it may be, but praise your children when they express their feelings in words. Commend them for venting themselves properly; then try to discuss the situation. Once children find that temper tantrums don't work but that talking does, they'll be more likely to discuss their feelings and less likely to throw a fit.

Put the brakes on backseat bickering.

When kids start fighting in the car, a trip down Easy Street can turn into a ride on the Highway to Hell. Next time the backseat becomes a verbal boxing ring, try this "when/then" strategy from Cynthia Whitham, a child-care expert at the University of California, Los Angeles, and author of *Win the Whining War and Other Skirmishes* and *The Answer Is NO*.

Pull your car over and say, "When you stop screaming, then I'll continue driving," Whitham says. Then keep busy until the fighting blows over, as it undoubtedly will. (Tip: Bring along a magazine that you can read until they settle down.)

And here's another suggestion from Whitham: Sometimes when the children *aren't* fighting, praise them for expressing themselves in words or getting along well in the backseat, Whitham says. A few kind words for good behavior may go a lot further than a few harsh words for misbehavior.

asked them to commit to one get-together a month for a year. They took turns planning activities—sleepovers, movies, dinners, book discussions, issue discussions, video reviews. Every three months they went away for the weekend. Once, they even took a European cruise, with the help of McQueen's small travel business. Sixteen years and five weddings later, the gang of 12 is still going strong.

You can modify both the size of your group and the form of your meetings. But, like McQueen, you'll find that your team is a fountain of energy that spills over into the rest of your life.

Join a class.

An interesting class can be a hotbed of energy, too. You can make it even hotter when you enroll with a partner—both you and the relationship with your loved one will benefit.

It's something leisure expert Margaret Carlisle Duncan, Ph.D., associate professor of human kinetics at the University of Wisconsin at Milwaukee and president of the North American Society of the Sociology of Sport, can talk about from experience. Her nine-year-old daughter signed up for a martial arts class, and, after a month of just watching from the sidelines, Dr. Duncan signed up, too. So did her seven-year-old daughter.

"It made an enormous difference in how we related to one another," says Dr. Duncan. "It gave us a bond, and we talked about the class quite a bit: 'How do you do this technique? How do you flip someone?' We developed a whole network of friends, a new vocabulary and a schedule shaped around our participation together."

Volunteer.

"The quickest way to help yourself is to help somebody else," says Dr. McGrath. And it doesn't matter what you choose as your social issue—the homeless, the elderly, the environment. "If you join a volunteer group, you become part of a collective with similar values," she says.

That mix of altruism and group energy is particularly potent. Research shows that life expectancy increases dramatically when you do regular volunteer work. "Working for a worthwhile social cause is deeply satisfying," says Dr. Staub. "And doing it as part of a group is further energizing. When you engage in social service together with other people, you can go beyond yourself; you can transcend yourself. And that's very exciting."

Relaxing
for Energy

Even machines need a little downtime for maintenance and repair. So you had better believe that the human body needs its R and R to function with ease and energy. Rest and relaxation—you simply have to gear down to tune up your body.

Here's what happens when you relax and why the process fuels your energy supply. "You breathe more deeply and take in more oxygen. Your heart muscle opens up and pumps more blood with each beat. Your blood pressure lowers. Your hands and feet warm up. And tense muscles begin to relax," explains Larry J. Feldman, Ph.D., a leader of workshops on stress and burnout and author of *Feeling Good Again*.

As your heartbeat slows, researchers have found, your mind focuses, and—even though you don't know it—your brain starts emitting alpha waves, brain waves that signal a state of wakeful relaxation.

Riding the Waves

You can bring on relaxing alpha waves in an endless variety of ways—sailing a sloop off the coast of Maine, losing yourself in the lives of your favorite soap-opera stars or climbing into a thick novel that gives you total escape into a fictional world. Everybody has a favorite time-out.

But there are also a number of techniques that you can learn specifically for the purpose of relaxation. Master these relaxation techniques and you won't be at the mercy of things like Maine weather, a bad soap-opera plot or a boring book. And researchers have found that you can achieve a relaxed state most efficiently with programs designed specifically for that purpose. Some of the best techniques include visualization, autogenic relaxation, yoga and biofeedback.

Even if you're skeptical and think that there are more tortuous twists in yoga than in pretzels, take heart: Many of these relaxation methods now have both hard science and firm evidence on their side. Visualization, for example, has been used in fighting chronic pain. If it can take on a pain like that, imagine what it can do with the comparatively simple process of helping you unwind and boost your energy level. And biofeedback is taught and monitored with the use of scientific equipment.

Visualization: The Eyes Have It

Imagine being able to boost your energy simply by picturing more energy in your mind's eye. Sound too good to be true? Advocates of visualization say it's not, and they're using the technique for everything from controlling pain to enhancing vitality.

How does visualization work?

"When people have a problem and they perceive that they can't operate because of it, it becomes a self-fulfilling prophecy," says Nicholas Hall, Ph.D., a leading imagery researcher, adjunct professor in the Department of Psychology at the University of South Florida in Tampa, adjunct professor in the Department of Biochemistry at the George Washington School of Medicine in Washington, D.C., and director of the Institute for Health and Human Performance in Orlando, Florida.

"Visualization allows a person to exert some measure of control over what they might view as being a hopeless situation. Done in a group setting, it may provide a source of social support."

It certainly seems to work when it comes to boosting your energy level. Just picture yourself in comfortable surroundings such as a warm beach or a lush garden.

Use this mental image to calm your body and mind. For example, if you envision a beach, feel warm sand beneath you, hear a distant pounding surf, smell the salt air. Make your image convincing—and relaxing.

If you're new to visualization, you may need to make an audiotape that talks you through the visualization process, says Maria Simonson, Sc.D., Ph.D., professor emeritus at Johns Hopkins University Medical Institutions in Baltimore and director of its Health, Weight and Stress Clinic.

Your tape should be 15 to 30 minutes long. During the last several minutes, you should talk yourself out of the relaxed state. Otherwise, you may get up feeling groggy.

When you make the tape, choose a mental picture that you find relaxing such as a beach. Then in great, soothing detail, describe the scene. Remember to appeal to all five senses in describing the scene and make it as realistic and relaxing as possible. Keep your voice soft, soothing and well-modulated. Listen to the tape with your eyes closed to help you create vivid, relaxing images.

Here's a sample narrative about a beach scene from Dr. Simonson.

"Close your eyes. You're very, very, very tired. You're on a sandy beach and you're all alone. There are no houses and there's no one around you. There are tall trees in the background and scrub pines on the sand dunes. You're lying there very tired with your eyes shut. You can feel the sun beating down on your cheeks. It's warm and your skin feels drawn. You feel tiredness seeping out of your body, down your arms, down your wrists. Your fingers are tingling with relaxation . . . "

Creating Images

Although results may vary, the usefulness of visualization is virtually unlimited. To fight fatigue, for example, try visualizing what your tiredness looks like, suggests Dennis J. Gersten, M.D., publisher of *Atlantis: The Imagery Newsletter*. It doesn't matter if the image makes sense, just let your mind and imagination create a symbol of your fatigue. "One patient of mine sees a huge boulder symbolizing her fatigue—that's her image," Dr. Gersten says.

You can then confront the image, talk to it or somehow symbolically deal with it, thus terminating your tiredness. For example, if your image is a large boulder, consider rolling it out of your life.

You can use a similar technique to shrink your stress by imagining that it just withers away and disappears. Here's a way to do that, adapted from the book, *Anxiety and Stress*, by Susan M. Lark, M.D.

Make yourself comfortable, either sitting or lying down. Then, breathe slowly and deeply. Picture the situation or person that makes you tense and drains your energy. Then, slowly begin to shrink the picture. When it's small enough to fit on your palm, hold out your hand and place the picture there. Shrink the picture even more, until it can fit on your finger. Watch it turn into a dot and disappear.

Find Peace, Piece by Piece

Used by itself or in combination with visualization, autogenic relaxation, a form of progressive muscle relaxation, is a useful and effective way to let go of tension. It relaxes you, body part by body part, inch by inch.

Created more than 50 years ago by doctors Johannes H. Schultz and Wolfgang Luthe in Germany, autogenic relaxation works by a process of mentally talking your body into a relaxed state. The word *autogenic* means "self-regulation"—that is, without outside influence—and that's exactly how you do it.

"Autogenic relaxation is based on visual mental images," explains Viviane Lind, M.D., assistant professor of psychiatry at New York Medical College in Valhalla.

According to experts, here's how to use autogenic relaxation to help banish the tension and stress that deplete your energy.

Be comfortable.

There's no special posture or position to magically relax you, but comfort is the name of the game, says David Edelberg, M.D., a facilitator of the American Holistic Center which has offices in both Chicago and Denver. Many people find that lying down and wearing loose clothing help them relax. Be sure to unplug the phone and find a quiet area.

Set the scene.

Begin with a visualization technique such as the one described earlier, suggests Dr. Simonson. "Take yourself away to that deserted beach," she suggests, "and as you're doing this, speak to yourself in a soft, slow modulated voice."

Find repose from head to toes.

Autogenic relaxation starts at one end of your body and progresses through each section, ending with the relaxation of your entire body. You accomplish this by imagining each body part feeling warm, heavy and thoroughly relaxed. According to experts, this is how to do autogenic relaxation step by step.

1. *Face and head.* Feel your facial and scalp muscles relax. Imagine that your face feels like a pool of calm water.

2. *Neck and shoulders.* Take extra time to focus on these commonly tense spots until you can actually feel the muscle tension unwind.

3. *Arms.* Work downward from your right shoulder to your right hand. Then do the other arm.

4. *Fingers.* Slowly relax each finger on your right hand, one at a time, until you feel your entire hand go limp. Then do the other hand.

5. *Chest.* Relax your entire chest and upper torso.

6. *Abdomen.* After relaxing your chest and arms, concentrate on your abdomen.

7. *Buttocks and back.* Release the tension in these areas to finish relaxing your entire torso.

8. *Thighs, calves and legs.* Do one leg at a time, making sure they're both entirely relaxed.

9. *Toes.* Relax the big toe on your right foot, then the other toes. Repeat with your other foot.

Activate your imagination.

Create descriptive images as you're mentally moving through your body. "Imagine feeling the tiredness sliding out of your body," says Dr. Simonson. "It leaves your head, comes down your neck and down your arms. Feel it slide into your fingertips and then drip out from your fingertips and out of your body."

Move on to other body parts, imagining that the tiredness is slipping out from your torso, your hips, down your legs and out through your toes. Continue doing this until your body is so limp that you feel complete tranquillity and peace.

Practice, practice, practice.

Although some experts suggest that you practice autogenic relaxation for two 20-minute sessions each day, Dr. Feldman finds more frequent, shorter sessions to be most beneficial, as they reduce the negative physical effects of stress.

As you practice and become more familiar with autogenic relaxation, relax your body in a way that is most comfortable for you, suggests Dr. Feldman. For example, if you are most comfortable starting with your toes and working your way up to your head, do that. The important thing is just to do it. "You can even relax your body and mind at a red light or while pumping gas," he maintains.

Yoga for Relaxation

Yoga is a discipline that combines stretching, meditation and breathing to induce relaxation and generate energy. The word *yoga* comes from the Sanskrit root word *yug*, meaning "to join together" or "yoke." And although yoga may take a lifetime to master, with regular practice you can start reaping the benefits even while you're still a beginner.

Yoga is also a marvelous way to turn around the low-energy, humdrum effects of a lifestyle of lassitude, says Alice Christensen, executive director of the American Yoga Association, which is located in Sarasota, Florida, and author of *The American Yoga Association's Beginner's Manual.*

"Yoga is an educational tool that can be used by anyone," Christensen says. "It gives you a rest from the intense mental demands you have."

Here are some of Christensen's tips for practicing yoga.

Keep it light and loose.

Your clothing should not restrict movement during yoga. Try wearing sweatpants or a stretchable exercise outfit, like a leotard. Also, wear socks, but not shoes.

Make time for yourself.

Practice regularly but have fun, Christensen says. Even if you can't do a full yoga routine, try a few stretches and breathing exercises in your spare time.

"You can practice in bed, in a chair or while watching TV," Christensen says.

Biofeedback for Stress Relief

Most of us know what feedback is. The boss tells you what's right or wrong with your report. Your spouse lets you know what's right or wrong with dinner.

*Bio*feedback can tune you in to what's right or wrong with your body in terms of stress.

When you get biofeedback, you're hooked up to a monitor that provides information about what's going on in your body. That's the feedback. Working with a biofeedback trainer, you can use the information to learn how to gain conscious control over bodily processes that you don't normally control consciously. In practice, biofeedback can teach you how to counteract the energy-depleting effects of stress on your body.

"When you're attached to it, a biofeedback machine feeds back to you information from your body about its state of tension," says Dr. Feldman.

Different biofeedback machines (or monitors) record different kinds of information with sensors. Some machines measure muscle tension—they measure it even before you become aware that the tension is there and before it translates into pain.

Other machines take the temperature of your skin. Chilly fingers or toes means that the blood is being pulled from your extremities to the core of your body, and that is one of the telling signs of stress. Stress makes the blood rush to vital organs to protect them—part of your instinctive, built-in response to danger.

Yet another machine determines the electrical conductivity of your skin: If you're nervous and sweating, your skin is saltier, and it conducts more electricity.

Benefits of Being Bionic

All of these biofeedback machines can alert you to energy-depleting stress in your body. You may think that you know when you're tense and stressed—they're large emotions—but that's not always so.

"Most of us are so out of tune with our bodies, we don't know what's going on inside until we get headaches, stomach problems, back and neck pain. We have no idea how to begin to relax, how to stop bracing those muscles," says Pam Ladds, R.N., a social worker who practices biofeedback in Philadelphia and is former president of the Pennsylvania Society of Behavioral Medicine and Biofeedback.

Yoga for Beginners

You don't have to be a contortionist to be good at yoga. Its benefits will come naturally in time. When you're just starting out, work slowly and steadily and don't be afraid to lean on a chair or table for balance when you're trying a difficult technique, says Alice Christensen, executive director of the American Yoga Association, which is located in Sarasota, Florida, and author of *The American Yoga Association's Beginner's Manual*. Also, never stretch to the point of pain—just to the point of resistance.

Here is a brief, easy yoga routine for beginners that Christensen recommends to fight fatigue. (Portions of this routine, which was reviewed and approved by Christensen for this book, originally appeared in her yoga *Beginner's Manual*.)

Do the routine daily in this sequence. Remember to breathe through your nose, not your mouth. Be sure to check with your doctor before starting any new exercise routine. Avoid doing the routine after drinking caffeinated beverages or eating a large meal.

Shoulder roll. Standing with your arms hanging loosely at your sides, lift both shoulders up toward your ears, then roll them forward, making small circles. Breathe normally. Do several repetitions forward. Then reverse your circles and do several repetitions backward.

Easy bend. Stand straight with your arms at your sides and exhale deeply. Now breathe in and raise your arms in front of you, keeping your palms facing up, until your arms are parallel to the ground. Breathing out, start to "dive" slowly forward into a slouched-over position, letting your head and arms completely relax. Bend only halfway. Inhale while raising yourself to the starting position. (Eventually, you can try the full bend, where you

"With a biofeedback machine, we can show a person that his body is under his physical control," she explains. "Gradually, once he starts doing relaxation exercises, he learns how to change his physiological processes—what's going on inside. And he learns what that feels like. The goal is to have him do it on his own without the machine."

Here's how to gain the maximum relaxation benefits from biofeedback.

Pick a practitioner.
Several different kinds of specialties use biofeedback as a stress-reducing tool. Psychologists and physical therapists are the most common practitioners. But psychiatrists, nurses and psychotherapists may use biofeedback, too, says Ladds.

continue leaning down until you can touch the floor.) Match your breath with your movement. Do three to five repetitions.

Folded pose. Sit in a chair, with your hips touching the back of the chair and your feet firmly on the floor. Separate your knees slightly and lean forward, placing your hands on your knees for support if need be. Lean down until your chest rests on your knees and let your arms dangle. (Or cross your arms on your knees for support.) Let your head and neck relax completely. Hold for several seconds, keeping your breathing normal. Repeat one more time.

Knee squeeze. Lie flat on your back with your arms at your sides and begin inhaling, while raising your right knee to your chest. Pull your leg toward your chest by grasping the inside of your thigh with both hands. Hold your breath, while pressing your leg in to your chest. Hold. Exhale as you straighten your leg. Do three repetitions on each leg, then repeat three times with both legs working in unison.

Easy bridge. Lie flat on your back with your knees bent and your feet slightly apart but in as close to your hips as possible. Keep your arms straight and against your body and your palms down. Exhale deeply and relax your body. As you inhale, raise your hips off the ground and gently arch your back so that your body forms a bridge. (Keep your shoulders on the floor and relax your neck muscles.) As you exhale, slowly lower your hips to the floor. Repeat three times.

"Always include at least three complete breaths and a few minutes of relaxation or meditation as part of your fatigue-fighting routine," says Christensen.

You may want to ask your doctor to recommend a qualified biofeedback trainer in your area.

Another excellent way to find a trainer is to write the Biofeedback Certification Institute of America, 10200 West 44th Avenue, #304, Wheat Ridge, CO 80033. Enclose a self-addressed, stamped envelope; you'll receive in return a list of certified specialists in your area.

Embrace technology.
When you visit a biofeedback specialist, he'll first teach you some basic breathing exercises and then hook you up to a biofeedback machine. The sensors, cords and wires may look intimidating, but you won't feel a thing, says Ladds.

Biofeedback Gadgets

Biofeedback intimidates a lot of people.

Many are put off by the notion of being hooked up to a machine that will tell them things about themselves that they don't know. Training sessions are not cheap. The process takes time.

If this sounds like you, take heart. Getting biofeedback about your body's state of stress doesn't always mean being hooked up to an expensive machine. There are also some inexpensive, lighthearted, but useful ways to experience biofeedback in action, says Larry J. Feldman, Ph.D., a leader of workshops on stress and burnout and author of *Feeling Good Again*.

Check Your Ring

Believe it or not, the vintage mood ring was one such biofeedback item, says Dr. Feldman. The mood ring changed color according to the temperature of your finger. Warm, relaxed hands colored the ring blue or violet. Cold, tense hands turned it black. You can usually find mood rings at novelty shops for about four dollars. Prices, of course, vary depending on the ring setting.

That's the same principle at work in other biofeedback products, says Dr. Feldman. Futurehealth, a company in Trevose, Pennsylvania, makes a product called BioDots that works much like the mood ring; it's sensitive to minute gradations of temperature. BioDots, also called stress points, are small circles that stick to your finger and change color according to your stress level. Dr. Feldman buys them by the bushel for the stress workshops he leads.

"They're a big hit when I lead people through relaxation techniques in a workshop," he says, "because they can watch the dots change color from the beginning of the workshop, when they're tense, to the end of the workshop, when they're relaxed."

Once you learn deep breathing or other relaxation techniques, you'll be able to change the measurements that the machine records. When that happens, the machine will signal you. Some machines hum or beep. Others may light up. Some merely move a needle.

Whenever you can make your machine respond, it means you're in control. The feeling of control is very stress-relieving, says Dr. Feldman. When this happens, something good is going on—you sweat less, your skin is warming up, your muscles are relaxing . . . and so is the rest of you.

"Stress cards," or "mood cards," are similar to BioDots. You press your finger against the dot on the card to record your color and check your stress level.

Both BioDots and stress cards are available through the Conscious Living Foundation, P.O. Box 9, Drain, OR 97435 and Futurehealth, 3171 Rail Avenue, Trevose, PA 19053.

Even simpler are tiny, handheld thermometers made solely for the purpose of monitoring stress. You can watch your temperature rise as you relax. They are available at some drugstores.

"Toys" to Enhance Self-Awareness

These things may all seem like psychology toys, but they actually have some value in helping you monitor and control your level of energy-depleting stress, says Dr. Feldman.

"You can get instant feedback in different circumstances with these devices," he says. "In the office, for instance, you can see what's stressful and what isn't. It's not always what you suspect. Then you can learn to bring that stress under control."

The biofeedback tools could also let you know which relaxation techniques—deep breathing, meditation, visualization and so on—work best and most quickly for you, says Dr. Feldman.

A couple of caveats about the mood rings and BioDots: You need a room-temperature environment to accurately gauge hand temperature. If the room is cold, your hands will naturally be cold, whether you're stressed or not. BioDots give false readings after meals, too, when your blood is busy with the digestive process. So don't use them when you have a full stomach, advises Dr. Feldman.

Give it some time.

Learning to relax enough to make the machine respond usually takes anywhere from three to six lessons with a trainer, Ladds estimates.

"First, we show a person how easy it is to change a reading just by changing her breathing," she says. "The change isn't significant at first, but it's enough to show the person that change is within her control."

The next step, says Ladds, involves learning a few simple relaxation techniques. These may involve muscle relaxation along the lines of autogenic training or some simple breathing techniques. Doing these techniques while hooked up to a machine helps you tune in to how you feel when you relax. You can see or hear yourself doing the very things with your body that will eventually bring you deep relaxation and renewed energy.

Do your homework.

After you learn the relaxation techniques while hooked up to the machine, Ladds suggests that you start practicing on your own without the help of the machine. She recommends five-minute relaxation breaks, three times a day at the minimum.

Monitor yourself.

In addition to regularly scheduled practice sessions, Ladds recommends doing what she calls a self-awareness check every hour to check for signs of tension. Are you tensing your shoulders? Clenching your jaw? Forgetting to breathe deeply? If you learn how to spot the signs of stress early on, she says, you can take an R and R break right when you most need it. That way you can banish the effects of stress before they put a major drain on your energy supply.

Scheduling
and Organizing
for Energy

*T*he house. The job. Kids. Family. Friends. Pets. Cooking. Cleaning. Laundry. Hobbies. Appointments. Obligations. Responsibilities. HASSLES. You certainly have it all . . . except for maybe the one thing you need most: energy.

"Who wouldn't be tired?" asks Redford B. Williams, M.D., director of the behavioral medicine research center at Duke University Medical Center in Durham, North Carolina, and the nation's leading authority on the type A personality and the harmful effects of stress.

Or rather, the question might be "Who isn't?" After all, statistics show that the rat race has become a marathon. The average jobholder now puts in 163 additional hours at work each year compared to 30 years ago—the equivalent of an extra month on the job. If you have kids or parents living with you, add another 50 hours each week in cooking, cleaning and other housework duties . . . and that doesn't include ferrying family members to *their* appointments and obligations.

Add it all up, and you might think it's downright medieval how busy you are. Actually, it's worse. Between work and home, you're working 330 more hours each year than the typical peasant did in the thirteenth century.

Looking Within to Energize

Something has to change, although it's not likely to be your workload. Leisure time has shrunk by 40 percent since 1973, and all indications are that it will continue to dwindle. So it's more important than ever to use your time wisely.

"It's as simple as this," says Pat Dorff, an organizational consultant in Minneapolis and author of several books on time management and organization, including *File, Don't Pile*. "If you don't plan, if you don't organize and schedule what you need to do each day, fatigue *will* happen."

The place to start is inside your brain, Dorff says. Give some serious thought to the kind of person that you really are. "I wish I could make a blanket statement that says doing one or two things helps everyone be better organized, but the truth is, everyone is different," she says. "The key is to know yourself, so you know what's best for you." Following are her suggestions for finding that out.

Do a personality profile.

"Everyone gets energy from different sources," says Dorff. "Extroverts get energized being around people, while introverts are just the opposite—they need quiet time alone. It's important to know if you're an extrovert or an introvert so that you can actually schedule yourself time to re-energize."

Well, what if you are an extrovert? "You might want to schedule yourself time to be around other people after work or just after finishing an activity that is particularly draining," Dorff suggests. If you're an introvert, "you'll probably benefit from some quiet time away from everyone immediately after work."

Don't assume that you need to organize.

Another aspect of knowing yourself is knowing your work style. "While being organized in the truest sense of the word is certainly more efficient for everyone, it can actually be fatiguing for certain personality types—especially creative, intuitive types," says Dorff. "If you're that kind of person, then you probably will be revitalized not by cleaning up and organizing your desk or home but by immersing yourself in it. While I'm not suggesting that a messy desk is efficient, it can be energizing for certain people—especially writers and artistic types."

Take hold—of yourself.

What exactly are your stressors? The way you react to certain responsibilities is a good indication of when you should do those chores. And if you look at the way you react, you'll also get a clue about what responsibilities you should delegate to other people.

There's actually a good way to gauge your reaction to situations that are causing stress. Bring your fingertips together so that just the pinkie of one hand is touching the index finger of the other—and vice versa. Do those fingertips feel cold?

"When you're under stress, blood vessels constrict. So if your hands or feet feel colder, it's a good indicator that stress hormones have been released that could affect your energy," says Steven Fahrion, Ph.D., a clinical psychologist and director of research at the Life Sciences Institute of Mind-Body Health in Topeka, Kansas.

When this test tells you that you're having a chilly reaction, you need to step back and take a clear look at what you're doing with your time, Dr. Fahrion suggests. Get a better of idea of the specific chores that might be zapping your energy so that you'll know how to deal with them.

Enlisting Lists

Of course, there's one thing that we all need—no matter whether we're introverts, extroverts, neatniks or the owners of closets so sloppy that they could hide Jimmy Hoffa's body: more time.

So how do we squeeze a few more hours into those precious 24 we are given each day?

The rule is: take some time to make time. Time-management experts say that you can save two hours of doing for every hour you spend in planning. The best way to plan? Write down schedules and stick to them, say the experts. Here are some of the top strategies for doing that.

Go by the book.
One body. One appointment book. That's how organization experts recommend that you balance time equations. If you have more than one book, you're likely to schedule something for work that conflicts with your home schedule. So a good appointment book is worth the search; it's your organizational right hand.

What you want is something small enough to carry in your purse or briefcase but large enough to hold both home and work entries. And you want to be able to write down as much as possible—everything from your grocery list to scheduled appointments.

An appointment book puts everything right in front of you so that you check it often. "Make it an integral part of your life," urges Stephanie Culp, author of *You Can Find More Time for Yourself Every Day* and other books on organization and time management.

Make a list for the next day.
"Each night, you should make a list of the most important things that you need to do the following day before going to bed," says Dorff. "This list doesn't have to be anything fancy, but it should include up to 10 to 12 items that you really should do. It's important to do this every night—even on weekends or if you know you won't complete everything—because it gives you a sense of direction for the next day."

Another advantage is: "Often I think of something right as I'm falling asleep," adds Judy McQueen, educational program coordinator for the Women's Resource Center at Michigan State University in East Lansing. "If I couldn't write it down, it would wake me up three times during the night."

Rank your activities.

You can set priorities by labeling your tasks in order of importance with an A, B or C, suggests B. Kaye Olson, R.N., an instructor and adviser in stress management at Lansing Community College in Lansing, Michigan, and author of *Energy Secrets for Tired Mothers on the Run.*

So, what gets done first? Common sense would suggest the A's, the most important jobs.

Generally, yes. "But if there's a job you especially hate—no matter how important it is—you should always do that one first," adds Dorff. In other words, even if the nastiest job is a B or C, do it before the A just to get the upper hand. "Once you get through that unpleasant job, whatever it is, it'll free you up. Same goes with days. If you have a bad project for the week, do it on Monday."

Log in.

Keep a time-activity log as one of your first organizational steps, advise both Olson and Culp. This way, you can see exactly where your time goes and you can identify your time wasters.

To organize the log, draw two lines down a sheet of notebook paper to divide it into three columns. Write the date at the very top of the paper. In the left column, enter the time of day; in the middle column, your activity; and in the right column, any comments. Keep this log for a week, noting your time wasters in the comments column. Then start thinking about ways to change them.

Write on the road.

If you're really on the go, you probably spend a lot of time in your car. So it's a good idea to have a dashboard pad and a pencil. You'll find these pads (with a suction cup or tape fastener) at any big hardware or department store that sells automotive products. Besides helping keep track of your schedule, these dashboard notepads help you keep track of creative ideas as they come up. Another way to capture those ideas is to keep a minicassette recorder in your car.

Refuse So You Don't Lose

All the scheduling in the world isn't going to help if you make the biggest mistake made by the overachieving overweary—biting off more than you can chew. Often, it's working women who do this, and frequently, the overcommitment is the result of guilt.

A Time for Everything

If you feel as though you're spinning your wheels and getting nowhere, it could be that you have been scheduling your chores all wrong—by not taking your body clock into account.

"We all have daily best and worst times for practically every activity in our lives, and this is all dictated by your body clock," says Maria Simonson, Sc.D., Ph.D., professor emeritus at Johns Hopkins Medical Institutions in Baltimore and director of its Health, Weight and Stress Clinic.

Researchers have found that your body clock is controlled by many factors including sunlight, work schedules and when you eat and sleep. Even your personality is a factor, says Donald P. LaSalle, Ph.D., a chronobiologist at Talcott Mountain Science Center in Avon, Connecticut.

Introspective people who prefer structure-oriented lives and put a big emphasis on achievement tend to be morning people, or "larks." Those who are more outgoing, creative and money-oriented tend to be night people, or "owls." Most of us fall somewhere in the middle, with a natural leaning toward being a lark or an owl, according to Dr. LaSalle. And while this leaning can change depending on our schedules, experts find that most people do have a best time to do certain chores. Here are some of the prime times in most people's daily rhythms.

To make decisions: Between 7:00 and 11:00 A.M., when depression and anxiety are lowest. The worst time for decision making is between 2:00 and 8:00 P.M., when they're highest.

To remember things: Short-term memory is sharpest between 10:00 and 11:00 A.M. Long-term memory is best in early- to midafternoon.

To do simple tasks: *(like housecleaning)*: Early in the morning for larks; immediately after lunch for owls.

To do complex tasks: *(like your taxes)*: Midday or early afternoon, when body temperature reaches its highest point.

To exercise: It's easiest in the morning, when your threshold for pain is highest, but overall athletic performance peaks around 1:00 P.M.

To have sex: Technically, the best time is between 5:00 and 9:00 A.M., when both male and female hormones peak, resulting in maximum pleasure and performance.

To visit the dentist: First thing in the morning, because your pain threshold is highest. It begins to sag after noon.

To reflect: Between 2:00 and 4:00 P.M., when body temperature begins to drop.

Winning the Chores Wars

It's a war out there—in the kitchen. In the bedrooms. In the family room. The fight: How do you get the rest of the brood to pitch in and do their fair share?

A lot depends on scheduling, which means everyone has to get together and agree on when they'll pitch in. But how do you get the initial agreement?

One way is to call a family meeting involving Mom, Dad and the kids. Sit down at the kitchen table for a brainstorming, problem-solving session. Here's how to approach this sit-down session so that you come up with positive, action-oriented results.

List every chore.

Lead off the meeting by making a complete list of household chores by category: shopping and cooking, laundry and vacuuming, pet care, telephone calls, child care. And don't forget the outside chores like mowing the lawn and washing the windows.

Let family members rotate and swap.

Different people like different things, of course. You can rotate unpopular chores weekly. Once the schedule is set up, it should be okay for one person to trade with another as long as the jobs get done.

Get a big weekly calendar.

Once you've listed each day's chore assignments on the calendar, hang it in a prominent place in the kitchen. Anyone wondering whose turn it is can just check the calendar.

"It's partly the way we're brought up—to feel guilty if we're not spending time on other people," says Marjorie Hansen Shaevitz, director of the Institute of Family and Work Relationships in La Jolla, California, and author of *The Superwoman Syndrome.* "We think time for ourselves is somehow illegitimate, but we need time to relax in order to feel energetic." Here's how to make that time.

Delay your response.

Good organization skills aren't the only reason why the same people continue to be flagged for every volunteer duty that comes down the pike—from heading up the Little League fund-raiser to taking control of Uncle Bob's retirement party. If you're being chosen again and again, maybe it's because you don't say no.

Or maybe you feel as though you *can't* say no. But you can—and without being rude—notes Shaevitz. Before agreeing to any request, give yourself some distance, she advises. "Say something like 'Thank you so much for asking, but I'll have to check my calendar and get back to you.' "

Then ask yourself two questions: "How much do I really want to do this?" and "How important is it, given everything else that is going on in my life?" If you answer "not much" and "not very" to those questions, "you have to be assertive and say no," says McQueen. "It's especially hard for mothers who work outside the home to say no because they feel guilty and the superwoman stuff comes out. They have to remember that it's their time they'd be using for other people's priorities."

Don't be afraid to call it quits.
Another problem that can lead to fatigue is refusing to throw in the towel—especially on projects or responsibilities that don't particularly excite you. "When something hangs over your head unfinished, it can be even more draining than actually doing it," says Dorff. "That's because lack of closure weighs on you and drains your energy. So either finish a job, delegate it or chuck it. In fact, sometimes making a decision not to do something can be more energizing than actually doing it, because you've made a decision and removed the stress of it hanging over you."

Divide to Conquer Fatigue

Passing the buck can help you bypass fatigue, so another key to organizing and scheduling for energy is to give some of your duties to another. "Delegation is the key to self-multiplication," says Dorff. "Unfortunately, those who could benefit the most from delegation are probably those least likely to do it."

That might be because delegation is a skill that must be learned—and learned correctly—in order to be done correctly. Here are some tips for mastering the energizing art of delegating.

Match the job with the person.
"Unfortunately, most people delegate what it is that they don't want to do," says Dorff. "But that's dumping. Delegating is matching the task with the person's ability and capabilities."

For instance, a seven-year-old child could help you set the dinner table, wash vegetables or even put together a simple salad—all jobs that could ease your meal-preparation duties—but you wouldn't want him hovering over a hot stove keeping an eye on dinner.

Give up ownership.
What separates a good delegator from a great one is the ability to pass ownership. "People want the freedom to do a job the way they deem fit," says Dorff.

"You should give them very clear instructions on what should be accomplished. But then say, 'I trust you will do it.'"

After that, says Dorff, you need to truly delegate the tasks, leaving them to the other people to do their own way. One reason why delegation fails is because the "boss" tends to get too wrapped up and can't let go.

Like yourself more.
"People who are the best delegators are those who tend to feel good about themselves," adds Dr. Fahrion. "If you feel you're at the mercy of others—for friendship, respect or whatever—you're not as likely to pass on tasks, and you're at greater risk of being fatigued." His advice: Remind yourself that you're not delegating "your" chores as a way to punish but as a way to get things done more effectively—for everyone involved.

Barter on your friendship.
Bartering is a good way to get chores done and to see your friends. Plus, a good barter involves trading a task that you don't like for a task that you do. Agree to do something you enjoy—whether it's gardening, cooking or babysitting. Offer to do that for a friend in exchange for a job that she enjoys for you.

Casting Out Clutter

Cleaning the house or office might seem like the least of your worrisome chores. Not a priority, you say? Maybe not. After all, some folks thrive in clutter, says Dorff.

But even if you're energized by having clutter around, it does cost time. And wasted time leads to fatigue. "You spend a lot of time in bits and pieces looking for things and being late for appointments, because you couldn't find the right clothes to wear in the morning, for instance," says Culp. "And that has a domino effect. All those two- to five-minute daily frustrations wind up as one great big wad of stress." Here are some suggestions for keeping your home less cluttered.

Toss the old when you get something new.
"Make it a rule that every time something new comes in, something old has to go out," says Culp. "It works for everything—toys, clothes, newspapers, magazines." In a clutter-free household, fewer items are misplaced.

Use it or lose it.
Your clothes closet is a thorn in your side on workday mornings—or anytime that you're in a rush. "Throw out everything you don't wear," says Culp. "If your closet isn't crammed, you'll cut down on the ironing."

The Forgotten Priority—You

Taking time for yourself may not come naturally in the context of your busy life. But a big part of scheduling and organizing is making time to relax. Once you've scheduled that time, you have to make sure to respect that schedule and relax when you plan to.

Some busy people tend to run until they drop from either exhaustion or illness and then are too tired to enjoy their free time. But it's in everybody's interest for you to feel happy and rested, says Shaevitz.

One way to protect some time is to mark your appointment book with at least 30 minutes every day for you, whether it's watching TV, talking on the phone with a friend or doing another activity to recharge your battery.

And here are some other tactics for free-time protection:

Try another kind of R and R.

Relaxation Response—unlike rest and relaxation—is an easy meditation-like technique that stills your churning mind. "You have to turn your brain off so it can rest," says Richard Friedman, Ph.D., professor of psychiatry and behavioral science at the State University of New York at Stony Brook. With your eyes closed and no outside distractions, pick a word or phrase, like "peace" or "love," and repeat it each time you exhale. Continue for 10 to 20 minutes. If a thought distracts you, try to ignore it and continue with your word repetition and your breathing. After a few weeks, this routine should become very natural.

Snatch your half-hour—on the road.

Olson has identified the optimum time for daily decompression: the time between when you leave work and arrive home. She suggests extending it for at least 20 minutes—to enjoy the silence, listen to an audiotape, stop your car and read or just think things through. This helps some who don't get quiet time at home because of interruptions from children or other family members.

Sleeping
for Energy

Well, even if you do manage to shoehorn everything into your crowded hours, what's the one thing that you really want to do? For many of us, the answer is sleep. The only trouble is that every night, when you finally crash into bed, sleep escapes you, chased off by the long "to do" list that keeps repeating itself in your mind.

Lack of sleep is a huge energy drainer. Often, you feel so dragged out during the day because of the shut-eye that you missed the night before.

A Nation without Sleep

"We're a nation of sleep-deprived people," says sleep researcher Wilse B. Webb, Ph.D., professor emeritus of psychology at the University of Florida in Gainesville. "We go to bed when we want. And we get up when we have to." Our sleep debt is so large that Congress established the National Center on Sleep Disorders Research, which is part of the National Institutes of Health, after a three-year federal commission reported that as many as one-third of us toss and turn with insomnia at least once a year.

Forty million of us have specific sleep disorders, like insomnia, where we're unable to sleep night after night, or apnea, where we stop breathing for short periods in our sleep. An additional 20 million to 30 million more people have occasional problems falling asleep, staying asleep or staying on a consistent sleep schedule.

But there's another deficit. Many of those who sleep well don't always sleep enough. On any given day about a quarter of us are drowsy and yawning. When you total up all the combined deficits, "well over a third of us don't get adequate sleep," says Michael Stevenson, Ph.D., clinical director of the North Valley Sleep Disorders Center in Mission Hills, California.

Our brains as well as our bodies need sleep, says Philip Smith, M.D., medical director of the Johns Hopkins University Sleep Disorders Center in Baltimore. "Sleep deprivation makes us moody and irritable and limits our ability to concentrate, make judgments and perform mental tasks."

Making Friends with Your Pillow

Since we know that we need sleep for mental and physical energy, how do we get so tired? "The two answers are we don't allow ourselves enough time to sleep. Or we're too tense to fall asleep," says Rosalind Cartwright, Ph.D., director of the Sleep Disorder Service and Research Center at Rush–St. Luke's Presbyterian Medical Center in Chicago.

Researchers have noted that more women than men are likely to have insomnia. There is evidence that an estimated 40 percent of all women over 40 are fighting insomnia.

"The menstrual cycle, pregnancy and hormone changes at menopause are all reasons why women have many more insomnia complaints than men," says Dr. Stevenson. "And, even in this day and age, women are still the ones who get up with little kids in the middle of the night. That's very disturbing to sleep."

If sleep eludes you so constantly that you can't do what you have to during the day, a visit to your doctor is mandatory, says Tedd Mitchell, M.D., medical director of the Cooper Wellness Program at the Cooper Aerobics Center in Dallas. Insomnia could be a symptom of something else, like depression. Yet if your sleeplessness is annoying but not debilitating, changes in schedule, exercise, diet and even eating habits can make you better friends with your pillow.

Catching a Few Zzzs

While sleep shortages can get to be a habit, some habits are meant to be broken.

"You have to court sleep," advises Dr. Cartwright. "Often, people can't sleep because they're too wound up. They rush around all day. They try to work to the last minute. Then they want to fall asleep quickly and they can't do it. You have to be ready for sleep."

To get ready, here are some top methods for attracting the sandman.

Steep in the tub.
"Take a hot bath. This is the best way I know to court sleep," says Dr. Cartwright. "It sounds so strange in this day and age when people take morning

When Snoring Is a Symptom

Snoring can be more than an annoyance. Loud snoring that ends with a snort or a gasp could be a symptom of apnea, a breathing disorder that occurs during sleep. The danger of apnea is that it deprives the body of energy-producing oxygen and can ultimately lead to heart attack, stroke and death. It's more common among men than women and more frequent among people who are overweight. It's also more frequent among people who have short, thick necks, but anyone can have the problem.

When someone with sleep apnea snores, his tongue falls back in his throat and plugs it up like a champagne cork. The sleeper stops breathing while his body struggles to unplug the cork. The person gasps for air, jerks—and then breathing resumes.

Someone with sleep apnea generally dozes through this action. But his heart pumps wildly to supply the brain with oxygen until the gasp of air finally comes. Sometimes that doesn't happen fast enough. Sleep apnea causes about 38,000 deaths a year.

People with sleep apnea feel sleepy all the time, even when they've put in enough bedtime hours. They're "pathologically sleepy," says sleep researcher Timothy Roehrs, Ph.D., director of research at the Sleep Disorders and Research Center at the Henry Ford Hospital in Detroit. People with sleep apnea routinely fall asleep in five minutes or less.

This problem is eminently treatable, according to doctors. Weight loss and a change of sleeping position make a big difference for some people. Sleep experts recommend sleeping on the stomach or side, never on the back.

For severe cases, doctors advise the use of a masklike breathing device called CPAP (an acronym for continuous positive airway pressure) that can clear up almost every case. This prescription device must be adjusted to the individual during a night's sleep at a sleep disorder center or by a pulmonary physician.

showers that people look at me in shock when I mention it. But once they try it, they adore it."

As with many sleep rituals and routines, timing is important. "Take the bath 2 hours before bedtime, so you have 1½ hours to do quiet things when you come out," says Dr. Cartwright. "Use bath oil—it floats on the surface of the water and retains the water's heat. Relax in the tub for 20 to 30 minutes. That relaxes your muscles, too. When you come out, you're as limp as a noodle."

Watch dumb movies.

After your bath, have a little quiet time before you climb into bed. "Do something mindless—nothing to wind you up, something to wind you down," says Dr. Cartwright. She suggests old Marx Brothers comedies if you like to laugh to release tension. "But don't watch any murder mysteries," she warns. "And don't watch a gory newscast. You want dumb movies."

Make some sleepy pudding.

Go to bed hungry, and you won't sleep. Go to bed full, and you won't sleep either, say sleep specialists. A good snack, on the other hand, can promote the production of serotonin, "the brain's own sedative and relaxant," says Phyllis Herman, a nutrition specialist certified by the American College of Nutrition and contributor to the *Encyclopedia of Sleep and Dreaming*.

What you want is some food containing the amino acid tryptophan, which triggers the serotonin-production process. Milk products, tuna and turkey are all good choices, says Dr. Cartwright.

One swift but soothing snack to summon sleep is instant pudding, says Peter Hauri, Ph.D., co-director of the Sleep Disorders Center and director of its insomnia program at the Mayo Clinic in Rochester, Minnesota, and author of *No More Sleepless Nights*. Choose the sugar-free variety and make it with skim milk to keep fat and calories down. (The calcium in milk is a natural relaxant, too.)

Favor vanilla.

The smelling and feeling centers in our brains are directly connected, says Alan R. Hirsch, M.D., neurological director of the Smell and Taste Treatment and Research Foundation in Chicago. Which one should we use? And certain scents can fill us with feelings of calmness and well-being—such as lilacs in spring or the smell of freshly baked apple pie.

Dr. Hirsch has been studying certain scents in detail. And he's found that some smells can lure sleep by lowering anxiety. Among the best soothers are the scents of lavender, green apple and vanilla.

"Since 90 percent of taste is really smell, one way to obtain the scent in a very concentrated way is to eat the food with the appealing smell," suggests Dr. Hirsch. So make vanilla pudding. Or slice bananas into nonfat vanilla yogurt. It's two sedative effects in one—the tryptophan in the milk and the calming taste, plus smell, of the vanilla.

Mind Games for Snatching Shut-Eye

You know the pattern. You turn out the light, and today's tiny traumas start replaying themselves in the dark. Or you run through tomorrow's lines for the presentation you're giving at work. You worry whether Junior will get into the college of his choice. You worry about your folks down in Virginia. And when you can't sleep, you worry about not sleeping.

"We bring yesterday and tomorrow into tonight," says Dr. Webb. "The greatest problem to getting to sleep is that we keep *thinking*."

But the experts have some sleep techniques to settle or sidetrack our thinking brains.

Write a worry diary.

If you're a worrywart, here's one way to defuse that prickly pastime.

Two hours before bedtime, make two columns in your worry diary, Dr. Cartwright suggests. "On the left-hand side of one page, write down what you're worried about," she says. "On the right-hand side, write down what you're going to do about it. Then close the book, put it away and say, 'Well, I took care of that.' *Finish* the day."

Count crickets.

If counting sheep is too corny for you, then count cats or dogs or crickets. But even if you have to resort to the old standby, sheep, as Dr. Webb does, it works. Here's why, he says: "It's a task to do. But it's a task that you want to give up. The counting distracts you from thinking about things. It interferes with whatever is interfering with your sleep."

Confine the clock.

Alarm clocks can be, well, alarming to poor sleepers. You tend to keep checking the time—and that only tells you how well you're *not* sleeping. "The more aware you are of what time it is, the harder it is to fall asleep," says Dr. Hauri.

You need a clock without a cord that you can stash under the bed or in a closet. Or "set the alarm and hide it in the top dresser drawer," Dr. Hauri suggests. (Don't forget to first test the alarm in its hiding place to make sure that you will hear it in the morning.)

When Sleep Pulls a No-Show

Writer F. Scott Fitzgerald called 3:00 A.M. the "real dark night of the soul." It's when you run out of crickets to count. Or give up before you reach five digits. Dr. Hauri once had a patient who counted 5,865 sheep before she called it a night on that technique. So here's what to do when all the numbers in the animal kingdom fail you.

Don't try to sleep.

"Trying to sleep keeps you awake," says Dr. Hauri. "Ninety percent of the people with insomnia spend too much time in bed trying to sleep."

Read or watch TV until you feel drowsy. Fight sleep, then turn out the light when you no longer can stay awake. But never turn out the light and *try* to sleep, he says.

Don't panic.
Panic turns insomnia from a one-night visitor into the Man Who Came to Dinner—and wouldn't leave.

"People with insomnia almost develop performance anxiety," says Timothy Roehrs, Ph.D., director of research at Henry Ford Hospital's Sleep Disorders and Research Center in Detroit. They turn out the light, and then the pressure to sleep banishes sleep. "They need relief from the idea that they have to sleep. Sleep is a natural process and it will happen."

If it doesn't happen fast enough some nights, Dr. Hauri says not to worry. "You can function quite well after one night of poor sleep, even if you don't think you can. Don't sweat it. Hang in there. Pass the night by reading."

Drift off with lavender.
The smell of lavender oil is known to have a light sedative effect. And a study by British researchers found that lavender oil was more effective than tranquilizers at helping nursing-home residents get a restful night's sleep. In that study essence of lavender oil was introduced into the air with an odor diffuser. But there's another way if you don't have a diffuser: "You can use a few drops of lavender oil on a handkerchief that you keep on your pillow," Dr. Hirsch says.

The Sandman Rules

Things we do or don't do—as well as the things we eat or drink—can add up to shut-eye problems before you know it. Exercise, caffeine, alcohol and cigarettes all jiggle our sleep systems. Here's what to do about them.

Schedule sleep.
Go to bed at the same time every night—and get up at the same time every morning, say sleep therapists.

"You can train the body to go to sleep at a particular time," says Dr. Cartwright. "But if you screw around with that time—two hours later here, two hours earlier there—the body doesn't know when to go to sleep. The more regular the pattern, the more solid the sleep."

Even if you do wind up blowing your bedtime, don't change the setting on your alarm. You can handle an occasional midnight fling. Just don't sleep in, sleep specialists agree.

Sleeping through the bright light of morning jars your body clock even more than lying awake in the darkness. So if you really must steal an hour, take one from night, not day. Otherwise, you'll find yourself going to bed later and later and wanting to snooze the morning away, says Dr. Mitchell.

Exercise for better snoozing.
"Exercise is absolutely the best thing you can do for good sleep," says Dr. Mitchell. "Exercise actually burns off adrenaline, the biochemical that keeps us ready for fight-or-flight and that ups our anxiety level."

A study done at Duke University Medical Center supports Dr. Mitchell's assertion. Researchers there looked at 24 men to compare their sleep patterns. Half of those men were sedentary types. The other half were fit walkers, joggers and swimmers who had exercised vigorously at least three times a week for a year or more. During the study both groups either exercised for 40 minutes or did no exercise.

It took the sedentary group an average of 27 minutes to fall asleep—but it took the active men an average of only 12 minutes. The inactive men also spent more time awake during the night. And the fit group slept better even on the days when they didn't exercise.

So aim for at least a four-day-a-week exercise program. Twenty to 30 aerobic minutes is a good target to shoot for, most experts say.

Check your meds.
Most poor sleepers know that too much caffeine will disturb sleep. You probably know some of the things that are loaded with caffeine—such as coffee, tea and cola.

But caffeine is also added to many of the drugs we use, both over-the-counter and prescription. Check product labels or prescription package inserts to find out whether caffeine is one ingredient.

Other ingredients in drugs can also disturb sleep, says Dr. Mitchell. Watch out for nasal decongestants that contain ephedrine, pseudoephedrine (Actifed, Tylenol, Sudafed) or phenylpropanolamine (Dimetapp) and bronchodilators containing theophylline (such as Quibron or Theophylline) or beta agonists (such as albuterol, found in Proventil or Ventolin). Antidepressants, weight-reduction drugs (such as phentermine, found in products like Adipex-P or Fastin), thyroid-replacement therapy, and methylphenidate or Ritalin, a drug used to treat hyperactivity in children, can also cause sleepless nights.

If you're unsure whether a medicine you're taking could upset your sleep, ask your pharmacist or doctor, Dr. Hauri advises. Even the very drugs given to induce sleep can ultimately disturb it, which is one reason to avoid any kind of sleeping pills, if possible.

Ax the alcohol.
Sure, a glass of wine at bedtime makes you sleepy. But you'll probably pay for it later when you wake up at 1:00 A.M. That's how alcohol works. First it's a de-

pressant; then three to five hours after you stop drinking, it leaves the body in withdrawal, and you become more alert. In other words, it wakes you up.

Alcohol wrecks sleep worse than caffeine does, according to Merrill Mitler, Ph.D., director of research for sleep medicine at the Scripps Clinic and Research Foundation in La Jolla, California. "Alcohol is a terrible sleep disrupter—particularly in people over 30."

Most sleep experts caution against drinking anything more than a glass of wine or beer early in the evening. Some experts caution against any at all for the poor sleeper. It's an individual thing, says Dr. Hauri. "Know your limits. If you sleep poorly after a glass of wine, take the consequences."

Bag the butts.

Here's one more reason not to smoke. The *British Medical Journal* in a series on sleep reported that the average smoker snoozes 30 minutes less than a nonsmoker. That's because nicotine is a stimulant. It raises your blood pressure, works your heart faster and speeds up your brain waves. And heavy smokers sometimes wake up during the night craving a cigarette.

Sleep soundly with your spouse.

Admittedly, this isn't always easy. If snoring keeps you awake, offer the offender a wedge-shaped pillow. Frequently, just the change of pillow puts an end to snoring problems. If your spouse's tossing and turning bothers you, invest in a king-size bed or twin beds. Or you can "sleep separately but be united during the day," advises Dr. Hauri.

Still those legs.

One strange but not-so-uncommon medical condition, restless legs, can cause sleep problems. If you or your spouse has this problem, be sure to tell your doctor. Sometimes it can be treated with small doses of the prescription medicine L-dopa, a drug used to treat Parkinson's disease, says Dr. Hirsch.

Avoid temperature tantrums.

Too warm is just as bad as too cold. If you like it warm while your partner likes it cool—or vice versa—get an electric blanket with separate heating controls, one for each side. Or let the chilly party have an additional blanket on just that side of the bed.

Block out sights and sound.

To block light, use a sleeping mask. But make sure that you try it before you buy it to see if the band holding it to your head is comfortable and if it fits well. Use silicone or foam earplugs to dampen noise. Or you can mask obnoxious sounds with white noise by setting your radio dial to the hum at the end of the radio band or by buying a white-noise generator, available at electronics stores or sleep stores.

Drape it dark.

Biologically, "you really need not to have light at night," says Dr. Cartwright. Good-quality lined drapes will keep the light out of your room. So before you buy your next set of drapes, first ask about their room-darkening capacity.

Pull-down shades come in room-darkening versions, too. Just make sure that the tube they come in has the words "room darkening" on it.

Make it quiet.

If you do choose lined drapes, the extra thickness of the lining will also help to absorb noise. Wall-to-wall carpeting serves the same purpose. Fans or air-conditioners can be used to mask noise, says Dr. Mitchell.

Position yourself properly.

If you have a bad back, sleep on your side with or without a pillow between your knees. If you get heartburn, sleep with your head elevated. You can do that by placing six-inch blocks under the head of your bed or if you sleep with someone, you can elevate yourself by using a wedge-shaped pillow. If you snore, sleeping on your side or stomach may help you. Snoring occurs because the muscles in your throat naturally relax during sleep. When you're on your back, this fleshy tissue partially blocks your airway and vibrates, says Dr. Roehrs. Other contributing factors for snoring are alcohol and sleep deprivation.

How Much Is Enough?

Maybe you're tired because you've cut corners on sleep time, and now you can't make up for lost snoozing. You go to bed late and you get up too early. But how much sleep do you need, anyway?

"Sleep is highly malleable," says Dr. Hauri. "Everybody needs a different amount. There's no use talking about averages."

Dr. Hauri once studied a nurse who slept only four hours a night but still felt perfectly fine. Another sleep specialist remembers a high-powered corporate executive who was so tired that he thought he had a sleep disorder, but didn't know why. "He was so busy working, working out and meeting his family obligations that he allowed himself only five or six hours of sleep a night. And he needed more," says David N. Neubauer, M.D., associate director of the Johns Hopkins University Sleep Disorders Center in Baltimore.

The range of sleep needs is wide, experts say—from four hours up to ten. While most of us do need at least eight hours or so, we often make do with about an hour less than we need.

"You've slept enough if you're not tired during the day and if you can watch TV at night or go out to a movie without falling asleep," says Dr. Hauri.

Say Ah

Y-a-a-a-w-w-w-n-n-n.

"Oh. Excuse me!"

For most of us, a yawn in public can spell embarrassment. Yawning is often taken as a sign of boredom in the midst of what should be an attention-grabbing event. An important business meeting. A special religious ceremony. A holiday family gathering.

Teachers typically take offense at students' yawning in class, but not Monica Greco, Ph.D., associate professor of psychology at Rowan College of New Jersey in Glassboro. "I'd much rather have my students yawn than fall asleep," she says. "If yawning gives them a little more energy to pay attention, I'm all for it."

Dr. Greco's appreciation for yawning is a special one. Her doctoral dissertation challenged previous research on the subject.

Despite a flurry of studies on yawning, doctors don't really know a lot about it, Dr. Greco asserts. Researchers have mostly confirmed what the rest of us already suspect. You usually yawn during the hour before bedtime and possibly after getting up in the morning.

We also know by experience that yawns can be contagious. But why are they contagious? No one really seems to know.

A commonly held belief that yawning occurs as a response to a lack of oxygen or the buildup of carbon monoxide in the body seems to be untrue, a study conducted at the University of Maryland concludes. But the question of what purpose yawning serves still remains a mystery. "Nevertheless, we know that people claim that yawning gives them energy, at least for the short term," says Dr. Greco.

In the search for greater energy and amid the plethora of hypotheses and the dearth of evidence concerning the nature and function of yawning, there is one question we might want answered: Is there a right way to yawn, a way to get the most out of it? "I think the important thing is not to stifle the yawn," Dr. Greco says.

Falling asleep at the drop of a hat does not mean that you're a good sleeper. It means that you're sleep-deprived. And many sleep experts say that use of an alarm clock is proof of that deprivation. A well-rested person wakes up naturally, without the need for that jolt.

Here are some ways to set your timing so that you beat the bleat on your handy alarm clock.

Calculate your sleep quota.

If you're one of the clocked and alarmed, and you're tired of being tired, you can figure out how much sleep you need.

Start by systematically adding a small amount of sleep to your schedule. "Go to bed a half-hour earlier for each night for a week. Then, if you're waking up spontaneously and maintaining your alertness throughout the day, that extra half-hour is what you need," says Dr. Roehrs.

But add the sleep at the beginning of the night, not in the morning, he suggests. That way, you won't throw off your natural body-clock rhythms.

If you're still waking to the alarm clock and falling asleep in your armchair, add another half-hour in the same manner. For most of us, an extra half-hour to an hour is what we need. But if you're what the specialists call a long sleeper—if you need nine to ten hours a night, as Albert Einstein did—keep adding the sleep that you need.

Nap away fatigue.

If you have a new baby, a heavy workload or a bedridden parent and you truly can't add any sleep to your nighttime schedule, napping may be the answer to your sleep deprivation, says Dr. Webb.

We're biologically programmed for naps—it's what causes the afternoon slump. But napping is a tricky proposition. Naps revive and refresh some of us. Other people feel groggy for hours after a nap. Some experts even contend that poor sleepers should avoid naps, which may further upset their night sleep, he adds. The only way to find out if naps will help is to give them a try.

For the nappers among us, Dr. Webb suggests, "Don't nap for more than an hour. And don't nap after 4:00 P.M."

But schedule your naps just like you schedule regular sleep, says Dr. Mitler. Regularity is sleep's best friend.

The Wages of Aging: Changing Sleep Patterns

As we age, we need to learn how to sleep again, too. It's not that we need less sleep. The fact is that we need just as much or almost as much, but we have to restitch our sleep patterns.

"Older people are less able to sustain prolonged bouts of sleep. They wake up more frequently and nap more often," says Donald L. Bliwise, Ph.D., director of the Sleep Disorders Center at the Emory University School of Medicine in Atlanta.

As we get older, sleep tends to come in segments. We rarely get our eight hours whole. And not only is sleep more fragmented, it's more shallow; we spend less time in deep-sleep stages as we age. Our patchy sleep is why we often wind up falling asleep when it's still light out and waking up when it's dark, says Dr. Bliwise. But there are ways to reset biological bad timing.

Welcome in the dusk.

Check the time of sunset in the newspaper or on The Weather Channel and time a 20- to 30-minute walk that ends right before the sun's last rays. "Exercise literally reverses the sleep problems we tend to associate with old age," says Dr. Mitchell. Along with the exercise, you get the fading daylight to help reset your body's sleep/wake cycle.

Turn up the lights.

Use your brightest lamps to light your evening activities. It's an informal light therapy that will prompt you to stay awake until bedtime, says Dr. Neubauer. And it helps to reset your body clock, so that you don't drowse away the evening in dim light. When you go to bed—and turn off the lights—you're ready.

Instant
ENERGIZERS

2

Affirmations

Ever wish you had more energy? Then you know that simply wishing won't make it so.

But there is a mental process that's definitely energizing, and it's one notch up from wishing. These energizers are affirmations—positive thoughts or ideas you focus on in order to produce a desired result. "They're more a statement of a goal or an intention," explains Douglas Bloch, author of *Words That Heal*.

Affirmations are designed to help change the often-unconscious stream of negative thoughts or emotions that go through our minds, explains Susan Jeffers, Ph.D., author of *End the Struggle and Dance with Life* and *Feel the Fear and Do It Anyway*. "Affirmations are a way to change the negative chatter that goes on in our heads all the time into something positive."

And positive thinking, experts say, is more than just a pleasant interlude. Studies suggest that the more you believe in your own abilities, the better you're likely to do, says Albert Ellis, Ph.D., president of the Institute for Rational-Emotive Therapy in New York City. "Affirmations may temporarily make people feel better about themselves, so they do better," he says.

Replacing the Bad with the Good

The reason affirmations work, says Dr. Jeffers, is that you can't think two thoughts at the same time. By putting positive thoughts in your mind, you automatically displace the negative—and that can have powerful effects.

Suppose, for example, you're constantly thinking to yourself, "Boy, I don't have enough energy to lift a finger." This is a negative thought that's reinforcing the problem: no energy. A better strategy is to replace that thought with an affirmation: "I am experiencing being tired and I can do something about it," or "I now have more energy."

This kind of affirmation can do two things, Dr. Jeffers says. "It opens up the possibility to you that you could have more energy, and it changes your mind's focus so that you start paying more attention to the things that actually can give you energy."

You can use affirmations to help reinforce all those good behaviors—like having better eating habits, getting more rest and relaxation, keeping up with exercise and so forth—that will provide more time and energy and let you enjoy life more.

One of Dr. Jeffers's favorite affirmations is "I let go and I trust."

"As soon as you let go—not feeling like you have to control everything, which you can't do, anyway—you have more energy. I mean . . . Phew! You're not fighting so hard!" she says.

To get the most from affirmations, here's what experts advise.

Focus on what you need and want.
For affirmations to be most effective, they must be specific and focused. Pick an area of your life that you want to address, decide what you want and formulate a concise statement that expresses the desired outcome, Bloch recommends. Let's say, for instance, that your eating habits are bad and you want to eat better—more fresh fruits and vegetables, less fat and sugar. Your affirmation could be "I eat only healthy foods that support my body."

Use the first person and present tense.
Affirmations are most effective when you say "I"—in terms of "I want" or "I need" or "I am," according to Bloch. "When you say, 'You are healthy,' it's as though you are talking to somebody else. When you say, 'I am healthy,' you're addressing it directly to yourself and you are owning it. It's more powerful," Bloch says.

By saying "I am" rather than "I will be," you're making a statement that's more immediate. "It's the only tense we ever live in—the here and now," Bloch explains. Saying "I am healthy" and imagining yourself that way can make your brain think it's so, Bloch says.

Be positive.
Which sounds better to you: "I am not poor" or "I am prosperous"? Because the subconscious usually doesn't hear the word "not," there's always the danger that an affirmation expressed negatively will send the wrong message. "You can use a negative, but only if you follow it quickly with a positive," Bloch says.

Try it on for size.
You may need to work through a few versions, but when you find a good affirmation, it will click and feel right to you. "The affirmation needs to be realistic, although you don't have to believe it 100 percent for it to work," Bloch adds. "It is okay to have doubts, you may be uncertain, but one thing is clear—you want it very much, and that's what you are affirming."

Letting Go of Doubts

Even though affirmations are a powerful tool for feeling better temporarily, they may not help resolve long-standing problems—unless, that is, you're willing to put in a little extra work.

"You need to delve into the negative thoughts that may continue to crop up to oppose your affirmations," says Albert Ellis, Ph.D., president of the Institute for Rational-Emotive Therapy in New York City.

Write down your affirmations on the left-hand side of a piece of paper, advises Douglas Bloch, author of *Words That Heal*. Then, "sit quietly and notice what bubbles up from your subconscious mind." Pretty soon, Bloch says, you'll probably find yourself thinking about all the negative beliefs and assumptions you hold regarding your affirmations. Write these down in the right-hand column.

Bringing negative thoughts into your awareness is the first step in getting rid of them. "You can say to them, 'I release you,'" Bloch says. Over time, you'll find that the affirmations will slowly crowd out the negative beliefs.

Make it a mantra.
Once you've settled on an affirmation that you like, repeat it again and again, like a mantra, until it becomes so automatic that you're practically saying it in your dreams.

"In the beginning the practice has to be intensive because your mind is so filled with negativity that you have to slowly recondition yourself to think more positively," Dr. Jeffers says. "It's breaking a habit, and that is very difficult."

So she tells people to say their affirmation every day for at least a month, or until the message becomes almost automatic. "It's like when you constantly hear the lyrics of a song," she says. "It starts to come into your mind much more freely and easily."

Say them out loud.
"There's something about hearing your affirmations in your own voice that makes them more powerful," Dr. Jeffers says.

Say them morning and night.
Early morning and late night tend to be when people are most open to suggestion—and, more destructively, when they tend to ruminate on negatives, Dr. Jeffers says. Say your affirmations when you wake up and before you fall asleep. These are almost always good times to repeat them, she says.

Surprise yourself.

Write your affirmations on bits of paper and put them in unexpected places, Dr. Jeffers suggests. Put them on your mirror and bulletin board and write them in your daybook. "Seeing your affirmation is a great reminder; it gives a jolt of positive energy."

Get them on tape.

Record yourself saying your affirmations, then play them back while you're falling asleep or driving—times when you're particularly open to getting the message, Dr. Jeffers suggests.

Hook up with a higher power.

Some people, including Bloch and Dr. Jeffers, believe affirmations become more powerful when they have a spiritual component.

"I find that when we put out affirmations that not only serve who we are but serve humanity as well, there is a different feeling in the body," Dr. Jeffers says. "We are bringing in higher thoughts that are very healing to the body and the mind. When we see ourselves above the petty and above self-involvement, we are lifted to a new dimension in thinking and it is really beautiful, powerful and energizing."

Here are a few affirmations that you may want to try.

- "I am creating a life that not only serves myself but serves the rest of the world."
- "I have much love to give to the world. I create warmth wherever I go."
- "Love and light are constantly being given to the world through me. I am a channel for God's love."

Even if you decide to affirm something more material—a desire for wealth or fame, for example—Bloch suggests that you turn the final outcome over to a higher power. Conclude your affirmation with "this or something better now manifests for me in totally satisfying and harmonious ways for the highest good of all concerned."

Altruism and Volunteering

*I*t's no secret that helping others makes you feel better about yourself. What may be less obvious is that it also makes you feel better. Period.

Besides giving your overall health a lift, giving someone a helping hand can also boost your energy levels—whether you're a Boy Scout helping grandmothers cross the street or a Little League coach helping budding ballplayers cross home plate.

"People who volunteer say that they are less likely to feel tired," says Alan Luks, a lifelong volunteer and author of *The Healing Power of Doing Good*, a book about the power of helping your health by helping others. "A big reason why people feel tired is because of stress. And one way to cut off stress is to help someone else."

Helper's High

People who do volunteer work on a regular basis report feeling what Luks calls a helper's high.

"This is similar to the runner's high that people feel during intense aerobic exercise—a sensation of well-being, more energy and possibly even a bolstered immune system," says Luks. "I don't know if it's a physiologic response or simply one that is imagined, but it seems to be consistent among people who volunteer on a regular basis. And, like exercise, the more you volunteer, the more benefits you'll get."

Volunteering can be particularly helpful in making you feel younger than your years. "As they get older, most people report a decline in health," observes Howard Andrews, Ph.D., an epidemiologist and statistician at Columbia

University College of Physicians and Surgeons in New York City. "But people who do volunteer work don't view their health as declining. And while their peers report feeling more tired as they age, volunteers see themselves as having more energy."

Although research into this area is relatively new, scientists have long speculated that altruism can help beat stress, which is among the biggest energy zappers. "Dr. Hans Selye, the original stress researcher, came up with the concept that we can only beat stress by helping one another," says Luks. "He called it altruistic egoism."

Studies on laboratory animals have examined the effects that a type of social interaction similar to volunteerism has on the brain. These studies were done by Jaak Panksepp, Ph.D., distinguished research professor of psychobiology at Bowling Green University in Ohio.

"No one has ever demonstrated that brain-chemical changes similar to a runner's high occur in humans from volunteering, because you need to get into the brain and measure cerebral spine fluid or get a PET scan, which measures brain function—and you can't study one's helping behavior while he's in a PET-scanning tube," says Dr. Panksepp. What Dr. Panksepp's research has done is demonstrate that social interaction does activate the production of "feel-good" chemicals in animals.

"In a logical and reasonable extension from that animal data, I would say that positive social interaction like volunteering could activate a large number of neurochemical changes that could increase your energy," says Dr. Panksepp.

Reaping Rewards

At the least, helping others can boost your self-esteem and feelings of self-worth, two proven energy boosters. And research does show that people who volunteer or engage in other social interaction are less likely to suffer from depression, says Dr. Panksepp.

But not all volunteerism can help you reap these personal benefits. So to boost your energy from helping others, here's what the experts suggest.

Get personal.
While donating clothes or painting your church's walls are noble efforts, they don't produce the same physical sensations and increased energy, says Luks. "It's the social interaction that makes people feel healthier and more energetic," he says. "I'm not saying those efforts aren't worthwhile and help you feel better about yourself, but you need direct contact with people to reap the physical rewards."

Help a stranger.

"Those who only help family members or neighbors do not report the same benefits as those who help people they don't know," adds Luks. "The theory is that a major way to cope with stress is to gain a greater sense of control in your life. And helping strangers gives you more control than the 'have-to' helping of a sick relative. That is often done more out of a sense of obligation than feelings of increased control."

Do it regularly.

Volunteering once in a while won't produce the long-lasting effects of continuous social service. "Those who reap the best rewards are what we call regular volunteers—people who do it at least once a week," says Dr. Andrews. "Of course, the more they do it, the better they reported feeling."

In a survey that Luks conducted, he found that most people who reported increased energy averaged two hours a week in volunteer work.

Find your niche.

Some people have the best intentions but quit their altruistic efforts because they find it too depressing. "I know two ladies who volunteered to counsel patients at a nursing home," says Luks. "One absolutely hated it—she couldn't stand the smell and found the whole experience to be very depressing. But the other thought it was the best experience in her life.

"The point is that not every type of volunteer work may be right for you. So if you try something and it doesn't feel right, don't quit volunteering. Find something else—as long as it's done on a regular basis and is helping strangers. And there are a lot of things to do out there."

Aromatherapy

It's as plain as the nose on your face: There's nothing like common scents to get you energized. Smell a plate of freshly baked cookies, and you'll start salivating like Pavlov's dogs. Take in a whiff of ocean air, and you'll immediately feel revived. And a snort of strategically placed perfume can jump-start the most idle libido.

That's because smell is the quickest of all senses for inducing a change in emotion, mood or even hunger, say researchers. And that's significant when you want a quick boost of energy.

But, some say, these everyday fragrances stink when it comes to *keeping* you going. "Incense, flowers, food odors and other smells can invoke a tiny mood switch because they are pleasant," says John Steele, an aroma consultant in Los Angeles. "But they come quickly and are diminished just as quickly, so there's nothing therapeutic about it. For lasting therapeutic effects, like boosting energy for the long term, you need the essential oils of aromatherapy."

Through the Ages

Odor therapy—the smelling of certain fragrances for medicinal or emotional wellness—was started by ancient Egyptians about 5,000 years ago. They (and later the Greeks and Romans) recognized that the nose knows—and used aromatic flowers and herbs for massage, bathing and medicine. The sages of antiquity also burned incense in religious ceremonies.

It wasn't until the eleventh century that European healers took it one step further and, in the process, discovered aromatherapy—a system of caring for mind and body with specific botanical oils such as lemon, lavender, rose and peppermint. These healers began working with what are called essential oils, potent liquids extracted from plants in extremely high concentrations through distilling or squeezing. Aromatherapists, who require no specific medical training, believe that it's specifically these essential oils—and not just nice fragrances—that have therapeutic powers.

Dealing with Essentials

"The advantage that aromatherapy has over just being exposed to fragrances is that essential oils are in such high concentrations. You would need about 100 pounds of basil to get the same effects that you would from one drop of basil essential oil," says Jeanne Rose, an aromatherapist and herbalist based in San Francisco, president of the National Association for Holistic Aromatherapy and author of *The Aromatherapy Book*.

Aromatherapists use these essential oils in several ways. Here are their favorite approaches.

Breathe deeply.
The quickest and most common way to use essential oils is to inhale them. "You can take a whiff directly from the bottle, put a few drops on a hanky and inhale it or even just place a few drops on your pillow before you go to sleep," says Rose. "What I prefer is to use a home diffuser, which is a machine like a vaporizer that emits the oils and costs about $45. I have mine connected to a timer, and that's what wakes me up in the morning."

Another advantage of diffusers, which are the best method for spreading essential oils in the workplace or other large areas, is that you can control the dosage, adds Steele. Using diffusers, Steele has created aromatherapy mixtures for the Miami Marriott Hotel and other businesses.

Time it right.
Although most aromatherapists say that essential oils can be used anytime, some believe they can have maximum effect during certain periods of the day. "Chinese herbalists say that your maximum breathing time, or 'lung time,' is between 4:00 and 6:00 A.M., so perhaps the best time to use the essential oils is first thing in the morning," says Rose. "If you're using essential oils for more energy, that's an especially good idea—so you can stay energized for the entire day."

Massage them in.
Besides inhalation, another energy-boosting way of using essential oils is to massage them directly into the skin. But before you do that, they should be diluted to a 3-percent solution, advises Steele. If you were making 100 milliliters for a whole-body massage, 97 milliliters (about 6½ tablespoons, or about 3¼ ounces) should be a vegetable "carrier" oil like safflower, sunflower or other cooking oil. Mix the carrier oil with 3 milliliters (¾ of a teaspoon, or ⅛ ounce) of the essential oil, and you have the 3 percent solution that you need. Or you can place about six drops of essential oil directly on the soles of your feet and massage it in, says Steele.

Take a bath.

You can also benefit from adding a few drops of oil directly to your bath. "I'd recommend adding about six drops to a full tub of warm bathwater, preferably while you're in the tub because most of the fragrance is released in the first 30 seconds this way," says Steele. "Be sure to stir it around so that it disperses."

Don't light up your lungs.

Besides the recommended methods of inhaling essential oils, there's one that is not a favorite of aromatherapists: placing a few drops on a lightbulb. Though the heat from the bulb burns the oil, emitting the fragrance, this method has many drawbacks. "I think that's a dumb idea," says Rose. "For one thing, the drops can roll down the sides of the bulb and ruin it. And the oil is really wasted on bulbs because it burns so quickly that you're getting the effect of incense, which is minimal."

Making Sense of Scents

There are literally hundreds of essential oils, and most are used for a specific purpose. Most essential oils sell for $5 to $15 per half-ounce (15-milliliter) vial, depending on the oil's purity and where it's produced. But some can cost as much as $75. They're sold in many health food stores or by aromatherapists; they can also be purchased through mail order. Luckily, most of the home-care oils that can boost energy are on the lower end of the price scale, says Michael Scholes, an aromatherapist who runs his own aromatherapy school in Beverly Hills, California.

How do you buy essential oils? And how do you know which ones to choose to boost your energy? Here's what Scholes and other experts recommend.

Read the label.

No matter what type of oil you're using to boost energy, make sure you're getting the real McCoy. "If the label says it's a fragrance, then avoid it because it's not an essential oil and it won't work," says Scholes.

Smell that citrus.

"Lemon, lime, orange, mandarin and grapefruit oils are great for overcoming a somber mood because they create a bright and uplifting environment," Scholes says. They're also among the cheapest, typically selling for around $5 for five milliliters. They work best in a diffuser.

Another citrus oil is bergamot, which helps provide long-term energy by relaxing you. But it might be harder to find, says Steele.

Love that lavender.

"If there's one oil that no home should be without, it's lavender," says Scholes.

Lavender boosts energy by helping you relax and overcome stress, adds Steele. It's also among the most available oils.

Get pepped with peppermint.

Peppermint oil energizes because it's a mental stimulant, so it's best for those days when you're mentally fatigued, says Scholes. Peppermint works well as a bath oil and sells for about $5 per five-milliliter bottle.

Find those florals.

Floral oils like rose and jasmine can be pricier but are considered the best for stress relief, but cheaper oils like geranium are just as effective, says Steele.

Think herbs.

Basil, rosemary, chamomile and other herbs are especially good for low-energy days because they have ingredients that are invigorating—one reason why they're used by many people who have chronic fatigue syndrome, adds Steele. Other good energizing oils include rosewood, sandalwood, melissa and black spruce.

Use caution if you're pregnant.

Because essential oils can have strong effects on the body, you should not use them when you're pregnant unless you consult your doctor or a practicing aromatherapist, cautions Steele.

Bathing

Physically and spiritually, water has traditionally been considered a giver of life. But just why that morning shower or evening bath feels so darned good is anybody's guess.

It could be the steam you inhale, the delightful sense of buoyancy, the enveloping warmth or simply the act of dissolving the day's grease and grime and letting your skin breathe again. (Yes, skin does breathe.)

Whatever the reasons, you've no doubt discovered the energy connection for yourself: Bathing can be both invigorating and relaxing, depending on how you go about it. Here are a number of tips from bathing experts on how to get the biggest energy payoffs from your daily encounter with soap and water.

Rev up right.

"Nothing beats a long, hot shower to get you going in the morning," says Jonathan Paul De Vierville, Ph.D., director of the Alamo Plaza Spa at the Menger Hotel in San Antonio. To get the most energy out of this pleasant experience, he suggests that you use a body brush and an herbal shower gel that contains rosemary, pine or juniper. Then, finish off with a quick splash of cold water.

"As you dry off, your body will flush warm as it generates heat and energy, and you'll feel ready for the day," he says.

Gear up with ginger.

In Chinese medicine, ginger is considered a super-octane herb, explains Mary Muryn, author of *Water Magic: Healing Bath Recipes for the Body, Spirit and Soul.* "It's used in many preparations to invigorate and rejuvenate."

Add an ounce of powdered ginger to your bathwater, she recommends. The herb will make your skin and genitals pleasantly warm. "Bathing in ginger is good for aches and pains, colds and flu or if you get up in the morning and feel yucky, tired and worn out," she notes. Soak for 15 to 20 minutes. But don't add ginger to your Jacuzzi; that may make you sneeze.

Revive with a contrast bath.

During the day, alternating warm- and cold-water baths is a good way to generate more energy, Dr. De Vierville says. He believes it's better—and less of a shock—to use contrast baths only on your arms or legs, not your whole body. "That way you can move blood through these limbs and back toward the heart."

Always start with water that is comfortably warm—just a little above body temperature. Around 100°F is ideal. "Warm up for 30 seconds to 2 to 3 minutes, until you feel a flush, then put your limbs into cold water that's 54° to 56°F for 10 to 15 seconds, or until you begin to feel a prickling sensation," Dr. De Vierville says. After you take your arms out, let them warm up naturally for a few minutes. "You'll feel them flush with heat, and that is where you get your energy," he says. Repeat the procedure two or three times in 15 to 20 minutes.

You can use two deep basins for arm baths, immersing your arms all the way above the biceps. Set up a deep, sturdy plastic dishwashing pan filled with water at one temperature near your kitchen sink, which is filled with water of the other temperature. You can purchase these pans at a restaurant-supply store or the housewares department of a home-improvement center or department store.

Dr. De Vierville recommends immersing your legs to just above the calves. Since most of us don't have basins that big, you can use two tall plastic kitchen wastebaskets. Before you buy them, measure the containers beside your calf to be sure that they're the right depth. Place the containers in your kitchen or in your bathtub. Sit on a chair or a tub stool so that you can have both legs in the warm container and then move safely to the cool container. You'll begin to see results after doing a contrast bath daily for at least a week, says Dr. De Vierville.

Have an herbal bath nightcap.

Take a relaxing bath in the evening for deep, restful sleep that leaves you fully energized in the morning, Dr. De Vierville says. He recommends keeping the water just above body temperature at 100° to 102°F, never more than 104°. Just before you get into the tub, add bath oils that contain calming herbs such as lavender, lemon balm, hops or valerian and soak for 20 to 30 minutes.

Get back to the earth.

Need to perk up quick before a busy evening? Try a clay bath, recommends Muryn. She adds about one-half pound of Aztec Secret Indian Healing Clay powder to comfortably warm water, stirring it in with her hand and reserving a bit to mix as a paste to apply to her face. About 20 minutes in this soup does the trick, she says. This clay is available at health food stores.

"When you are exhausted, and your brain doesn't work and you are wondering how you are going to get through the evening, this bath brings your body back to life again," she says.

Scent away stress.
It is possible to unwind and energize with a lemon-lavender bath, according to Muryn. She recommends adding ten drops of lemon essential oil (not the same as lemon juice) and ten drops of lavender essential oil to the bathwater.

"When you are stressed but have to get yourself going, the lavender will get the stress out, and the lemon will wake you up," Muryn says.

Clear Thinking and Decision Making

Surf or turf? Skirt or slacks? Used car or new? Comedy or drama?

Each day, you're faced with literally hundreds of decisions—everything from choosing those important directions that your life will take to deciding on the videos that you want to rent.

But whatever options you choose, one thing remains the same: Making decisions takes a lot of energy. Each time you need to ignite that proverbial lightbulb between your ears, the energy must come from somewhere. Unfortunately, it doesn't end there, since most of us tend to second-guess ourselves and even agonize over the choices made—or ponder if we made the right decision. This process can cloud your mind and de-energize your body worse than the Seattle weather.

But the way to more energized decision making is clear—or rather, clear thinking. "Clear thinking takes more work than muddling at first, so it requires more energy . . . in the short run," says Carol R. Ember, Ph.D., an anthropologist at the Human Relations Area Files, a research agency at Yale University. "But once you begin to clear up your thinking, you'll see the energy benefits."

Decide How You Decide

The first step to clearer thinking and better decision making is to decide how you decide. There are four types of decision makers, according to Dorothy Leeds, a New York City consultant who teaches executives how to be better decision makers and is author of *Smart Questions: A New Strategy for Successful Managers.* She describes them this way.

Commanders, by nature, are impatient. Their eagerness leads them to make quick (and sometimes foolish) decisions.

Convincers are the persuader-promoter types. They tend to act on their emotions, deciding quickly what "feels good."

Carers decide on the basis of their feelings but are concerned with others. Since they don't want to hurt others, they tend to take a long time to make decisions.

Calculators want all the information that they can get before making a decision. Their problem is that since they can never get all the information that they need, they tend to take way too long to make a decision.

Leeds has advice to help all four types of decision makers make better choices and cut down on energy-depleting second-guessing. "If you're a Commander type, force yourself to slow down and bring your proposed decision to a Carer, who would consider all sides. If you're a Carer, set a time limit on your information-gathering stage and find a Commander to assess your judgment. If you're a Convincer, bring it to a Calculator. And if you're a Calculator, find a Convincer."

Mind over Matters

No matter what your decision-making style, experts say that certain rules apply to everyone. And here's what they suggest for making better decisions and clearing up that muddled, energy-draining kind of thinking.

Ask a lot of questions.
Before you can make any good decision, you have to assemble as many facts as possible, with a little detective work, and that comes from asking questions. "Mistakes are usually made because someone has insufficient or bad data," says John C. Johnson, M.D., regional director of Unity Physician Group in Valparaiso, Indiana. In the emergency room he faces life-and-death crises daily and has come to rely on his ability to ask as many questions as possible to make decisions that save lives.

Dr. Johnson describes the case of a badly wheezing child brought to the hospital. If the attending doctor isn't thinking clearly, he might assume the child is having an asthma attack and treat her as the symptoms suggest. But a sharper doctor, he says, will first ask questions (When did the wheezing begin? Under what circumstances? Had the child been playing with small objects?) and may discover that the child is choking. So before making any decision, ask yourself every conceivable question.

Then ask one more.
After you ask all the questions, ask yourself one more, advises Dr. Ember: "What's the central question, issue or point?" True, there may be more than one

What Color Is Your Thinking Cap?

People commonly confuse innate intelligence or IQ with the ability to think. But clear thinking is not the same thing as being smart, says Edward de Bono, Ph.D., author of numerous books about more effective thinking, such as *Lateral Thinking, Six Thinking Hats* and *Masterthinker.*

"Good thinking is not a matter of intelligence, not a gift; it is a skill that can be practiced and developed like any other," says Dr. de Bono. Among the ways he encourages people to think more effectively is by using the image of six hats: Think of them as thinking caps of different colors, each representing different questions to help you make better decisions. Here's the rainbow of hats you might use.

White hats represent facts, figures and information. (Think of a scientist dressed in a white lab coat.) The white-hat questions you ask yourself are "What facts will help me make a decision? Where and from whom can I get them?"

Red hats symbolize emotions and feelings, hunches and intuition. (Think of a red heart.) The red-hat questions: "How do I really feel about this? What's my gut reaction to the situation?"

Black hats represent a negative outlook, playing devil's advocate, using your judgment and thinking why it won't work. (Think of a judge robed in black.) Ask yourself: "What are the possible downside risks and problems? What is the worst-case scenario?"

Yellow hats symbolize opportunities, optimism and constructive thinking. (Think of bright yellow sunshine.) Questions: "What are all the possible advantages? What would be the best outcome?"

Green hats represent creative, fertile thinking. (Think of green sprouts from newly planted seeds.) Questions: "What completely new, fresh, innovative approaches can I come up with? What creative ideas can I dream up to help me see the problem in a new way?"

Blue hats are for the coolness of control, thinking about thinking. (Think of the blue overarching sky under which you find everything else.) The blue hat is to allow you to review your thoughts and sum up what you have learned.

---

answer, but most situations have a single "crux of the matter."

To find that crux, try to put the issue or problem into a single declarative sentence. "The problem or question must be one sentence long and no more," she says.

Put your thoughts in order.

Most of the time we don't put our assumptions in logical order, adds Dr. Ember. "I ask people to put their thoughts and ideas on separate index cards and then reshuffle the cards until they are in some sort of order where one assumption leads to the next," she says.

Look for hidden answers.

Another common problem is that we tend to make many decisions with an either-or attitude. This limits our options when, in reality, there are usually more answers facing us.

The cerebral world of chess is a perfect example. According to Michael Valvo, one of America's top-rated chess masters, the downfall of many players in chess, as in life, is that they "concentrate on only two or three moves while at least seven or eight are usually available."

Trust your gut—with guidelines.

One of the most energy-draining aspects of decision making comes from within—not trusting your own instincts. Although your gut feeling isn't always your best, it often is, as anyone who has ever taken a multiple choice test can attest. Sony president Akito Morita went with his gut when he wanted to market what became the wildly successful Walkman portable stereo—even though it meant ignoring the reasoned advice of his sales experts who predicted that it was a mistake.

But you must temper your instincts with logical analysis, advises Donald MacGregor, Ph.D., a psychologist with Decision Research in Eugene, Oregon. So do what Ben Franklin did when he made a decision: Write all the positives of your gut feelings on one piece of paper and the negatives on another. The paper with the most reasons is the action to take.

Drop your "musts."

Besides trusting your gut, you should listen to the little voice inside your head. If it's saying, "I must have this . . . . I must do that . . . .," ignore it. People are born with a tendency to take their important desires and turn them into musts, says Albert Ellis, Ph.D., president of the Institute for Rational-Emotive Therapy in New York City.

But this limits your ability to think objectively and, as a result, clearly. So instead of saying, "I must," he advises asking yourself, "Must I?" You'll realize that, often, you don't really have to follow the instructions of that insistent little voice.

Decide what's important.

Use your values to help decide what's important enough to think about and work through and what you should let go. "Nit-picking and thinking about things that really aren't very important to you are definite energy drainers," says Dr. Ember. "A lot of energy gets wasted thinking about things that are insignificant in relation to what we really value. But if you know what's important, you can focus your thinking on these things."

Keep a log.

Get used to starting each day with some mental organization, urges Dr. Ember. Many people find that it's helpful to have a daily "to do" list of activities and things to be accomplished. "I have a running memo book where I organize, then carry over from the previous day. I check things off as I get them done," she says.

This log can also help you prioritize, which helps clear your thinking. "When you make a list, ask what you really have to do today," she says. But beware because, if you're compulsive, you may spend too much time just making your list. "List making should free up your mind, not bog you down," she says.

Coffee

There's been a lot of controversy brewing along with that French Roast over the health benefits of coffee. Over the last 30 years, health researchers have studied—and have tried to link—our most popular wake-up drink with everything from bladder cancer and high blood pressure to ulcers and birth defects.

So far, most coffee-related studies have been inconclusive. Experts tend to agree that most people face little risk from the typical U.S. coffee consumption—which is up to six cups a day. But there's no question about coffee's effect on our energy levels: It's darn good stuff.

"Coffee can energize you in just a few minutes; usually, you start to feel the effects within five to ten minutes," says Manfred Kroger, Ph.D., professor of food sciences at Pennsylvania State University in University Park and an authority on the effects of caffeine and coffee. "That's because the caffeine is a central nervous system stimulant. It interferes with some neurotransmitters in the brain that would normally cause sleep.

"On a cellular level," Dr. Kroger adds, "caffeine causes chemicals that would normally cause fatigue to 'go to the unemployment line.' When you drink a cup of coffee, your pulse rate and heartbeat accelerate. Your eyelids open. Fatigue is gone. You're more alert, and your motor skills improve. In layman's terms, coffee wires you."

That Racy Feeling

And we love that feeling. Sure, there are other sources of caffeine—it's in all colas (unless they say "caffeine-free," of course) and in sodas like Mountain Dew. You also get a bit of caffeine from teas (except herbal kinds), chocolate and many over-the-counter pain relievers. But Americans get 75 percent of their caffeine from the Big Daddy: coffee. "A typical 6-ounce cup of coffee contains about 100 milligrams of caffeine, but if you drink out of a mug like I do, you're getting closer to 200 milligrams," says Dr. Kroger. "By comparison, most colas have only 50 to 60 milligrams in a 12-ounce can. And teas are very low, containing only about 25 milligrams. To feel the energizing effects of coffee, most people need about 100 milligrams, so coffee is the best way to get caffeine."

Americans consume about 45 million pounds of coffee beans each year, making it second only to oil in international commerce. About 50 countries produce coffee beans, including Egypt. In fact, Egypt is where this mania for java probably began. About A.D. 850, a local goatherd named Khaldi noticed that his herd hadn't come home as usual. The next morning, legend has it, he found his normally docile goats dancing around a half-eaten coffee bush. He nibbled some of the berries himself—coffee beans—got a quick boost and joined in the festivities. The beans found their way to some local monks, so the story goes, who used the discovery to stay awake during their endless prayer sessions.

Thus, java and its jolting reputation were born.

A Little Dab Will Do You

Today, caffeine is still used as an energizer—and sometimes abused—by as many as eight in ten Americans. We all know about its mind-energizing effects. But studies also show that the amount in one good-sized mug of coffee can help you exercise longer. That's why some endurance athletes such as marathon runners frequently drink coffee before a race, although coaches advise against it because its diuretic effects may interfere with athletic performance, says Dr. Kroger.

Caffeine may also help you burn more fat during exercise, says Matthew Vukovich, Ph.D., assistant professor of exercise physiology at the Human Performance Lab at Wichita State University in Kansas. And the longer you work out, the better your long-term energy levels will be.

"The caffeine in coffee stimulates the heart muscle by speeding pulse and heart rate," says Dr. Kroger. "This is why older people appreciate coffee, because it 'kicks on the old motor,' as they say. They have a cup of coffee and come to life."

But when that cup becomes more than six in a day, you can get *too* energized—a syndrome known as caffeine buzz or coffee nerves. "It can happen at any dosage for some people, after one or two cups, even. But for most people it occurs after about 600 milligrams in a several-hour period," says Dr. Kroger. "You have jittery nerves, your body may vibrate, and you can't fall asleep. Because coffee keeps you awake, too much can cause insomnia, which eventually leads to fatigue."

Benefiting from Brew

Despite its drawbacks, though, coffee is a definite battery charger if you sip it strategically. Here's how to get the most from your favorite blend while you go about your daily grind.

Schedule your coffee break.
You can time your "fix" to reap the most energizing effects from caffeine. "We know caffeine is quickly absorbed," says Roland Griffiths, Ph.D., professor of neuroscience at the Johns Hopkins University School of Medicine in Baltimore, who has spent years studying caffeine and caffeine withdrawal. Although its energizing effects begin within 10 minutes of your first sip, the full force kicks in about a half-hour later, lasting about 30 minutes.

"Then, about half of the caffeine has been absorbed in your body and the effects start to diminish," adds Dr. Kroger. "After another 30 minutes about one quarter of the caffeine is left. After another 30 minutes only an eighth, and so on—a condition known as a half-life. After about three hours the energizing effects of coffee are pretty much gone, and you crave another cup."

Watch your water.
Caffeine can boost your energy, but it can also become an energy demon because it's a diuretic. "Caffeine has a dehydrating effect," says Nancy Clark, R.D., director of nutrition services at SportsMedicine Brookline in Brookline, Massachusetts, and author of *Nancy Clark's Sports Nutrition Guidebook*. So it's particularly important for athletes to drink plenty of water if they are coffee drinkers—especially during hot weather.

Crush out the smokes.
Smokers may especially savor a cigarette with their joe, but the one-two punch of caffeine and nicotine—another central nervous system stimulant—may put your system into energy overload. Because it acts like caffeine, nicotine combined with caffeine can give you coffee nerves and fatiguing effects faster than drinking coffee alone. Also, if you smoke and drink a lot of coffee, and do it frequently, you could be stressing your heart too much, according to medical experts.

Increase your sensitivity.
You can get more bang from your cup by reducing your body's tolerance for it. That means if you cut back your coffee consumption, eventually, you'll get the same energizing effects on less caffeine, says Dr. Griffiths.

If you drink between two and three cups a day, however, there's really no need to cut back, adds Dr. Kroger.

Don't go cold turkey.

For those who want to cut out caffeine completely, slow and steady wins the race. "It's best if you gradually give up caffeine over the course of several weeks," says John Hughes, M.D., director of the Human Behavior Pharmacology Lab at the University of Vermont in Burlington. "I recommend a 10 to 30 percent reduction every few days. So if you drink 3 cups of coffee a day, drink 2 to 2½ for three or four days, then decrease by another ½ cup a few days later, and so forth."

Don't mis-treat yourself.

Either too much or too little caffeine can cause an energy-zapping headache, especially during withdrawal. Unfortunately, many folks don't know that some headache pain relievers can contain as much as 130 milligrams of caffeine per dose. So read the label first, advises Dr. Griffiths. Better choices are aspirin and acetaminophen.

Abstain if you're pregnant.

While moderate consumption poses no significant health risk for most of us, pregnant women are advised to abstain from coffee and other caffeinated products altogether. That's because although the half-life effects diminish in adults after a few hours, they can continue all day in a fetus—keeping the developing child too wired, says Dr. Kroger. Coffee has not been shown to cause physical birth defects in humans, but heavy use has caused them in laboratory animals, so the jury's still out.

Daydreams
and Fantasy

Sex symbols beg for your body. Intellects yearn for your mind. The kids do what they're told and the boss brings *you* coffee. As you might imagine—and probably have—anything is possible in that space between your ears.

Including more energy.

"For many people daydreams and fantasy just occur, and we let them run their course—like nighttime dreams," says Harold Roger Ellis, Ph.D., a psychologist in Hicksville, New York, who publishes *The Dream Switchboard*, a national newsletter for connecting people who want to share their nighttime dream experiences. "But you can make a conscious effort to control the content and outcome of your daydreams and fantasies. Unlike nighttime dreams, you basically decide what it is that you're daydreaming about and what the outcome will be . . . which can include more energy."

Just Your Imagination

This process described by Dr. Ellis is known as guided imagery—a method of healing the body with the power of the mind that's been used for thousands of years. But it wasn't until the 1600s that physicians started taking it seriously and even believed that imagery could influence embryos in pregnant women.

Although it never was embraced by Western medicine, imagery as a healing tool was practiced by such notables as Sigmund Freud, Carl Jung and other European psychiatrists. But in the 1970s, a California oncologist began using guided imagery to help cancer patients—with encouraging results. Since then, other studies have shown that imagery can help overcome cancer and other diseases.

"Guided imagery is a directed use of the daydreaming or fantasizing faculty," says Martin L. Rossman, M.D., co-director of the Academy for Guided Imagery in Mill Valley, California, and one of the nation's foremost authorities on imagery's healing potential. If you want to get more liveliness in your life, you can direct your imaging ability where you want it to go. Here's how.

Think down memory lane.

"If you want to feel as energetic as possible, try to think of a time in your life when you were particularly energetic," says Dr. Rossman. "Imagine going back to that time and try to remember what it was that made you so vital."

Use all your senses.

Once there, Dr. Rossman says that you need to use all of your senses to recapture the feeling. "Try to notice what you see. What you hear. What it feels like. What you smell. Pretend that you have a volume control, like on a radio, and turn it up and down."

Focus on the positive.

"Sad or morbid thoughts are energy-depleting, so make a conscious effort to focus on the positive aspects of your life," says Francis X. Clifton, Ph.D., co-director of the Center for Mental Imagery in New York City and a psychotherapist who specializes in expanding the use of the imagination. If a negative thought pops into your head, he suggests distracting yourself with a memory or idea that makes you happy.

Do it in the morning.

Although it's a good idea to consciously daydream whenever you need a quick boost of energy, Dr. Clifton advises doing it first thing in the morning. "I recommend that people spend 20 to 30 seconds each morning imagining that they are on the beach, getting taller and taller until they can reach the sun. Imagine that you're able to reach out and grab the sun and feel its warmth going through your arms and then your entire body. Picture yourself smiling and dancing on the beach and having an aura of energy around you."

Get the right chair.

To make the most of your daydreams, you need the right environment—some place that's comfortable and free of excess noise. "It's best to sit in a straight-back chair with armrests so that your hands aren't resting in your lap," says Dr. Clifton. "You want to turn your energy inward." If you place your hands on armrests, he points out, you're likely to keep them still, in a restful position, so that you don't distract yourself with hand movements.

Deep Breathing

When you're relaxed, you breathe slowly and deeply, inhaling sumptuous streams of vital, energy-producing oxygen.

When you're tense, however, you breathe lightly and rapidly, delivering less oxygen to your body's cells. In addition, hormones that your body produces when you're tense and under stress constrict your blood vessels, further cutting down the amount of oxygen that reaches the cells.

To a blood cell, stress is suffocation, says Larry J. Feldman, Ph.D., a leader of workshops on stress and burnout and author of *Feeling Good Again*. "When you're tense, your brain increases its demand for oxygen," he says. "But your shallow breaths decrease the intake of oxygen. Anxiety is the expression of each cell in the body suffocating."

That's bad news on the pep and vitality front. Since each of us requires about 5,000 gallons of air every day, good breathing is important.

The Power of Positive Breathing

The good news is that by learning how to breathe correctly, you can increase your energy level, according to Dr. Feldman.

In fact, the first step to controlling your energy-depleting reaction to stress is to control your breathing. Since the brain under stress is begging for more oxygen, taking a deep breath will help that anxiety go away, says Dr. Feldman.

Can stress control and energy enhancement really be as easy as breathing?

"It sounds so simple—just take fairly deep, comfortable breaths and long exhalations, and you'll relax," says Martin Pierce, director of the Pierce Program, a yoga center in Atlanta that teaches stress-reduction, and co-author of *Yoga for Life*. But even though breathing *seems* automatic, studies suggest that 80 percent of us don't really know how to breathe properly. "The main problem is that many people think good breathing is good inhalation," he says. "The key is long, slow exhalations and breathing out completely."

Here's the full technique you'll need for breathing for stress relief and maximum energy.

Make a balloon.
"This analogy isn't anatomically correct, but it works if you imagine there's a balloon in your torso somewhere below the middle of your chest," says Pierce. "Now inhale and fill up the balloon in all directions—top, bottom, forward, backward. That's the ideal inhalation." Breathe in until you feel comfortably full, but not too full.

Blow it off.
Exhaling is more important than inhaling, and there's an ideal way to do it. "When you exhale, pull the lower abdomen in first, then the upper abdomen," says Pierce. "The rib cage comes in from the sides and down from the front. Make the exhalation just a little bit longer than you think it should be. Hold it for a half-second before you inhale again. That should be very relaxing."

Practice to get the feel of it.
The power of proper breathing is something you have to experience for yourself. "Reading a book about how to breathe isn't the same thing as actually doing it," says Dr. Feldman. Ideas have to get out of the head and down into the body or we won't change.

Stagger your practices.
You don't need to shoehorn in 30 minutes of deep-breathing practice at the end of a time-crunched day, says Dr. Feldman. "A short exercise several times a day for 3 to 4 minutes is probably more effective in terms of tension control than one long period."

Let off steam, too.
The next time your hair dryer blows a fuse just before you leave for work, take about 15 slow, deep breaths. You'll feel calmer, and you'll unwind all that energy-depleting tension before it has a chance to build.

Breathe before answering.
Establish cues that will remind you to breathe deeply. One expert recommends using the telephone for this purpose.

"When the phone rings, don't answer it right away," suggests stress expert Emmett E. Miller, M.D., founder of Source Cassette Learning Systems in Menlo Park, California. "Nobody hangs up before three rings. So you have three rings to relax. Whatever you're doing, stop. Close your eyes and take a deep breath. Let go of all your mental and physical tension. On the third ring pick up the phone." This pause gives you a chance to relax completely.

Forgiveness

Carrying a grudge is right up there with carrying the weight of the world on your shoulders. It's enough to exhaust anyone. That's why a grudge is something you'll want to drop—the sooner the better. And the way to do that is by forgiving.

The word *forgive* comes from the Greek language. It means "to let go of." And that's exactly what forgiveness is, says Susan Jeffers, Ph.D., author of *End the Struggle and Dance with Life* and *Opening Our Hearts to Men*. It's working through and resolving your thoughts and feelings about an incident or a person so that you don't have to keep replaying it over and over in your head and letting it control you.

A Gift You Give Yourself

"Forgiveness is something you do for yourself, not for the other person," says Dr. Jeffers. Forgiveness does not mean that you need to forget about the incident or the set of circumstances that made you angry or hurt you. In fact, once the issue has lost its emotional impact, you may remember it more clearly.

And forgiveness does not mean that the person who offended you was justified or is getting away with something. "If anything, forgiving helps you drop the role of being the victim and take real steps to protect and assert yourself," she says. "A victim mentality brings only upset and is an incredible waste of valuable energy."

If visions of sweet revenge still tinge your thoughts, Dr. Jeffers says, consider this: "The best revenge is being happy—and forgiveness lets you be that." But it's also important to do something about your anger. Anger can mask the fear and pain that you need to address, she adds. "It's easier to be angry and to blame than to take responsibility for your life and say, 'Wait, what do I have to do to change this?' " So feel your anger, learn from it and then let it go, Dr. Jeffers suggests.

Here are steps that can help you deal with the anger and leave that grudge behind.

Have a good holler.

Chances are, you feel angry and hurt with the person and the situation—perhaps rightly so. So some screaming and crying may be in order. Do this alone or with a close friend, not the perpetrator of the offense, Dr. Jeffers recommends.

"I suggest that you drive your car someplace isolated and scream your head off 'at' that person to get the rage out, because it is a poison in your body," she says. "Once you do that, you will feel an incredible sense of lightness."

You can start your scream therapy gently by saying, "I'm angry." From there work up to a crescendo until you feel it coming from your deepest self, Dr. Jeffers advises.

Have a good cry.

Often, after you've let go of some of the anger, hurt and disappointment will emerge, resulting in tears. "Let the sadness come over you, like a sense of warmth," Dr. Jeffers says.

Adopt a forgiving pose.

A branch of psychological research called bioenergetics suggests that certain body postures can evoke specific feelings, says G. Frank Lawlis, Ph.D., psychology professor at Southwestern College in Santa Fe, New Mexico, and author of *Transpersonal Medicine*. These postures are adapted from ancient religions and cultures.

For a pose that generates feelings of security and forgiveness, put your left hand over your heart and your right hand over your navel, he suggests. Do this in a sitting position if you are feeling confused or standing if you are feeling confronted, he says. Or you can do it lying down, which according to Dr. Lawlis, generates feelings of self-love.

"This pose can help you bring up images of people you need to forgive, such as parents," he says. "Stay in this pose as you go through the process of letting go."

Go over the details.

Forget the old saying "Forgive and forget." The real process is remember fully and forgive, says D. Patrick Miller, author of *A Little Book of Forgiveness*. "While we do eventually forget some things that we've forgiven, that kind of forgetting takes care of itself. Trying to forget is just another means of denial."

Remembering fully helps us take note of what we do not want to see repeated. Though we're forgiving that person, we don't want to give anyone inadvertent permission to commit the same mistakes again and again, Miller says.

If you can, review the event like a slow-motion movie, two or three times, until you can observe it without getting emotionally caught up in it, suggests Dr. Lawlis. "You want to review it enough times so that you begin to feel that you are observing it as an outside witness. You may still not totally understand it, but you'll have a different perspective." Ideally, ultimately, you'll feel detachment and acceptance.

Trade places.

Try putting yourself mentally in the offender's place. This is crucial to the process of forgiveness, Dr. Lawlis says. "Switch places with the person who wronged you so that you can get an understanding of that person," he says. In fact, you can get an inner dialogue going that may give you some insights into what went wrong. As that person, you can answer questions addressed to you and explain your actions.

Forgiveness is "a decision to see beyond the limits of another's personality," explains Robin Casarjian, director of The National Emotional Literacy Project for Prisoners and author of *Houses of Healing: A Prisoner's Guide to Inner Power and Freedom*. "Forgiveness requires recognizing that if a person is acting insensitively, then implicit in their behaviors and attitudes are fear, anger and hurt, and the need for respect, acknowledgment and love," Casarjian says. Putting yourself in the other person's shoes may bring a sense of understanding and compassion.

Explore your own role in the incident.

Pick up a mirror, not a magnifying glass, Dr. Jeffers says. "Do this, not to blame yourself, but to understand yourself. Instead of saying, 'Why did he do it?' ask, 'Why did I react this way? What could I have possibly contributed to this? What made me choose someone who did this?' "

Your continuing anger may come from an obsessive need to have someone else make you happy when you are not creating happiness for yourself, Dr. Jeffers explains. "Usually, people who are angry in relationships haven't built a very rich life for themselves," she says. "They don't understand that they are important and make a difference."

To avoid future replays of the same incident, you may have to give up wishing for that other person to make you happy. Pursue things that make *you* happy, and you're more likely to break the pattern of anger.

Project love.

Sit quietly, eyes closed, and envision the person you would most love to hurt, Dr. Jeffers suggests. Then, practice sending that person thoughts of "I love you."

"In the beginning this is almost impossible," she says. "Ultimately, however, the anger melts away and you start to realize that this person did do the best he could." If you're having trouble with self-blame, send yourself the same caring "I love you" thoughts, Dr. Jeffers recommends.

Let go.

Hold in your mind the image of whoever is to be forgiven, then let it slowly recede, Dr. Lawlis says. Let yourself detach emotionally from the image so that it no longer controls you.

Miller suggests saying, "I release you from the grip of my sadness, disapproval or condemnation."

Take action.

Just because you've forgiven someone doesn't mean you have to trust them. "Trust must be earned back," Miller says.

You also don't have to let that person back into your life, Dr. Jeffers says. "When you forgive someone, you might become more clear about not putting up with their nonsense anymore," she says. "We can't blame anyone for walking all over us. We can only notice that we are not getting out of the way."

You may find it helpful to write down the things that made you decide a particular person is not good for you. "That way," says Dr. Jeffers, "you don't let the part of you that is needy let you go back to a person who doesn't treat you right."

Gratitude

Do you have to wait for a cosmic kick in the pants . . . for something awful to happen to you before you feel grateful for what you have?

"Many of us feel like that," says G. Frank Lawlis, Ph.D., professor of psychology at Southwestern College in Santa Fe, New Mexico, and author of *Transpersonal Medicine.* "We get so wrapped up in our lives and personal concerns that we become isolated and disconnected from the rest of the world."

Taking things for granted can affect us in subtle, energy-sapping ways. When we expect to receive more than the world is giving us, we're likely to feel anger and resentment and the weight of our obligations. Taken to extremes, we end up feeling like we always need to be doing and acquiring, instead of enjoying what we have. If you recognize this pattern as your own, you may be surprised to discover how much energy you can find when you can start saying thanks (even to yourself) for what you have.

Lessons for Living Fully

Being grateful isn't an inherited talent, says Susan Jeffers, Ph.D., author of *End the Struggle and Dance with Life.* "We can learn how to acknowledge the gifts in our lives. We can teach ourselves how much there is to be grateful for in this world despite any negative circumstances that surround us."

It's very simple, she says. "When we focus on abundance, our lives feel abundant. When we focus on lack, our lives feel lacking. It's simply a matter of focus."

The reward of all this? "Having gratitude allows us to reap in the bounty that lies all around us, to scoop up the rewards, to live life fully," Dr. Jeffers says. What could be more energizing than that?

So what can you do to stay focused on what you have, rather than dwell on what's missing? Here's what the experts recommend.

Cultivate the habit of saying thank you.

"When we say 'thank you,' we are acknowledging a gift we were given," Dr. Jeffers explains. "If we don't say thank you very often, it is a sign that we are taking things for granted—sleepwalking our way through life. Giving thanks is one way of waking ourselves up."

Besides thanking the usual people—bus drivers, waitresses, secretaries and the like—it's vital to thank the significant people in our lives: parents, spouses, children, even bosses and co-workers, Dr. Jeffers says. This can be difficult to do, especially when you feel as if you're giving more than you're receiving. "Gratitude is one of the most powerful ways of healing the many understandable hurts that may be hampering your ability to truly enjoy your life," she says.

Make a ritual out of it.

"Rituals can help us embrace the beauty and transcend what is painful in our lives," Dr. Jeffers says. You can develop your own personal rituals or add a few that are tried-and-true: Say grace over meals, say a few words of appreciation at sunrise and sunset or when you get up and when you go to bed.

These rituals don't need to be elaborate or theatrical. "Just say, 'I am thankful for the food I am about to eat,' " she says. This gives you pause before gulping down your food mindlessly and without appreciation. Or you can get a little more elaborate and hold hands around the table, just letting the blessings roll over you.

Make it habit forming.

Our general habit as a culture is to be ungrateful, Dr. Jeffers says. So it may take some effort to establish the habit of being grateful. You may even need to put a sign on the table as a reminder to do some form of thanksgiving before the meal.

Create a book of abundance.

Place a journal by your bedside, and each night before you go to sleep, jot down at least 50 wonderful things that happened to you that day, Dr. Jeffers suggests.

Fifty? That's right. "This exercise helps you look mindfully and deeply at the blessings in your life," she explains. "It helps you spend the day looking for them and takes your focus off the bad."

Need some help getting started?

Start small, Dr. Jeffers suggests: "My car started. I am able to walk. I have food to eat. The sun is out. I'm breathing. My toothbrush is in the same place I left it last night." The idea is to recognize each moment as extraordinary.

Find ways to give back.

Some of us may feel guilt when we realize how much we have taken without giving anything in return. "I call this healthy guilt," Dr. Jeffers says. "It can motivate you to begin giving back and, as you do that, your guilt disappears."

Make it a daily ritual to express gratitude by including one payback item on your daily "to do" list, she suggests. The payback item can be extremely simple—picking up paper that's cluttering the street, contributing to a charity or writing a letter of thanks. But those kinds of gestures go a long way toward building energy.

Take time to do things you enjoy.

Whether it's sitting down to play the piano, going for a long walk in the woods or smacking a little white ball around with a stick, take time to do things that give you pleasure. These actions can shift your perspective, making you more grateful for your abundance, says Dr. Lawlis. "That's what fishing is all about," he says. "It's not about catching fish. It's about not having to do anything else."

Keep "gratitude" reminders around you.

These could be rocks from the shoreline of some heartbreakingly beautiful lake, religious objects such as a cross, a card or a gift from a friend or quotes that remind you how awesome the world really is, Dr. Lawlis says.

Strike a grateful pose.

A field of psychology called bioenergetics postulates that certain body postures can evoke specific feelings, Dr. Lawlis says. These postures are adapted from ancient religions and cultures.

For a pose that generates gratitude, stand straight, then arch slightly backward and extend your arms above your head in a V-shape, "like a football referee signaling a touchdown," Dr. Lawlis explains. (Yoga fans will recognize this as step one in the sun salutation.) Hold the pose for a few minutes. If your arms get tired, drop them and press your hands into your lower back.

"This pose is good for generating a sense of accomplishment and high self-esteem, of celebration and victory," Dr. Lawlis says. "The whole stance invites being appreciative not only of your self but of the world."

Take ten to be grateful.

Take time during the day to cultivate your sense of gratitude—to reconnect with the world and to realize that you are part of something greater than yourself, Dr. Lawlis suggests.

You may want to go outside and commune with nature, pray or meditate or tune in to the love that comes to you from other people and that you extend to others. "It's critical to take time during the day to do this," he says.

Hugging

*I*t all started back in the early 1980s, when researchers first confirmed what grandmas have known all along. Babies who get lots of warm physical contact thrive better and score higher on mental tests than children who aren't cuddled. Researchers also found that these children have better sex lives and less illness when they're adults.

The bumper stickers first asked, "Have you hugged your child today?" Soon, bumper stickers came to include just about anything that would hold still long enough to get your arms around it—dogs, cats, trees, you name it.

But seriously, what's it all about? Can a bunch of good hugs really charge up your energy cells?

Squeeze Out Some Energy

We all know a sincere hug can make us feel loved and protected. The question is, how does that translate into more energy?

Researchers say that, like other forms of caring touch, hugs help banish stress, the number one energy drainer. Studies show that a calming touch can reduce stress hormones, increase the body's production of natural killer cells (which are important for immunity), reduce pain and normalize heart rate and breathing, says Tiffany Field, Ph.D., professor of pediatrics, psychology and psychiatry and director of the Touch Research Institute at the University of Miami School of Medicine. What better reason to be sure you get—and give—at least one hug a day?

Here's how experts say you can get comfortable doing that.

Just do it.
Look for opportunities where a hug is exactly the right thing to do, suggests Stanley E. Jones, Ph.D., professor of communication at the University of Colorado in Boulder and author of *The Right Touch: Understanding and Using the Language of Physical Contact.*

He tells of a nurse's first meeting with a suicidal female patient who had recently tried to slash her wrists. "The nurse took one look at the sad expression on the woman's face and immediately embraced her," he says. "No one had come near the woman since her suicide attempt, and the uncalculated and spontaneous touch was exactly what was needed. It said not only 'I care' but also 'You are touchable, someone I want to reach out to.'

"That hug was the first step in establishing a relationship in which the nurse could guide the woman back to physical and psychological health," Dr. Jones says. Among adults such occasions are uncommon. Trust your instincts to recognize them.

Cuddle your kids.

Babies, even animal babies, need touching just as they need food, Dr. Field says.

Try a skin-to-skin "kangaroo hug" with your baby, suggests Gene Cranston Anderson, R.N., Ph.D., professor of nursing at the Frances Payne Bolton School of Nursing at Case Western Reserve University in Cleveland. Lie down and place the baby so it's lying on its bare belly on your bare chest. Keep your hands on the baby's body. "Even newborn babies in this position will put their arms around their mothers as far as they will go. They really connect," she says. "We have some absolutely beautiful photographs of this." Dads can do exactly the same thing.

If you'd like to hug a toddler or older child, it's best to take it slow, especially with a child you don't see all the time, Dr. Anderson says. "It's not that they don't want to be hugged, but they are rightly cautious initially. It's just natural."

Try to get down on their level, relax, be friendly and let your affection take its course, Dr. Anderson recommends. The hug will come.

When in doubt, ask.

If you've never hugged a particular person before or if you're not sure how a person will respond, ask before you hug, Dr. Jones recommends. "You can say, 'Would you feel comfortable giving me a hug? I like to do that.' "

It's okay to ask for a hug in some situations. Asking for or giving hugs at work, however, can be risky business, Dr. Jones adds. It may be perceived as sexual harassment. The exception is the corporate congratulatory hug, which usually occurs when an entire group, "the team," acknowledges a co-worker's accomplishment.

Don't stroke unless you're serious—very serious.

Moving your hands around on someone's back while you're hugging is almost always perceived as a sexual overture, Dr. Jones says. Don't do it unless that's the message you want to convey.

Avoid below-the-belt contact.
Full-body hugs should be reserved for sexual relationships, says Dr. Jones. "For supportive or congratulatory hugs you'll want to stick with the so-called A-frame hug, where the chests come together, but that's it."

Adapt to size differences.
Short people often feel uncomfortable being drawn into someone's breasts or stomach, Dr. Jones says. So the taller person will need to bend over. "And a short person should avoid moving in on a tall person if that person does not accommodate him by bending down some," he adds. "Side hugs—an arm across the shoulder or around the waist—are safer when there's a big size difference between people."

Take it easy.
Don't squeeze hard, even in fun, and don't pick someone up while you're hugging him, Dr. Jones says. It's aggressive and it can hurt.

Respect ethnic differences.
Some countries—Russia, for example—are big on greeting with hugs and kisses. In other countries such behavior could get you in trouble, especially with a member of the opposite sex. Your best bet? On foreign turf let the other person initiate a hug, advises Dr. Jones.

Consider alternatives.
If hugs make you squirmy, stick with other kinds of body contact. "A friendly hand on an arm or back can communicate your goodwill as well as an embrace and may be more acceptable between men," Dr. Jones says. It's fine to save hugs for special occasions.

Journal Writing

No doubt there's been a lot written about, and maybe even a few knife fights over, which can do mightier damage—the pen or the sword. But there's little argument over which is better for healing.

When pen hits paper, you get answers as your deepest thoughts and feelings are opened and pour forth. The result: a host of benefits, including more energy.

"Whether you're keeping a diary, writing poetry or doing some other type of journal writing, as soon as you begin to write things down, you begin to get control—and that's very energizing," says Nicholas Mazza, Ph.D., associate professor of social work at Florida State University in Tallahassee, who has been teaching writing therapy for more than 25 years.

Writing Your Way to Health

Experts have long understood that writing down your problems can help relieve stress and result in a more positive attitude. But the benefits go beyond your emotional health. Studies show that people who express their deepest thoughts and feelings in a journal can bolster their T-cells, specialized, disease-fighting cells that help keep immunity strong.

The benefits of keeping a journal begin almost immediately and can persist for weeks, says James Pennebaker, Ph.D., professor of psychology at Southern Methodist University in Dallas and author of *Opening Up: The Healing Power of Confiding in Others*.

What's more, some of these benefits are far-reaching. Dr. Pennebaker has found that unemployed people who keep journals find new jobs faster than those who don't. "Writing helps people organize their thoughts and put things in perspective," he explains.

Many people use journal writing as a form of therapy, a way to confront their innermost feelings and fears. "When you write, you are literally taking a thought or feeling and putting it in a physical form—and that's very therapeutic," says Kathleen Adams, director of the Center for Journal Therapy in Denver and author of *Journal to the Self*.

"Many people who want to learn about journal writing are trying to cope with a serious illness or traumatic event," Adams adds. "Keeping a journal can help speed the course of treatment. At the very least it can help you know yourself better."

There are no rules when it comes to journal writing. Don't worry about grammar, spelling or punctuation—the point is to get thoughts on paper, not write a graded report. "There is no best type of book or writing instrument, no best method or subject. It all depends on what works best for you," says Adams. "But writing down your feelings does have an advantage over talking into a tape recorder or other methods because most people are more expressive in their writing than in talking."

Here's what the experts recommend for getting started.

Make it a habit.

Although it's not necessary to write in your journal every day, most experts do advise making it part of your regular routine. You'll probably start feeling its energizing effects after about ten minutes, although you may want to write longer, Adams says. "A longer session might be more relaxing, which in turn can give you more energy, but it doesn't have to take a lot of time."

Focus on the significant.

Although writing down any thought or feeling is helpful, Dr. Pennebaker finds that those who reap the best rewards, including more energy, are those who concentrate on their innermost feelings of love and pain—the big emotional issues that most people have a hard time discussing.

"It may be painful at first and even fatiguing, but it's definitely better than just writing about whatever just pops into mind," says Adams. "The most common misperception about journal writing is that you should sit down and start blasting away. Actually, for most people, it's best to focus on a particular issue that's really bothering them."

Keep an energy log.

Our lives are packed with potential de-energizers. If you don't make the effort to identify them, one by one they'll continue wearing you down—and you'll never be sure what, exactly, is doing the damage.

"If you're just feeling a little run-down, and your fatigue isn't related to a bigger issue, a great place to start with journal writing is to keep an energy log," advises Adams. "Ask yourself questions like, 'How does my energy level rate on a one-to-ten scale?' or 'How does it correlate to my sleeping habits, diet or exercise levels?' "

Over time, you can look back at your journal and see what events in your life took away your energy—and, just as important, what kinds of things made you stronger and more invigorated.

Do it when you're drained.

"For most people it doesn't matter what time of the day they practice journal writing. But from the standpoint of energy, I would advise people to write in their journals when they're feeling most depleted," says Adams. "That way, they can probably be more tuned in to the reasons why they don't feel energetic."

A journal is a great reference point, agrees Dr. Mazza. "It gives you a visual history of how you were feeling at that particular time—angry, frustrated, even fatigued—so you can gauge if you're making progress." Check it often to see how you're doing and whether you need to be doing more.

In fact, Adams suggests leaving a blank page after every few pages you write on. When you look back at your journal—days, weeks or even months later—you can give yourself some feedback. "Ask yourself, 'Am I getting the results I want?' " says Adams. "If not, ask yourself what you need to do to achieve those results and go for it."

Laughter

You won't find the names of comedians Milton Berle, Sid Caesar and Jay Leno in the American Medical Association membership directory. But according to some who actually are listed, maybe you should.

It's long been know that shtick—or any form of comedy, for that matter—can help the sick. Hippocrates recognized the importance of a good laugh to help keep you healthy. And since the thirteenth century, when French surgeon Henri de Mondeville proposed that laughter be used to help speed recovery after an operation, humor has been prescribed by some cutting-edge surgeons and rehabilitators nearly as much as Tylenol.

But more recently, scientists have discovered another health-helping aspect of laughter: more energy.

No joke.

Emotional Energy

"There is no research I know of that addresses laughter specifically as a way of boosting your energy," says Steve Allen, Jr., M.D., son of the famed comedian and an authority on the health benefits of humor, who is associate dean for student affairs at the State University of New York Health Science Center in Syracuse. "But there is plenty that shows laughter can do other things associated with increased energy—relieve stress, boost immunity, improve creative thinking and problem solving and help people recover faster from disease."

"Besides," adds Dr. Allen, "laughing makes you feel better about yourself. And when you feel better about yourself, you tend to be more energetic."

A Quick Fix

Research also shows that laughter has a physical effect that can boost your energy.

"When you laugh, you get an immediate increase in the heart rate, circulation and blood pressure, so the blood is more efficiently and forcibly distributed throughout the body—which, of course, can energize. When you exercise on a rowing machine or stationary bicycle, it takes about ten minutes to achieve the same results," says William Fry, M.D., associate clinical professor emeritus at Stanford University School of Medicine and one of the nation's top authorities on gelotology, the science of laughter. "Of course, you can exercise a lot longer. If you laughed continuously for ten minutes, you'd be exhausted . . . but well-conditioned."

"Laughter is aerobic," adds Clifford Kuhn, M.D., professor of medicine at the University of Louisville and a psychiatrist who specializes in teaching terminally ill patients to use laughter to help deal with their pain. "In fact, when you laugh for 20 seconds—the average length of a good, hearty laugh—your body gets the same aerobic workout as it would from running or doing any other aerobic exercise for the same time."

When you laugh, your heart rate actually doubles—unless you're a highly conditioned athlete to begin with. Then your heart rate stays elevated for three to five minutes once the snickering subsides—similar to the energy-boosting effects of exercise. And while you're chuckling along, the body releases endorphins, painkiller chemicals that can induce a feeling of well-being and boost immunity, making you more resistant to disease. Over time, regular laughter can also help drop the resting heart rate, making you more resistant to heart disease.

Let Out Your Inner Child

The trick, of course, is to get enough yuks to reap heart-healthy benefits—about 30 minutes each day. "That's actually a lot and takes more discipline than most people are used to—even if you have a great sense of humor," says Dr. Kuhn. "But it can be done, since laughter is natural. The typical 5-year-old child laughs about 250 times a day, but the average 35-year-old adult laughs only 15 times a day. The reason? We teach ourselves to suppress our laughter. But we make it natural again if we allow ourselves to become as playful as children."

And here's how.

Journalize those jollies.
One key to unleashing your slap-happy inner child is to rediscover what makes you laugh. Some things, of course, are obvious. But other good moments may be slipping by without grabbing your attention. To get a handle on humor, a laughter diary might help.

"I have my cancer patients keep a 10- to 14-day diary of images that occur to them during the day that they find funny," says Dr. Kuhn. "By doing this, they can recognize the type of situations that cause them to laugh and concentrate on getting more of those things in their lives."

A laughter diary helps you track the roots of your humor history for a better understanding of why certain things and not others make you laugh, says Dr. Kuhn. And knowing what tickles your funny bone can help you build a humor library of things that make you laugh. Start with a box full of funny books or magazines and just grab something from the box when your energy is ebbing. A pause, a distraction, a few yuks, and you'll find yourself powered up again, adds Dr. Fry.

Sit for sitcom.
Another way to get an instant laugh is to switch on the TV. "The Comedy Channel is a great source that's always available—and not only because it runs my father's old reruns," says Dr. Allen. "If you don't have that, try a sitcom." If TV isn't your thing, try some favorite humor books, like those by Erma Bombeck, Dave Barry and Lewis Grizzard. Go to movies. Or get humor compact discs or tapes from your local library.

For a hoot, watch D.C.
For real laughs—especially during an election year—there's always the spectacle of the government in action on C-SPAN. Tune in anytime, and you'll see comedy in action in the nation's capitol. "Trying to see the lighter side of serious issues—like the budget—is a great way to improve your sense of humor and get more laughs," says Dr. Fry.

Pepper your life with props.
"I recommend that you absolutely litter your daily path with silly props—anything and everything that encourages amusement, if not outright laughter," says Dr. Kuhn. "This includes items like putting a humorous calendar on your desk or hanging funny items on bulletin boards to even wearing or carrying funny things—even if it's secretly.

"For instance, I wear silly ties for all to see, but underneath I also have funny boxer shorts and keep a rubber clown's nose in my desk drawer. Having props out in the open helps others see humor, which in turn helps you laugh. But when I reach in my desk drawer and see the clown's nose, it gives me a secret delight that causes a snicker."

Turning Sadness to Gladness

Of course, laughing is sometimes easier said than done. When you're feeling down—by illness, mood or fatigue—your sense of humor can disappear faster than Jimmy Hoffa. So how do you manage then?

Practice laughter meditation.

Just as you would meditate to relax, you can also use quiet time to make your-self laugh. Just sit in a relaxing environment with no outside interruptions and think funny thoughts.

"I have my cancer patients focus on amusing images—anything and every-thing that they have found funny," says Dr. Kuhn. "Some doctors recommend doing this for 40 minutes or so, but I've found that 15 minutes, three times a day, is sufficient. Besides teaching you how to laugh when you don't feel like it, laughter meditation reinforces the internal images of what's funny when you think there's nothing to laugh at."

Force a smile.

Even stretching the muscles in your face that control smiling can release endor-phins and turn around your mood—as well as your frown. "First, raise your eyebrows as high as possible, hold them there for 15 seconds and then release," suggests Dr. Kuhn. "Then close your eyes as tightly as possible for 15 seconds and release. Next, grin as though you were trying to touch the corners of your mouth to your earlobes and hold that position for 15 seconds before releasing. Finally, try to pull the corners of your mouth downward toward your chin for 15 seconds and release."

Doing this every morning—or several times a day when you're in the dol-drums—can improve your ability to smile and even trigger endorphin release. Dr. Kuhn also suggests some simple stretching exercises, such as shoulder and neck rolls, to release tension so that you're less stressed and better able to laugh.

Keep funtime fun.

If you have a competitive type A personality, it's especially important that you don't take this funny business too seriously. "I find that juggling is a great way to induce laughter—both in yourself and others—but you have to be able to keep it lighthearted," says Dr. Allen, who teaches juggling in humor-building work-shops. "I have one physician friend who I taught to juggle to release his stress, and he became obsessed with it. His wife called me and said he hadn't gone to work for three days and had developed the worst case of tennis elbow you ever saw. He took this far more seriously than I intended and only added to his stress. So keep it casual."

Join the crowd.

Laughter is contagious, and if you're around people who are prone to laughter, it's bound to affect you—even when you're in a down mood, says Dr. Fry. "Seek out humorous people and just try to be near them. When other people are in a playful mood, it spreads," he says.

When Laughter Isn't Funny

Laugh at yourself, and the whole world laughs with you. But laugh at others, and you could be asking for a world of trouble.

"There's no doubt that the healthiest form of humor is that which is directed at yourself," says Steve Allen, Jr., M.D., son of the legendary funnyman and a humor-building specialist, who is associate dean for student affairs at the State University of New York Health Science Center in Syracuse. "Teasing others is not recommended unless you know that person very well and know he'll also find it funny, because it can lead to hurt feelings—and, as a result, decreased energy for both of you."

Even when you know your targets extremely well, some forms of humor are strictly taboo.

Ethnic jokes. "My grandparents' generation were Irish-Catholic folks who were hysterically funny, but bigoted against every other ethnic group," says Dr. Allen. "They had wonderful wit, but great hatred. So their humor was more destructive than constructive."

Sexual innuendo. Another form of humor that must be avoided is anything that can be construed as sexual harassment, since there's nothing energetic about a possible lawsuit. "This is especially true in the workplace," says Dr. Allen. "It's so common to hear her saying, 'It's harassment,' and him saying, 'But it was only a joke.' Maybe it was only a joke, but it doesn't mean it's not harassment."

Victim humor. Everyone has been a victim of some sort—whether of a crime, disease or tragic situation. So jokes about rape, cancer and other serious topics tend to offend, no matter the intention.

Mince words.

You could also play word games—take a word and try to make new, funny words by switching around the letters or even creating silly new words. "Everyone has enough of a vocabulary to play with," says Dr. Kuhn. "And this can be fun if you think of words as toys for adults that are just waiting to be played with."

Looking out the Window

The first time Jim Lovell looked out the window of an Apollo spacecraft at Earth's cold, gray moon was Christmas 1968. Lovell, Frank Borman and Bill Anders were the first men to lay eyes on the moon up close and then gaze back at the Earth from a quarter million miles away. As they emerged from the moon's dark side and the sun rose over the barren, pockmarked surface below, they pointed a camera out the window to offer the whole world their exhilarating view of a crescent earth as seen from Apollo 8.

One hundred million households looked out that window with them while the astronauts took turns reading from the creation story in Genesis—of Heaven and Earth, of light and darkness, of the waters and the dry land.

"The loneliness up here is awe-inspiring," said Lovell, as he gazed outside. "It makes you realize just what you have back on the Earth. The Earth from here is an oasis in the vastness of space."

Twenty-eight months later, Lovell once again looked out a spacecraft window at the Earth. His Apollo 13 mission to land on the moon had been aborted. An apparent meteor collided with the craft's service module, ripping its guts to shreds. Once again, Lovell pressed his face against Apollo's window. This time, he recalls, "I drew a breath and began to suspect I might be in deep, deep trouble."

In the three days between the mishap and their triumphant return to Earth, there were touch-and-go moments when it was not clear that Lovell and his crewmates would make it back. He looked out the window often. Often he looked anxiously. Nearer to home he looked out with anticipation and exhilaration.

It may be hard to top the view Lovell saw from his spaceship, but looking out the window at work or at home is surely safer. And, apparently, it's just as energizing.

Room with a View

Over the past 40 years scientists have been looking into the effects that windows have on people. In prisons they compared those whose cells looked out onto farmlands and forests with those whose did not. They found that inmates with nature views were less likely to report for sick call. Those with views of prison walls, buildings or other cells suffered more frequently from stress symptoms like headaches and stomach upsets. (Chances are, when Dr. Hannibal Lecter, the brilliant, cannibalistic, psychiatrist-killer in *Silence of the Lambs*, asked for a cell with a window, it was not mere fancy on his part. He probably knew the facts about a room with a view.)

Of course, you don't have to be in prison to get the health benefits of a view. A study conducted by researchers at the University of Delaware in Newark showed that hospital patients whose rooms looked out onto scenes with trees recovered more quickly than those whose views were without vegetation.

Several other studies have shown that short periods of time—as little as ten minutes—in front of a window with a nature view or even in front of a wall mural can promote recovery from stress in acutely stressed hospital patients. Stress, of course, is a major source of fatigue, and fatigue is the opposite of energy, notes Ronald L. Hoffman, M.D., medical director of the Hoffman Center in New York City, in his book *Tired All the Time*.

Whether your fatigue is brought on by stress or by any number of other sources, a starting point for a renewed vitality may be as near as your own window, says Roger S. Ulrich, Ph.D., associate dean for research and professor of landscape architecture and urban planning at Texas A & M University in College Station. Dr. Ulrich studies the influences of environment on psychological well-being and is an authority on the benefits of looking out the window.

"We have isolated what we call restorative influences," he says. To take advantage of the restorative influences—including boosting your energy level—that come from looking out a window, here's what Dr. Ulrich recommends.

Look for the unspectacular.
There's no need to have the Grand Tetons or the Grand Canyon outside. Most of nature is not grand at all. It's not how majestic your view is that makes you feel great. Nature alone does the job.

Plant a tree.
Many of us live in cities where nature seems far away. Having a tree in view amidst the brick and concrete of urban life has a dramatically positive effect. If you can, put some green foliage, even a single tree, in view. Research suggests that the untouched, natural desert environment did not have as positive an effect on well-being as the same environment did after some grass was added.

Get wet.
Water—trickling, running, shimmering, fresh water—has universal appeal as a source of refreshment. Research shows that even the sight of water has the power to enliven. If there is no babbling brook outside your window, consider adding a small fountain. The sight of a fountain has been shown to be restorative.

Help for the Windowless

What if you cannot get that corner office with a window overlooking Central Park? Or your townhouse looks out onto a crowded parking lot? Here are some next-best options.

Picture the country.
Having a nature picture within view is a good second choice if there is no green outside your window.

Dr. Ulrich recommends that the picture be a photograph or a realistic artist's rendering rather than a more stylized, abstract image. "The more real, the better, it seems," he says. In fact, studies have shown that those who are cut off from nature and surrounded by abstract and geometric art may suffer greater stress and may even become more aggressive.

Choose wide open spaces.
Not all green nature pictures are equally relaxing, refreshing and soothing. Environments that are more "savannah-like"—meaning flat and grassy—seem to have the most positive effects, says Dr. Ulrich. When you're selecting a picture, pass on the rain forest or dense woods in favor of a meadow or grassy lake view.

Looking out the Windows of Your Mind

For many people looking out the window or at a favorite nature picture also means daydreaming. Like looking out the window, daydreaming by itself can be energizing, says Eric Klinger, Ph.D., professor of psychology at the University of Minnesota in Morris, who is an expert on fantasy and inner experience and author of *Daydreaming*.

Daydreaming has been shown to have wide-ranging benefits, says Dr. Klinger. It can make you more relaxed and help you organize your life and increase your self-understanding. It can aid in problem solving and allow you to explore and rehearse life situations. "People in boring jobs often plunge themselves into daydreaming, not for relaxation but to keep their minds stimulated, sometimes even to keep themselves awake," he says.

Dream a little.

Done together, the benefits of daydreaming and looking out the window can be compounded, says Dr. Klinger. In daydreaming you are letting your attention wander in a very free, natural kind of way. It is the opposite of work, where your attention is focused on a task. "Work, which is not without its benefits, of course, leads to what is called operant fatigue," he says. "Daydreaming is what naturally seems to follow work as a restorative."

Take the pause that refreshes.

"If you look out the window, you're looking away from whatever you were doing—unless it reminds you that there's yard work to do. The window means that what's outside is a neutral space. Therefore, if you're daydreaming while looking out the window, you are choosing not to focus your attention on the task at hand but to let your mind do what it does naturally," says Dr. Klinger. And nature, it seems, is naturally energizing. After a few minutes you should, in fact, have more energy for your work.

Meditation

What do you think of when you hear the word *meditate*? Some sort of swami in the lotus position, eyes closed, levitating above a bed of nails? Or do you have a 1960s flashback to the Beatles' guru, the Maharishi Mahesh Yogi?

The Maharishi's particular brand, transcendental meditation, is but one of a wide number of different types of meditation. In fact, almost anything that you do with proper awareness can be considered meditation, says David Harp, a lecturer on meditation and co-author of *The New Three-Minute Meditator*.

Even cooking a meal or mowing a lawn can be viewed as moving meditation, if you maintain an awareness of your breathing while you do it, adds John Harvey, Ph.D., director of psychological services at Allied Services Rehabilitation Hospital in Scranton, Pennsylvania, and a contributing author for *The Big Book of Relaxation*.

And almost every religion has a meditation component, according to Janet Messer, Ph.D., a psychologist in private practice in Eugene, Oregon.

Enhancing Energy with Mind Power

All types of meditation, however, offer one key benefit: No matter what guise it appears in, meditation relaxes you, dissipates stress and increases your energy.

"Meditation promotes more than simple relaxation and energy," says Dr. Messer. "It can reduce your stress level. And you experience that change in functioning almost immediately. So if you meditate regularly, you'll find your normal functioning much healthier and calmer. It will move you to a whole new state of health, even a spiritual dimension."

"One of the essential ingredients of meditation is to be present in the moment, not thinking about the future or the past," says Dr. Messer. To do this, you have to focus your mind, often by concentrating on a single word or image. But another way to help focus is with deep, regular breathing—the kind that moves your whole abdomen, not just the top of your chest.

"Meditation isn't complicated. The simpler it is, the better it is. It's a very approachable practice that anybody can do," adds Dr. Harvey.

Getting into the Present

If you'd like to try meditation to relax and boost your energy, here are a few easy techniques to start with.

Focus on breathing.
"This exercise may be done sitting, lying down or even standing, as long as your back is relatively straight," says Dr. Messer. "And your eyes may be open or closed.

"Breathe in and out through your nose and allow your breathing to slow down slightly, letting it be natural and comfortable. As you breathe in, feel your lungs fill from the bottom to the top. Breathing out, empty your lungs from the top to the bottom.

"Put your attention on a spot in the center of your belly, about an inch below your navel and in the center of your body. This is the most important part of the exercise. It helps you feel grounded and connected to your sense of inner strength. As you inhale, feel your diaphragm—the sheet of muscle between your lungs and your abdomen—being pulled down toward the center of your belly. As you exhale, feel your diaphragm return to its natural position.

"Continue the exercise as long as you like. Do it for ten minutes at a time. Or five minutes if that's all you have. And do it several times a week." You can do this meditation in your car or on the subway or at your desk—any situation where you have a little time, Dr. Messer points out.

Count your breaths.
Another easy meditation is a traditional one from Zen Buddhism—with some additions from Dr. Harvey.

Breathe according to the directions above, but then begin to count your breaths. On the first breath, count "one" as you inhale and "one" as you exhale. Then, on the next breath, count "two" as you inhale and "two" as you exhale. Continue counting in this manner up to the number ten. After that, start all over again, from one to ten.

This exercise can bring you a feeling of great peace, says Dr. Harvey. It's a good one for beginners and people with active, busy minds who have trouble concentrating. He suggests doing this meditation for at least ten minutes.

Walk and breathe.

Another easy meditation to try is a favorite of Harp's. To begin, "walk a bit more slowly than usual, focusing your attention on the ins and outs of your breath," says Harp. Begin each inhale and each exhale with a mental label of "In" or "Out."

Without trying to control your breath too much, see if you can begin each in- and each out-breath exactly as a foot hits the ground. (Depending on how fast you're walking, each in and each out may begin every few steps or so.) Notice how many steps you take during each inhalation and how many steps you take during each exhalation, suggests Harp.

"Then count each step as you walk and breathe so that in your mind you are saying, 'In, two, three, four . . . Out, two, three, four.' Continue to substitute 'in' or 'out' in place of each count of 'one,' " says Harp, "to help you stay focused on the breathing as well as the walking.

"Your own personal breathing rhythm may be different—your exhales may take longer than your inhales. Or your inhales may take longer than your exhales. The step count may vary from one breath to the next. Just pay close attention so that you can accurately count your steps during every inhale and every exhale."

Clearing Your Mind

An important component of any meditation, whether you're doing it for relaxation and energy or for some other purpose, is mental focus. But no sooner do you start counting your breaths than your thoughts are off and running, "Oh, did I forget to turn off the stove?" or "Hmmm, did I send that memo today?" or "Where on Earth did Sophie get that lava lamp?"

In other words, little buzz bombs of distraction dart across your tranquil mind screen just when you're trying to clear it. In fact, the more you try to empty your thoughts and meditate, the more those thoughts buzz.

That's exactly what happens when you consciously try to clear your mind, says Larry J. Feldman, Ph.D., a leader of workshops on stress and burnout and author of *Feeling Good Again*. Meditators have been dealing with stray thoughts for centuries, and they've developed some of ways of dealing with them. Here are two ideas to help you meditate.

Watch your thoughts.

"Just allow your thoughts to happen," says Dr. Feldman. "The more you resist them, the more trouble they'll be. Imagine that your thoughts are cars in a traffic jam in the Holland Tunnel. But you're a traffic cop, and you simply wave them on through."

Focus on feelings.

If you're doing a meditation that involves doing something physical, like breathing, you can turn your mind back to the sensations involved.

"If you find yourself thinking about anything except the feel of your breath and the number of that breath, return to focus on the sensation of breathing and on the number of the breath," says Harp. "If you are not absolutely sure what number breath you're on, immediately begin again. 'In, two, three, four . . .'"

It's important to do this mental shift in focus without judging yourself, says Harp. Instead of thinking, "I blew the count," he suggests simply shifting back into "In, two, three, four . . ."

Music

Need some instant energy? Before you can say, "Bebop doowap," music can have you snapping your fingers, tapping your feet and waltzing around the kitchen, feeling as though life isn't so wearisome after all.

Aerobics instructors know all about music's energizing, motivating effects. Industry-based productivity specialists have shown that music can set the tone for a happier, more productive workforce. And the world-weary among us know that music can calm and revive after an energy-draining, stress-filled day at the office.

"Studies show that music can increase breathing and heart rates, increase your potential for muscular fitness and improve gait, coordination and control. It allows you to exercise longer, with less sense of effort," says Len Kravitz, Ph.D., adjunct professor of exercise science at the University of New Mexico in Albuquerque. "And if that's not enough, surveys show that music can help you stick to an exercise program over the long run."

While most of us think of hard-driving, fast music as energizing, it's not your only choice. Indeed, listening to it too much can produce the musical equivalent of "coffee nerves," says recording artist Steven Halpern, Ph.D., founder of Inner Peace Music in San Anselmo, California.

"It's true that you can get highly energized for a short time from this sort of music," says Dr. Halpern. "But if it's all that you listen to, your body is being constantly excited and never allowed to relax and come into balance. You end up more tired than before."

Tune In to Work Out

The same music that makes you want to shake, rattle and roll can be put to good use when it comes to exercise. Jazzercise founder Judi Missett built an aerobics empire based on that same thinking. "I pick music that speaks to my soul," she says. "And if it's speaking to me, I know that it's going to reach others as well."

Besides "soul" music, here are some other things that you'll want to consider when picking tunes for the workout room.

Make sure it's got rhythm.

Music with a prominent, predictable beat—usually a strong drum or bass—helps you match your movements to the music and spurs you on, says Cheryl Dileo Maranto, Ph.D., professor of music therapy at Temple University in Philadelphia and president of the World Federation of Music Therapy.

"I lived in New Orleans, where people marched for 12 miles in Mardi Gras parades without getting tired," she says. "I'm sure they wouldn't have done this so easily without their traditional ragtime marching music with its irresistible beat."

Pick music that matches your pace.

Most exercise music starts at 80 beats per minute and gradually increases to 120—or even as high as 140 beats per minute for the fast-moving set. If you're running, walking, biking or doing aerobics to music, this is a good range for getting a good workout and reaching your target heart rate.

Some people, however, prefer to use customized music that more closely matches their natural pace and rhythms. The Medical and Sports Music Institute of America in Bloomfield, New Jersey, offers walking tapes with music paced for 20-minute, 17½-minute, 15-minute or 12-to-13-minute miles. "These tapes tend to work like cruise control, helping you maintain a pace that produces the desired speed," says James Sundquist, director of the institute. For information about walking tapes, contact The Medical and Sports Music Institute of America, P.O. Box 1177, Bloomfield, NJ 07003-1177.

Listen for the human beat.

The relentless, computer-driven drumbeat found in some music these days stresses the heart, says Dr. Halpern. But "real drumming simulates the human heartbeat; it's organic and has subtle fluctuations in rhythm that your heart recognizes and responds to." In other words, it's "soul" music that makes your whole body want to watusi.

Look to rock 'n' roll groups such as Santana and early Motown such as Martha and the Vandellas for classic examples of this sort of drumming, Dr. Halpern suggests. Or check out contemporary African musicians. Two of his favorites are Babatunde Olatunji and Suru Eken. "These rhythms are played with hand drums and have layer upon layer of rhythm, which I find very stimulating and easy to move to."

Pick music with a positive message.

When it comes to working out, forget the somebody-done-somebody-wrong songs, Dr. Maranto says. "You want music that provides a pleasant distraction

Mood Music

If you would like to use music to give you more energy but don't know where to begin, try these picks from the experts. Many music stores will let you listen before you buy.

If you don't want to purchase the music, look for a library with a good audiotape selection. Or simply call your favorite college or public radio station. Radio stations often publish guides that tell you what type of music will be playing, and at what time.

Music for Energy
- Music by the Beach Boys
- *Breezin'* by George Benson
- "Respect" by Aretha Franklin
- Ragtime music by Scott Joplin
- Big band music by Glenn Miller, Benny Goodman, Duke Ellington and the Dorsey brothers
- *Abraxas* by Santana
- *Santana* by Santana
- *Graceland* by Paul Simon
- Marching music by John Philip Sousa
- *Fresh Aire* by Mannheim Steamroller
- "Pas de Deux (Black Swan)" and other selections from *Swan Lake* by Pyotr Ilich Tchaikovsky
- *Chariots of Fire* soundtrack by Vangelis

Music for Relaxation
- *Crystal Meditations* by Don Campbell
- *Waterfall Music, Music for Airports, The Pearl* by Brian Eno

and is associated with positive experiences in your life."

Missett's favorites in this genre include show tunes and big band sounds, like "In the Mood," "Sing, Sing, Sing," "Come Rain or Come Shine" and "I've Got the World on a String (Sitting on a Rainbow)."

Make the music fit the workout.
When you're going for a long, slow burn—a 10-mile ride on the ol' stationary bike, for example—you may be most comfortable listening to laid-back melodies, according to B. Don Franks, Ph.D., professor of kinesiology at Louisiana State University in Baton Rouge. "The relaxation brought on by the soft music may

- *Sacred Earth Drums* by David and Steve Gordon
- *Silk Road, Oasis, Silver Cloud* by Kitaro
- *Music of the Angels* by Gerald Jay Markoe
- *Canyon Trilogy* by R. Carlos Nakai
- *Sweet Memories* by Willie Nelson
- "Canon in D" by Johann Pachelbel
- *Adagio* and *Largo* by Relax with the Classics series
- *The Fairy Ring* by Mike Rowland
- *Winter into Spring* by George Winston

Music for Concentrating
- "Violin Concertos No. 1 and No. 2" and "Brandenburg Concertos" by Johann Sebastian Bach
- *Chant* by the Benedictine monks of Santo Domingo de Silos
- *Angels* (side 2), *Cosmic Classics* by Don Campbell
- "Nocturnes" by Frédéric Chopin
- "Cello Concerto" by Antonín Dvořák
- *Music for Your PC, Comfort Zone* and *Spectrum Suite* by Steven Halpern
- "Symphony No. 4" by Gustav Mahler
- "Sonata for Two Pianos in D Major" by Wolfgang Amadeus Mozart
- *Songs of the Indian Flute* by Ranier
- *Andante* by Relax with the Classics series
- "Symphony No. 6" ("Pastoral") by Ludwig van Beethoven
- *Sun Singer* by Paul Winter

make the exercise seem less difficult—enabling you to keep going longer," Dr. Franks says.

Of course, when you're pushing hard and fast, such as for a sprint on the treadmill, you'll probably want more rousing sounds, he adds.

Make your own music.
It's not just recorded music that can spur energy—you can put your own voice to work as well, says Don Campbell, founder of the Institute for Music, Health and Education in Minneapolis and author of several books about music, including *Music and Miracles*.

"Hold a bright E tone—'E-e-e-e'—and you'll be charged for exercise," he says. Hold the tone for as long as you can with each full breath, for a total of no more than two minutes.

"This tone vibrates faster and sharper than other tones, sending sound waves throughout your body," Campbell says. "If you are in a slothful mood, it gives you a sense of movement and attentiveness. It's like sonic caffeine."

Use music to imagine.

People who are unable to exercise—bedridden with injuries, for instance—can use music to help visualize themselves moving. And that actually improves blood circulation, Campbell says. "Close your eyes. See yourself running to the music. It does affect the body."

Mellow Melodies

If life is a pressure cooker and stress is taking its toll, you'll want to tune in to tones that help you fully relax. After all, if you want to call on your energy reserves when needed, you need some chill-out time. "Studies show that music can lead you into mental and physical relaxation, reducing blood pressure, heart and breathing rates and even levels of stress hormones such as cortisol," Dr. Maranto says. Unlike pharmaceutical sedatives, music does not induce sleep, only feelings of peace and serenity. And those feelings help you gather your energy forces to face the new day.

Here's how to select music that can muffle stress and help keep your energy high.

Choose songs without words.

"Lyrics force your brain to sort out the words, to make sense of them," says Dr. Maranto. Even instrumental versions of songs that have words can be a problem since you'll be thinking the words in your head. "It's a cognitive process that could interfere with your attempts to relax," she says.

Select music that's familiar.

It's a lot like hiking: You'll be more at ease on a trail that you have hiked a half-dozen times than on one that you have never before set eyes or foot on. "A piece of music you have never heard before is new terrain that your mind will be busy analyzing," notes Dr. Maranto. Listen to a new piece of music a few times before you try to use it for stress reduction, she recommends.

Choose music with no emotional baggage.

Some tunes are so closely linked with memories that you'll never be able to listen to them without getting worked up. "Even happy memories may be too stimulating for a relaxation response," says Dr. Maranto.

Choose music that's "complete."

If you want to drive a musician crazy, sing an eight-note scale and leave out the last note. The mind screams to have the last note sung and the tune completed. "You want music that resolves regularly and that harmonizes nicely," Dr. Maranto says. Music that fits this bill includes most kinds of baroque music (Bach, for instance) and some kinds of New Age music by performers like Aeoliah, R. Carlos Nakai and Brian Eno.

Hum a few notes.

Pick a note that really gets your chest vibrating, take a deep breath, then hold it as an "A-h-h-h" for as long as you can, then repeat, Campbell suggests. "Do that for two to three minutes when you feel stress, and it's going to change your world. It will affect your blood pressure, skin temperature, muscle tension and brain waves. It literally massages your body from the inside out."

Look for the signs.

You'll know that you're getting relaxed when you automatically take a deep breath, Dr. Halpern says. "If the music helps you to breathe more completely and deeper, you'll get relaxed and energized, just like that."

Tunes for Toil

The men who laid the first railroad lines across America coordinated their efforts with a song that's still popular, "I've Been Working on the Railroad." "Bodies move and work longer with music, and the body is stronger when you have a beat underneath it," Campbell says.

It's not just physical labor that gets easier with music. Anyone doing tedious tasks, like filing at the office, can use music to keep going while keeping the energy high. The same goes for mind muscles. The right music can help keep your brain humming.

Seek your own beat.

The same upbeat, rhythmic tunes that help you exercise longer can get you through long hours of many kinds of repetitive work, whether you're entering data or reviewing reports, experts say. The trick here is to listen to what you like, not the boss's hand-picked favorites.

According to researchers in the Department of Business Administration at the University of Illinois at Urbana-Champaign, personal headphones are a good solution. They found that employees allowed to listen to their choice of music on headphones had significant improvements in job performance and satisfaction, were less likely to say that they felt tired or sluggish and spent less idle time chatting with co-workers.

But Campbell warns against playing music too loud, especially if you're wearing headphones. It's easy to damage the delicate hearing apparatus in your ears with headphones that literally blast these cells.

Go with the flow.

When doing brain work, look for music with a gentle rhythm—no loud drums—and without lyrics, strong melody or structure, Dr. Halpern recommends. You want music that doesn't distract you, that keeps your mind focused.

Studies have shown, for example, that gently rhythmic music, which often includes flute or piano, is able to evoke alpha brain-wave states, Dr. Halpern explains. And that's a big bonus, because alpha waves have been associated with enhanced concentration. Dr. Halpern's own music is used by accelerated-learning centers around the world to enhance learning.

Naps

You're not a big baby if you need a nap in the afternoon. In fact, you might be the most energetic, good-natured person around if you follow your body's natural instinct to curl up and check out for a short snooze while the sun's high.

Midday napping is a preprogrammed part of our circadian rhythms—those neural timekeepers in the brain that regulate everything from hormone levels to waking and sleeping times, says Claudio Stampi, M.D., Ph.D., associate director of the Institute of Circadian Physiology in Cambridge, Massachusetts. "Napping is apparently a holdover from our tropical origins. In those regions a siesta is mandatory because the intense midday heat drains your energy if you're out running around."

These days, in temperate climates, people are more likely to use napping to catch up on the sleep they missed at night. Studies show that many people either don't get enough time to sleep or that they sleep poorly. Both lead to daytime sleepiness, which peaks about eight hours after our morning wake-up. For most people, that means a craving for shut-eye hits between 1:00 and 3:00 P.M.

The Pause That Refreshes

Most people can give themselves a quick jolt of energy by taking a nap, even a short one. Researchers at the University of Pennsylvania in Philadelphia found that when pilots flying intercontinental routes took a nap of about 20 minutes early in their 9- to 12-hour flights, they stayed more alert during the flights than if they did not nap. They also did a better job of landing the planes hours later.

It's your mental energy—the ability to focus, make decisions and solve problems—that perks up after you've taken a nap, Dr. Stampi says. A well-timed nap can also reduce stress and make you less likely to fill up on coffee or sweets in an effort to revive.

Many people maintain that an afternoon nap improves their energy levels during the evening hours. Winston Churchill, a famous napper, said a midday snooze let him cram 1½ days' work into 24 hours. That's not bad.

Here's how to nap for maximum energy.

Plan ahead.

If you know you're facing a short night with fewer-than-usual hours allotted for sleep, try to get in a nap that afternoon. "Studies show it to be more effective than trying to catch up on your sleep afterward," says James Maas, Ph.D., professor of psychology at Cornell University in Ithaca, New York, and developer of "Asleep in the Fast Lane" business seminars. "If you're going to have a long drive up to your cottage on Friday night, for example, the best thing you can do is to take a nap during the day on Friday," he says.

Make it short and sweet.

Some experts say that a 15- to 20-minute nap—certainly no more than 30 minutes—provides enough of an energy boost. Others stretch that ideal nap time to 1½ to 2 hours. But all agree that too long a nap can be counterproductive.

"Long naps can cause intense grogginess, known as sleep inertia, so that you take a long time to really wake up," Dr. Maas explains. A long nap also interferes with nighttime sleeping. If you find yourself wanting to sleep more than an hour or so in the afternoon, it means you need more nighttime sleep, he says.

Stretch out like you mean it.

Instead of dozing off in your easy chair, take your nap in bed or on a couch. This allows you to reach a deeper stage of sleep and awaken with the feeling that you slept much longer than your usual nap time.

If you can't sleep, rest.

Don't worry if you don't actually fall asleep during your nap. Merely lying down and resting can be almost as restorative as napping, according to researchers at Texas A & M University in College Station. "It's especially helpful for seniors who have trouble maintaining longer periods of sleep at night," Dr. Maas says.

Time it right.

Aim your nap for midafternoon, since the ideal nap time for most people is about eight hours after waking and eight hours before nighttime sleep. If you're up at seven in the morning, your body temperature changes at about three in the afternoon. That's when you feel most sleepy, Dr. Stampi says.

If you begin your nap after 4:00 P.M., you're more likely to remain groggy afterward and to push bedtime later, which becomes a problem if you have to get up with the birds. "People who fall asleep after dinner in front of the TV are especially likely to upset their sleep," Dr. Stampi says.

Sleep on the job.

"Napping is no longer equated with laziness," Dr. Maas says. "We can demonstrate a positive effect on the bottom line in terms of increased productivity and fewer industrial accidents. Why not take a nap instead of taking a coffee break?"

Pets

*O*kay, so maybe you're a little tired of your finicky feline's all-day standoffishness—and even more fatigued when you finally get TLC from her at 3:00 A.M. And Fido's unbridled appreciation for fire hydrants and playing catch can leave you . . . well, dog-tired.

Still, it seems as though man's best friend earns his reputation—at least when it comes to boosting your energy. And dogs are not the only animals with this special talent; it doesn't seem to matter whether your pet swims or slobbers or has fur, fins or feathers.

"There are plenty of hard data that show pets have an energizing effect on people," says Alan Beck, Sc.D., head of the Center for Applied Ethology and Human-Animal Interaction at Purdue University School of Veterinary Medicine in West Lafayette, Indiana, and author of *Between Pets and People*. Dr. Beck is considered by many to be the nation's foremost authority on the therapeutic uses of animals for boosting our emotional and physical health.

Studies pioneered by Dr. Beck in the 1970s and 1980s and continuing today show that owning a pet, or just being around animals, can boost energy levels by easing the burdens of this dog-eat-dog world. Pet ownership can even make you physically healthier and help you live longer. Pets have been found to reduce high blood pressure and improve symptoms of diabetes and other medical conditions that can zap your energy.

Need to Be Needed

When novelist George Eliot pointed out that "animals are such agreeable friends—they ask no questions, they pass no criticisms," she probably wasn't thinking about her health. But scientists know that the unconditional love these four-legged friends offer us can help boost our chances for longer and more energetic lives.

"There isn't a single reason why pets help us, and there are different things for different people—probably multiple reasons," says Dr. Beck. "But there is no doubt that pets make us feel better about ourselves, both physically and emotionally. They make us feel needed and improve our morale and feelings of self-worth. I think it's safe to say, and research will back me up, that anything that improves morale and feelings of self-worth has an energizing effect on us. One of the problems with having low morale and depression is that you feel tired and can't get things done."

Besides making us like ourselves more, pets help others like us. "Studies show that people react more positively to people who have animals," adds Dr. Beck. "Why? It's a good question, but across the board—from children to the elderly—it's been shown that pet owners are more popular, get invited to parties more often and are just perceived to be nicer and more likable people. And when you know that you're liked, you tend to have more energy."

Heartfelt Support—And More

Many of the nation's 236 million pets (that's about one for every man, woman and child living in America) play a significant role in improving the physical well-being of their owners. "People without pets react to life's stressors more often and more intensely than pet owners," says Judith M. Siegel, Ph.D., professor and associate dean of the University of California, Los Angeles, School of Public Health and researcher on the health-boosting effects of pets. "They also go to the doctor more often than those who own pets, sometimes because of their reactions to stress, but also sometimes because of loneliness—and because they want the companionship."

Since stress is not only an energy robber but also a major contributor to heart disease, this may help explain why pet owners tend to have fewer cardiovascular problems. But it's not the only reason: In an Australian study of nearly 5,800 people, pet owners consistently had lower blood pressure and lower cholesterol and lower triglyceride (blood fats) levels than non–pet owners—even when the pet owners ate more fast food and meat than non–pet owners.

In addition, diabetes researchers say that pet ownership helps keep blood sugar levels lower because there's a connection between blood sugar levels and stress. Also, elderly people prone to anorexia—a common problem in this age group—are more likely to eat if they own pets. "Eating is a social activity," explains Dr. Beck. "So when they feed their animals, they're more likely to eat themselves."

And studies indicate that pet owners reap more than heart-helping benefits. "There was a study in Wales of old retirees who were suffering from hypothermia because they were hoarding their money and not heating their homes," says Dr. Beck. Hypothermia is a potentially fatal condition in which the body's vital processes begin to shut down in response to cold. "But when they were given parakeets as pets and told that the birds would die if it were too cold, there were fewer instances of hypothermia among the pet owners."

Call on Animal Power

When it comes to using pet therapy for boosting energy, here's what the experts recommend.

Opt for a dog.
Although any pet is better than no pet, and most any pet can provide benefits, researchers say it seems as though dog owners reap the most energy-boosting benefits compared to people who care for cats, birds, fish or other animals.

"Our studies show that dogs offer the most stress-buffering effects," says Dr. Siegel. "Also, dog owners tend to think that there are more advantages to having them than do owners of other pets—probably because dogs are more responsive to their owners than are other animals."

Baby those critters.
One of the benefits of pet ownership is that regardless of the species or their age, they fill the role of children in the household, says Dr. Beck. "When people are around animals, they tend to talk baby talk—more slowly, sweeter and in a higher voice. This not only relaxes the animal but also the people. Pets allow us to be nurturers, which helps reduce anxiety and therefore boost energy."

Time it right.
"Our research implies that pet ownership is most beneficial in times of particular stress—such as a death in the family, the loss of a job or a divorce," says Dr. Siegel.

But that's not to say that you should run out and get an animal when tragedy strikes or impose pet ownership on others going through hard times. If you spot some clouds on the horizon, such as an elderly person who may be facing a personal loss in the near future, you might want to suggest that that person consider a loving pet to care for. "People who benefit the most from pets are those who have had a pet in the past or some connection to animals," adds Dr. Siegel.

Go fish . . . or to the birds.
Don't want the hassles of daily walks or changing cat litter? You can still benefit from the "second string" of pets—birds, fish or even snakes or lizards. "Looking at an aquarium is very therapeutic because there's enough randomness to hold

your attention," says Dr. Beck. In fact, studies show that watching fish swim lowers blood pressure and helps reduce anxiety—two factors that can boost energy.

Can't Own? Try "Visiting"

Of course, pet ownership isn't for everyone. One in four people with allergies is sensitive to dogs and cats. That means about 1½ percent of the overall population can't tolerate having these popular pets around. There are also lifestyle factors to consider: Some people live where pets are not allowed except for birds or fish. And others travel too much to make good pet owners.

But even if pet ownership isn't for you, here's how to keep your energy from going to the dogs.

Get a bird feeder.
"Having a bird feeder outside your home gives you some of the same rewards of pet ownership without the responsibility. This may be why the majority of bird feed in America is sold to people who don't own birds," says Dr. Beck. "There's the ability to nurture and validate the life process, and it also relaxes you and holds your attention. All of these things make you feel better about yourself and your surroundings and can be an energy booster."

Watch the Discovery Channel.
"If you live alone in a one-room apartment and work 18 hours a day, then having a TV is probably better than having a dog," says Dr. Beck. Watching wildlife documentaries can have an effect similar to that of watching fish in an aquarium or birds on a feeder—only with a little more action.

"When you see a lion rip apart a gazelle, it's understood that there's nothing personal and it's for food. That's not the same when you're watching the O.J. trial. When killing is done in the animal kingdom, there aren't the same negative feelings as when it's done against man," says Dr. Beck. Because of this—and the action—Dr. Beck says many people feel energized after watching wildlife documentaries.

Go to a zoo.
There's a good reason why more people go to zoos each year than to all spectator sport events combined. "It's not to learn zoology," says Dr. Beck. "It's because, in part, zoos make us feel safe. When you're in a zoo, you feel more positive about the other people there as well. Studies show that when you start a conversation with a stranger, he tends to be more defensive when you're talking to him in a park than when you're talking to him in a zoo. Plus, the animals make it easier to strike up a conversation."

Prayer

Wherever you find the poorest of the poor, the dying and those with AIDS, you're likely to find Mother Teresa.

The frail, wrinkled, diminutive nun travels around the world. Even today, well into her eighties, she helps younger sisters as they work in the streets from Calcutta to Rome, from New York to Kampala.

A recipient of the Nobel Peace Prize and heralded as a saint in her own lifetime, Mother Teresa presides over the Missionaries of Charity, the worldwide congregation of sisters she founded in Calcutta in 1950.

Where does she get her energy?

"Prayer," she says.

"In Christ we can do all things," Mother Teresa asserts. "Without him we could do nothing."

At a time when many other groups of religious sisters have cut back the time that they spend praying, experience has taught the Missionaries of Charity that regular prayer throughout the day beginning with Mass provides the energy boost they need to do what is often physically grueling and seems to many of us to be heartbreaking work.

The Missionaries of Charity are not alone. Throughout time, around the world and in many faiths, the energizing benefits of prayer have been understood.

An Energizing Relationship

"Our energy comes from our souls," says Lisa Aiken, Ph.D., a clinical psychologist and co-author of *The Art of Jewish Prayer*. "We have to eat to sustain us. We have to sleep to sustain us. But how we approach those things has an enormous effect on the energy we receive. We can go through our lives without any awareness of our souls, and so we receive only the physical effect of what we do. But when we connect everything physical to our spiritual source, it's that much more energized."

Prayer is much like exercise in that there are many different forms, styles and ways of praying. And, like exercise, it is possible to pray more or less effectively, with different kinds of prayer yielding more or less noticeable benefits. But teachers of prayer agree that, like exercise, prayer's most noticeable and lasting benefits come from developing a regular regimen.

"What relief prayer, made into a regular practice, can bring after a day when we have been beset by problems, harassed by noise, by the trite content of a persistently blaring radio, by advertising that assaults both our ears and our eyes," says Jean-Marie Cardinal Lustiger, Catholic Archbishop of Paris and author of *First Steps in Prayer*.

While definitions of prayer vary in the Judeo-Christian traditions, there are common themes. They typically define prayer with reference to a vital, loving relationship between God and people. "Prayer is an encounter with God," says Dr. Aiken. "It's talking to God from our hearts and telling him what we need, what we feel, and sharing our deepest selves with him."

"Prayer is keeping company with God," says the Reverend Simon Tugwell, a doctor of sacred theology, professor of theology at the Pontifical University of St. Thomas in Rome and author of *Prayer: Living with God* and *Prayer in Practice*. "Understood at its simplest, prayer is a straightforward talking to God."

The Reverend M. Basil Pennington, Ph.D., is a Trappist monk of St. Joseph's Abbey in Spencer, Massachusetts, and author of *Centering Prayer*. Father Pennington is a leader in the movement to reclaim the ancient Christian tradition of quietly "centering," or finding the revitalizing stillness of the heart that comes from quietly being alone with God.

"Prayer is love," Father Pennington says. "It is a communion and union in love. Besides this, everything else is secondary and inconsequential."

Finding the Energy to Pray

Chances are, you are leading a busy life already. Finding the time to pray may seem to be a luxury you cannot afford. Where can you possibly find the time and energy to pray?

In the seventeenth-century spiritual classic, *The Practice of the Presence of God*, monastery dishwasher and author Brother Lawrence tells the story of how he took advantage of his time at the sink to pray quietly, keeping company with God, as he did dishes.

Here are some proven ways to get praying.

Make any time sacred.
Brother Lawrence was neither the first nor the last to discover that prayer is one of life's most versatile activities. "An encounter with God can take place in any

arena of life—between husband and wife, at table in the way we eat, when we speak to people and when we are alone in an intimate encounter with God—when there is no one but the Almighty and ourselves," says Dr. Aiken.

Try formal prayers.

For most people some formal structure is likely to help them pray. "If a person doesn't have any structure, they are much less likely even to begin praying," says Dr. Aiken. "So using a prayer book not only gives us a place to start, it also gives us a focus and a direction to strive toward."

Let God speak.

Jews, Christians and Moslems are often referred to as "people of the book" because of the importance of *the book*, the Bible, in their common heritage. All three religions believe that God has spoken through their sacred writings. Therefore, prayerful Bible reading, which monks call *lectio divina*, or sacred reading, can be an important part of effective prayer for people who practice those faiths.

Turn to the Psalms.

For Christians and Jews alike, the Psalms, found in the Old Testament, has been the prayer book of preference throughout the ages. Much of its appeal is based on the wide range of subjects that the 150 particular Psalms cover. Some are for facing times of trial and difficulty with faith. Others praise the Almighty and his attributes. Still others extol the peace and joy that comes from right living.

"Memorize some Psalms and repeat them to yourself regularly," Cardinal Lustiger recommends. Whatever your situation may be, try using the Psalms to invoke God, and God can speak to you.

Take a one, two, three approach.

Besides using the Bible, the Psalms and formal, ritualized prayers, many teachers of prayer encourage more spontaneous praying. Dr. Aiken offers a three-step method.

First, recognize who God is and praise him. "God's not an egomaniac," she says. "The idea of praising God is to recognize his greatness, that he is all-powerful; he has the ability to provide whatever we need, and he has the knowledge of what's best for us. Also, we have something to strive for because everyone needs a role model. Our role model is God."

Second, ask for something. "We especially ask for that which will further our spiritual growth. By asking, we acknowledge that God has the wherewithal to help us in our daily lives," she says.

Third, give thanks to God. "One of the functions of prayer is to help us appreciate. The idea of generating a sense of gratitude is part of what helps us to uncover the divine image in us," she says. "By seeing what we have been given, we are more likely to become greater givers ourselves."

All three—offering praise, asking for things and expressing gratitude—are uplifting, energizing acts, Dr. Aiken says.

Create a sacred place.

Shrines are sacred places, and most religions have them. Pilgrims to shrines throughout the world have long reported how energizing the experience of visiting a place set aside for prayer can be. In our everyday world today, however, the importance of sacred places has largely been lost.

"Setting aside a place for prayer, a place where God is the point of focus, can lift up our hearts and minds to Heaven," says Mark Miravalle, a doctor of sacred theology, theologian and professor of spirituality at Franciscan University in Steubenville, Ohio.

"At home it may be a corner of the room where you and your family gather. At work it may be a spot on your desk where you have an icon, incense, a crucifix or a holy picture," says Dr. Miravalle. "Turn there as a place where you regularly meet God."

Set sacred times.

Mother Teresa's sisters have set times for prayer. But the practice of observing regular prayer times is far from new. Its roots are deep in the Judeo-Christian tradition. In ancient Israel there were seven appointed times during each day to turn to God. Likewise, Christian monks throughout the ages have followed the rhythm of *ora et labora*, prayer and work, by punctuating work throughout the day with the observance of seven prayer times.

A more common practice among Jews is to pray three times a day as King David did.

In Western monasteries and churches twice-daily prayer is observed by priests and devout laypeople. Known as the hinges on which the entire day turns, Lauds and Vespers are prayers as the day begins in the morning and when the day's work has ended in the evening.

Take a one-a-day prayer break.

Cardinal Lustiger encourages at least a once-daily routine of prayer, preferably for a half-hour first thing in the morning, as an energizing focus before the day's activities become too hectic.

He cautions against the possibility of a too demanding regimen, doomed to drag you down. "Before deciding if you are going to pray two, three, four, five, six or seven times a day, you should heed this practical suggestion: Associate the times of your daily prayer with regularly scheduled duties."

Punctuate the day.

"Set aside intervals for prayer, however brief, just long enough, perhaps, to give a nod of recognition to God," Cardinal Lustiger recommends. "But make it a strict obligation, no matter what happens, to consecrate a prayer to God at that specific time, even if you have no more than 30 seconds free."

Cardinal Opportunities

For busy people who have trouble finding times for prayer, Cardinal Lustiger offers these ideas.

Use the commute.
If you are on foot, in your car, on the subway or on a bus—why not use that time to pray? "If you are on your way to work, you may find yourself thinking about your colleagues there or of the difficulty you have to face in an office shared with one or two other persons. Ask God, before the workday begins, 'Lord, help me to live today's contract with my fellow workers in a spirit of true fraternal love,' " he suggests.

Plan a power lunch.
For most of us, lunchtime is a regularly scheduled break in the day's activities. Why not transform part of this break in your schedule into an occasion for brief energizing prayers? he asks.

Consider chauffeuring and carpooling.
"Maybe you're a mother who stays at home, but you have young children to take to and pick up from school at set times each day. Use those breaks in your activities for prayer," he recommends.

Combine exercise and prayer.
What could be more energizing than aerobic exercise combined with prayer? Cardinal Lustiger suggests an invigorating after-work walk to a nearby place of worship for a few moments of prayer, followed by a healthy, prayerful walk home.

Scientific research is beginning to make the connections between religion and health. So far, the emphasis has been on longevity. For example, one study among Jews in Israel has shown that those who are devout are likely to live longer than those who are not religious. To date, no scientific studies on the effects of prayer on personal energy have been published, but for centuries practitioners have sensed its benefits. One of these benefits is the liberating, and therefore energizing, sense you can get from prayer.

"What freedom we can experience in those intervals when we turn our being—soul, heart, intelligence—toward something greater than ourselves," Cardinal Lustiger says. "The result is that we ourselves become greater because of our attention to the One who is the source of all life and all love!"

Sex

Walk into any junior high school boy's locker room, and you'll hear some highly energized discussions about sex. But turn to someone who practices sex in the bedroom instead of talking in the locker room, and you'll more likely hear how their fantasies of "More!" have turned to "Chore!" . . . or even snore.

"It takes a lot of energy to have sex because it's not just your brain and genitals working—it's your whole system," says Carol Cassell, Ph.D., a psychologist and certified sex therapist who has her own consulting firm in Albuquerque, New Mexico and who is regional president of the Society for the Scientific Study of Sexuality. "When you have sex, it's a complete physical and psychological experience: Hormones are pumping, blood is circulating, you are tightening your muscular structure, and you're getting a pretty good aerobic workout, too," says Dr. Cassell.

"But sex is also directly linked to higher energy levels," she adds. "Having a healthy, active sex life can also give you more energy. A lot more."

From Glands to Groin

The act involves a lot more than just blood-engorged regions below the waist. Actually, sexual physiology is under the control of the endocrine system, the network of glands and organs that secrete and distribute hormones, including the energizing hormones like adrenaline.

"People with high energy levels tend to have, or at least want to have, a lot of sex. And part of the reason is because of the endocrine system," says Dr. Cassell. "The more sex you have, the more your endocrine system is pumping out these hormones. And the more hormones pumping, the more energy you'll have. If you're not having a lot of sex, the system shuts down, and you have to keep restarting it. But when you have sex frequently, which for people in their fifties would be at least a couple of times a week, the system is already 'well-oiled.' "

Of course, there can be too much of a good thing. "If you feel like you're having excessive sex—and that's a questionable term—it can sap your energy, and you won't have a whole lot of strength for anything else," adds Sheldon O. Burman, M.D., director of the Male Sexual Dysfunction Institute in Chicago, the nation's oldest and largest practice devoted exclusively to the diagnosis and treatment of male impotence. "But that's not a problem for most men."

Gender Differences

While a healthy sex life can energize both men and women, the act itself can fatigue men. And because of that, both sexes can find it an emotionally draining experience.

Unfortunately, many couples use more energy worrying, arguing or complaining about sex than actually having it—especially after middle age. Just about the time of life when men start to lose their sexual appetites, many women—free of the worries of pregnancy—want more sex, says Dr. Cassell.

And when couples do have sex, it often ends with men falling asleep just minutes after reaching orgasm. So *she* may be emotionally charged, but *his* snoring isn't exactly in energetic harmony, says Dr. Cassell. Well, rest assured, the blame doesn't lie with either men or women. It belongs to Mother Nature.

"Men don't roll over and go to sleep because they're insensitive clods. They do it because it's a physiologic response: The function of a man's body, after reaching orgasm, is to rest," says Dr. Cassell. "Women, on the other hand, don't need to rest after reaching orgasm, unless they ran a marathon beforehand. They tend to be more alert and energized immediately after the act."

Because a man's orgasm is so intense, Dr. Cassell notes, the climax can bring with it a quick end to energy levels as well. "Men need to have a rehabilitating period, and the typical response is to go to sleep," she says. "Women could endlessly orgasm, technically. The only thing that keeps them from doing so is their fatigue or, more likely, the fatigue of their partner."

How-To for High Energy

So here's what the experts recommend to keep both of you in high gear and to reap highly energized sex for high energy.

Do it in the morning.
"Since you need energy to have sex, the morning is the best time because that's when you tend to be most rested," says Arlene Goldman, Ph.D., coordinator of

the Jefferson Sexual Function Center at Jefferson Medical College, Thomas Jefferson University, in Philadelphia. "This is especially important for older couples or for people who tend to run out of energy toward the end of the day."

Other advantages of early-morning sex: "That's when a man's testosterone level is highest, and testosterone is what controls desire," says Dr. Burman. "Also, the stomach tends to be empty first thing in the morning. Food diverts blood from the groin and toward the stomach for digestion." Blood is needed in the groin to get an erection and maintain it.

Try an energizing position.
Certain sexual positions can result in more energized and frequent sex because they fatigue you less than others. "Many men find that the woman-on-top position is good because it doesn't require them to expel a lot of energy," explains Dr. Cassell. "And a position that's good for both partners is rear vaginal entry and clitoral stimulation while you're lying on your side. It's good for women because they can feel the thrusting of the penis especially well, while a man doesn't have to use his upper body to hold himself up."

Compare notes.
"The key to continued interest in sex is diversification," says Dr. Burman. "When things tend to be the same—same place, same positions—it certainly doesn't lend itself to highly energized sex. You need to tell your partner what you like, what feels good and what you think would feel good. And then you have to do what your partner likes and wants done."

Ban the booze.
If there's one thing that's almost certain to drown sexual performance—and appetite—it's drinking. "It's very clear that if you want a lot of energy as well as an energized sex life, you can't drink alcohol," says Dr. Cassell. "It depresses your whole system, including hormones. So, besides being less alert, you can't function as well sexually."

Don't smoke.
Smoking constricts blood vessels, hampering blood flow to the groin, adds Dr. Burman. In a study conducted at Johns Hopkins University in Baltimore, researchers found that smoking results in the inability to get or maintain an erection. This explains why frequent smoking can ultimately lead to impotence.

Take your vitamins.
While sex releases hormones that can boost immunity, a man loses stores of zinc and other immune-building vitamins every time he ejaculates. "I'd advise that you make sure your diet is high in zinc, B-complex vitamins and vitamin E—or take a high-potency vitamin/mineral supplement pill," says Dr. Cassell.

"Besides keeping immunity strong, these vitamins also help keep the glands necessary for sex in good working order."

Good food sources of zinc include oysters, beef, lamb and crab. The B vitamins—folate, niacin, riboflavin, thiamin, B_6, B_{12} and biotin—are in a wide array of meats and seafood as well as cooked dried beans and whole grains. And vitamin E, which is not in many foods, is found mostly in cooking oils and wheat germ. If you go the supplement route, ask your doctor about a B-complex vitamin containing all B vitamins. And if your doctor okays it, take between 15 and 25 milligrams of zinc and 200 to 400 international units of vitamin E.

Smiling

*I*nstant happiness, anytime you want it. Think that would perk you up and give you more energy?

No, it doesn't come in a bottle. But consider this: Psychological research suggests that people who have been trained to produce a reasonable facsimile of a genuine smile can trigger in their brains some of the same responses associated with positive feelings—the kind of brain waves that a baby produces when it sees Mom coming, for instance.

The problem here, researchers say, is that while all of us can fake some sort of smile, "few people can produce a genuine smile, on demand, with ease," says Richard J. Davidson, Ph.D., professor of psychology and psychiatry and director of the affective neuroscience laboratory at the University of Wisconsin at Madison.

Dr. Davidson's research on facial expressions was done with college students. Most of the study's participants needed "extensive muscle-specific instruction from an expert coach who was monitoring their facial muscles on closed-circuit video" before they could manage a passable fake. Those few students who didn't need much coaching were questioned extensively about how they did it, he says.

With findings from these studies as a guideline, here are a few smile-producing pointers from the experts.

Don't let your eyes lie.

To produce a sincere, deeply felt smile, you have to simultaneously contract two muscle groups, those that extend from the corners of your mouth to your ears and those that circle your eyes.

The mouth muscles are fairly easy to control, Dr. Davidson says. "But it is not the corners of the mouth that are the critical muscles signifying a genuine smile. It is the eye muscles that are the key, and they are much more difficult to control than the mouth."

Raise your cheeks, part your lips and let your lip corners come up. Contract your eye muscles to produce crow's-feet and a slight droop in the skin directly above your eyes. If the result is a tightened and raised lower eyelid and slight lowering of the fold of skin over the eye, you have the right muscle. You'll probably have to practice this in front of a mirror.

Do something that makes you smile.

Pleasant films of puppies gamboling in flowers and the like can produce sincerely happy smiles, researchers have discovered. "Finding or thinking about something that really makes you smile without effort is, for most people, a much easier way to go about it," Dr. Davidson says.

Get yourself on tape.

If your nickname is Old Stoneface, there's no doubt about it: You're as likely as a marble bust to crack a smile.

But if you're unsure how expressive your face is, set up a movie camera and videotape yourself for an hour or so while you interact with other people, suggests Stanley E. Jones, Ph.D., professor of communication at the University of Colorado in Boulder and author of *The Right Touch: Understanding and Using the Language of Physical Contact.*

"This can be very revealing, especially to men who are not used to being expressive," he says. "If you're really happy, you should let your face know about it."

If you can't tape yourself, ask friends if you smile much or show happiness, or look at photographs of yourself in candid shots, Dr. Jones suggests.

Know that practice makes perfect.

Some people who initially have a hard time making certain expressions—such as an angry face—find it easier over time as they practice that expression, Dr. Jones says. "Same goes for smiling. The more you do it, the easier it becomes."

Project what you want to get.

Flash an ear-to-ear grin to the world and that's what you'll get back, Dr. Jones says. "It's contagious. And I know that when other people smile back at me, it makes me even happier." (For best results also look the other person in the eye.)

Snacks

Feel the urge, nibble some chips. Flip on the TV, reach for the cola. Take a break at work, drop a couple of quarters in the vending machine. Satisfying? Chances are, you don't even notice. Energizing? Hardly.

"Snacking is part of the American way of life, and it's one reason why people overeat foods that don't offer much nutrition," says Wahida Karmally, R.D., director of nutrition at the Irving Center for Clinical Research at Columbia–Presbyterian Medical Center in New York City.

People eat between meals because they're hungry, of course. "But they also often turn to food because they're tired and trying to perk up," says Elizabeth M. Ward, R.D., a nutritionist at the Harvard Community Health Plan in Boston. Studies suggest that well-timed nibbling may, in fact, boost mental alertness. But there's a difference between snacking that charges your engines and the nothing-better-to-do snacking that's just a munching mania.

Energy by the Handful

Here's what nutrition experts recommend snack-wise for maximum alertness and energy.

Time your snack to count.
Afternoon noshing—between 2:00 and 4:00 P.M.—is the only snack time that's been proven to improve mental skills such as memory, arithmetic reasoning, reading speed and attention span, Ward says. "Any kind of snack during this time period will boost energy."

Eat after you exercise.
Eating carbohydrates soon after you exercise is important for boosting recovery and replenishing the sugar stored in muscles, says Ward. It's crucial for serious athletes who work out every day.

Keep fruit handy.

Snacking is a good opportunity to get in those recommended two to four daily servings of fruit. Fruit provides carbohydrates for a quick energy boost, plus important nutrients such as magnesium, vitamin C, folate, beta-carotene and fiber.

Apples and oranges hold up well and can be stashed away in your desk drawer until you're ready to eat them. Or try dried apricots, prunes or raisins, Karmally advises. Keep a bowl of washed fruit on your kitchen counter or a fruit salad in the fridge. "Children, especially, are more likely to snack on fruit if it's ready to eat," she says.

Go for the grains.

Complex carbohydrates, starches, are considered the ideal food choices for an energy source because they supply vital vitamins and minerals needed to keep you going.

Among the good guys for high-starch snacking are bagels, low-fat crackers and muffins, whole-wheat bread, baked potatoes, rice cakes, baked corn chips, popcorn, pretzels, cereal and instant oatmeal. Just be sure to steer away from high-fat versions of these snacks—such as buttered popcorn—since you'll slow down a lot if you load up your fat cells.

Covet leftovers.

Just about any food will perk up your brain if you haven't eaten for hours, says Ward. That includes cold pasta, cold pizza made with low-fat cheese, half a tuna sandwich or the three-bean salad you didn't have room for at lunch. "Leftovers can be a great snack, provided they aren't loaded with fat," explains Pat Harper, R.D., a Pittsburgh nutrition consultant.

Don't be afraid of chocolate.

Just about everything chocolate—cookies, cakes, ice cream—now comes in tasty, low-fat and even nonfat versions. That's great for people who consider chocolate the ultimate energizer. "Although chocolate may not be the most nu-tritious snack, it is fine on occasion," Harper says. "I just ask that people con-sider it a treat and limit their portions." One good way to do that, she says, is to dole out one portion at a time and wash it down with a big glass of skim milk (which is virtually fat-free).

Savor soup.

Soup is handier than ever, thanks to all the instant mixes available. Some in-stant brands even come with their own cups. "Soup fills you up fast and, if loaded with vegetables, provides an array of nutrients," says Harper. Read la-bels, though, to make sure that you're not getting more than three grams of fat per serving.

Mix 'n' match.

Have an apple and some low-fat cheese, some fat-free fig bars and a glass of skim milk, fat-free refried beans and tortillas, veggies and nonfat yogurt dip or a slice of cantaloupe and a scoop of low-fat cottage cheese. "All provide a balance of carbohydrates, protein and nutrients, without much fat," Karmally says.

Treat yourself before bed.

Call it dessert or call it what you want. If diet-imposed hunger is keeping you awake, aim for a late-night light snack that combines carbohydrates and protein, Harper says. That could be gingersnaps, graham crackers or vanilla wafers washed down with skim milk. Other possibilities are low-fat or nonfat frozen yogurt, instant pudding, hot chocolate or yogurt with your favorite cereal.

Sunlight

*D*o dreary days drain your batteries? Does being cooped up in a dark dungeon of an office numb your neurons? Do winter's brief days make you burrow into the sofa in a lame attempt at hibernation?

Despite the invention of the electric lightbulb—a recent occurrence in evolutionary time—our bodies still respond in amazingly creaturelike fashion to diurnal (day/night) cycles, says Dan Oren, M.D., a program chief in the Mood, Anxiety and Personality Disorders Research Branch at the National Institute of Mental Health (NIMH) in Washington, D.C.

When Winter Gets You Down

Like most animals, we depend on exposure to light and dark to regulate our bodies' internal clock, says Dr. Oren. This clock controls our bodies' natural daily and seasonal cycles, which include changes in body temperature and hormone secretion.

"Research shows that our exposure to light and dark can affect our energy levels more than previously realized," he says. That's because light and dark cycles can affect when and how well we sleep—and daytime alertness, mood, appetite and reproductive cycles.

Many people find themselves getting a little sluggish as winter settles in. And some people get downright depressed. That's because winter's abbreviated days can cause changes in brain chemistry that lead to less energy, increased appetite, weight gain, difficulty concentrating, sadness and withdrawal. When these symptoms are severe, the condition is known as seasonal affective disorder (SAD).

Let There Be Light

People with SAD usually feel their worst in January and February, when days are already lengthening again, says Michael Terman, Ph.D., director of the Light Therapy Unit at Columbia–Presbyterian Medical Center in New York City.

"But most people begin to perk up by March or April."

In the meantime, adjustments in exposure to both light and dark may help energize people with SAD or a milder case of winter blues, Dr. Terman says. Here's what experts recommend.

Take a stroll in the sunshine.
Aim for a daily 45-minute walk before you leave for work in the morning or at lunchtime, Dr. Terman says. "This is certainly the first thing I'd suggest for most people with mild winter blues. For some, it's all they need to do." People with severe symptoms will still benefit from a sunlit saunter but may also need to see a doctor who can prescribe further treatment such as artificial light therapy or even antidepressant drugs, he adds.

Walk through the rain.
Don't let the rain stop you from an outdoor excursion. "Even cloudy skies offer substantially more light than you can get from standard indoor lamps," Dr. Terman says. And the aerobic exercise has its own exhilarating effects.

Save sunglasses for the beach.
To reap sunlight's energizing benefits, you must let the light reach your eyes. So unless you have vision problems that require you to protect your eyes, wear sunglasses only when you're going to be outside an hour or more, Dr. Terman recommends. "While some sunglasses are designed to reduce the harmful ultraviolet light, which increases the risk of cataract formation, they also block beneficial visual wavelengths."

Be cool in yellow shades.
If you feel that you must wear sunglasses, select ultraviolet- and blue-light-blocking glasses. Ask your eye doctor about yellow-tinted lenses or clip-ons that block sunlight's harmful rays but not other visible wavelengths of light, suggests Seymour Zigman, Ph.D., professor in the Departments of Ophthalmology and Biochemistry at the University of Rochester School of Medicine in New York. For more information on the yellow-tinted lenses, write to Sphere-One, 20 Easedale Road, Wayne, NJ 07470. Lens blanks cost approximately $45 per set.

"These lenses make the world seem brighter, especially on cloudy days," he says. "They're great for people who want to enjoy sunlight but worry about eye damage."

Yellow-tinted lenses don't just remove excess light like regular sunglasses do, according to Dr. Zigman. Because they block short-wavelength blue light, they also reduce glare and enhance contrast, especially in dim light. This makes them ideal for people who have early cataracts or night vision problems, he says.

Wear a hat with a visor.

Even though you're aiming for more exposure, you don't want the sun shining directly into your eyes, Dr. Terman says. "It's simply too damaging."

Your best bet? Wear a hat with a brim that shades your eyes. This allows reflected light to reach your eyes but blocks direct sunlight from overhead.

Get a jump on dawn.

Some people can benefit by using high-intensity indoor lights to get a hefty dose of light early in the day, says Dr. Terman. Most high-intensity units are simple tabletop models that you sit in front of while you read the morning paper.

One model, called Dawn/Dusk Simulator, mounts over your bed and slowly brightens in the morning, mimicking the rising sun. It works—even when you're still sleeping—because your eyes are more sensitive to light after they've been in the dark all night long, Dr. Terman explains. Its advantages: You wake up effortlessly, and by then, you already have your daily prescription of rays.

For more information on the Dawn/Dusk Simulator, write to SphereOne, 20 Easedale Road, Wayne, NJ 07470. The entire system costs about $800. You don't need a prescription to use one, but if you have a condition that warrants its use, some insurance companies may provide reimbursement, says Dr. Terman.

See a doctor for a firm diagnosis of SAD, however, before you invest in therapeutic lights on your own, suggests Dr. Terman. And if you are diagnosed, the lights should be used under your doctor's supervision.

The Case for Hibernation

People with SAD sometimes say that they'd like to hibernate. Although getting more sunlight is helpful to people with SAD, some people apparently benefit from paying particular attention to darkness and sleep, Dr. Oren says.

"Many people with SAD say that they'd do just fine if they could get the sleep they'd like and if other people would leave them alone and not pressure them to do all the things that they might normally do at other times of year," he says.

Research, in fact, suggests that long periods of darkness in the winter months can energize some people, even those who are not sleep-deprived.

Research conducted at NIMH found that people kept in the dark for 14 hours a day—the equivalent of a winter night without artificial lighting—reported feeling happier, less fatigued and more energetic within a few weeks, says Thomas Wehr, M.D., chief of the Clinical Psychobiology Branch of the National Institute of Mental Health.

During their long nights people's sleep was broken into two periods, explains Dr. Wehr. Between the periods was a time of quiet wakefulness characterized by prominent and sustained alpha brain-wave rhythm—the kind of brain wave that occurs during meditation. These people also had higher-than-normal nighttime levels of two important hormones: prolactin and melatonin, he says.

While all these things could potentially produce more daytime energy and better disposition, "we don't know the significance yet of these findings," Dr. Wehr says.

Here are some things that you can do to benefit from the dark side of your daytime/nighttime cycles.

Hit the sack earlier.
Has your internal clock gone haywire? "For the minority of 'owls' who stay up very late in the winter and then find themselves glued to the mattress in the morning," Dr. Terman suggests, "going to bed earlier may be of help. What's important is getting plenty of light exposure upon awakening."

Go gently into that good night.
Try dimming the lights for a few hours before you go to bed, suggests Diane Boivin, M.D., Ph.D., researcher in the circadian, neuroendocrine and sleep disorders section of the endocrine division at Harvard Medical School–Brigham and Women's Hospital in Boston. This practice could help you nod off faster when you do hit the hay and help you wake up at your target time, she says.

Researchers used to think that only very bright light affected people's internal clocks. Now they know that while bright light has a strong effect, even normal indoor lighting can cause unwanted shifts in the body's internal clock, Dr. Boivin explains. Too much bright light at night delays a drop in body temperature associated with sleepiness; it also delays an early-morning rise in body temperature that helps you wake up.

The result? You fall asleep later and later each night and then have increasing trouble waking up at your regular time in the morning, Dr. Boivin says.

Don't expose yourself to very bright light as you go to bed, says Dr. Boivin. If you can, try dimming the lights around the time that you brush your teeth, put on your pajamas or take a bath. "Keep just enough light on so that you can see to do things," she advises. Be especially wary of reading to induce sleep. Keep lights dim for that, too.

Burning the Midnight Oil

People who get the winter blues or who have SAD are not the only ones whose energy gets depleted from lack of sunlight. People who work at night—typically an 11:00 P.M. to 7:00 A.M. shift—develop something akin to chronic jet lag. "Their internal clocks stay in sync with real time, not the artificial time zone created by their work schedules," Dr. Terman explains.

For many shift workers, this results in short, fitful bouts of sleep during the day and a terrible wave of fatigue from 3:00 A.M. to 6:00 A.M. That's about the time when some nuclear-power plant employees are lowering the radioactive fuel rods into place or drowsy long-haul truckers are trying to make up time to get to their destinations, Dr. Terman says.

"Their internal clocks are telling them to sleep when they have to be alert," he explains. Perhaps the name graveyard shift could take on new meaning because of the many industrial mishaps that occur during these hours.

Whether or not you need to shift your internal clock to stay hard at work, sometimes we all have special demands that keep us burning the midnight oil. Here's how to stay up and energized through those long nighttime hours without falling asleep at the switch.

Crank up the wattage.

Even a modest boost in brightness in your workplace can increase alertness and productivity all night long, Dr. Terman says. This lighting strategy doesn't try to permanently shift people's internal clocks, so it causes fewer problems on days off, he says.

Keep all the lights on in your office while you're working or add more lights to your work area if you can.

Get illuminated early on.

Research shows that workers exposed to bright lights for a few hours soon after their shifts begin tend to stay more alert during the shift than those not exposed to bright lights, Dr. Terman says. The lesson? If you're just getting to work at night, turn those lights up right away.

Wear shades on the drive home.

If you have been working all night and you have to drive somewhere at dawn, be extra cautious. "For people working the night shift, early morning is the equivalent of dusk, a time when they should be getting ready for bed," notes Charmane Eastman, Ph.D., director of the Biological Rhythms Research Laboratory at Rush–Presbyterian–St. Luke's Medical Center in Chicago.

Studies have found that wearing dark goggles during this time helps increase the duration and quality of your daytime sleep, says Dr. Terman.

"In our study we used welder's goggles, but this can make it difficult for people to distinguish the color of traffic lights," Dr. Eastman says. So try a dark pair of sunglasses, preferably wraparounds.

Sack out in darkness.

Once you're through with your all-night or late-night work, go straight to bed in a room as dark as you can make it, suggests Dr. Eastman. "One of the ways that we make bedrooms dark is with thick black garbage bags taped over the windows."

Light-stopping drapes are also an option. Even with your eyes closed, exposure to light can disrupt and shorten your sleep, says Dr. Eastman.

Jettison Jet Lag

Even if you don't have to stick to the old grind all night, you get to experience the equivalent of shift-work hangover every time you travel long distances. It's called jet lag, and its infamous energy-draining effects have everything to do with your sleep/wake cycles and your exposure to sunlight.

You have to cross at least two or three time zones in one day to experience the full force of jet lag's energy-draining effects. That's how business travelers find themselves struggling to stay awake during important presentations in Taiwan or prowling the streets of Prague at 2:00 A.M. looking for a restaurant that will serve them breakfast. And the leisure traveler who crosses several time zones on a long-anticipated vacation has an even tougher time since there's an element of excitement and anticipation that rings the internal alarm clock loud and clear.

"Your body clock is still synced to whatever time zone you came from," explains Tom Houpt, Ph.D., a research scientist at the Bourne Laboratory at the New York Hospital–Cornell Medical Center in White Plains. "And unless you take special measures, it won't adjust more than three hours a day toward the time zone you're currently in."

Exactly what measures to take depends on whether you're flying east or west and how many times zones you have crossed, Dr. Houpt says. Here are some details.

Fly east . . . jump forward.
If you have flown east across fewer than six time zones, you'll want to set your internal clock forward. This means that you'll need to spend some time outdoors the first morning and afternoon at your destination.

If you're flying from Newark, New Jersey, to London, England, leaving at 8:00 P.M., for example, you'll want to seek light the next day in London. When you arrive in London, try to spend some time outdoors from about 10:00 A.M. to 5:30 P.M., getting your maximum exposure from 11:00 A.M. to 2:00 P.M., Dr. Houpt says. At about 6:00 P.M., go inside even if it's still light outdoors, so that your "night" begins at that time.

The day after that, your ideal light-exposure times will be 7:00 A.M. to 1:00 P.M., with maximum exposure from 8:00 A.M. to noon. Again, you'll want darkness by 6:00 P.M.

Fly east . . . jump backward.

If you have flown east across six or more time zones, you'll need to set your internal clock backward, says Dr. Houpt. You can do this by avoiding morning light at your destination and by trying to catch some rays late in the afternoon.

Fly west . . . jump backward.

If you fly west across a few time zones, don't worry about jet lag. (Flying west is almost always easier than flying east, because it's easier for most people to stay up late than get up early, Dr. Houpt says.) If, however, you have flown west across 6 to 12 time zones, you need to set your internal clock backward, he adds. This one's tricky and requires the use of artificial lights.

Ideally, flying from New York City to Tokyo, leaving at 8:00 P.M., this would involve exposure to lights on the plane from midnight to 6:00 A.M., with maximum exposure from 2:00 to 4:00 A.M. Then the next day, in Tokyo, you'd need light exposure from 5:00 to 10:00 P.M., with maximum exposure from 7:00 to 10:00 P.M. You're not likely to get the light you need on the plane, but you have a good chance of exposing yourself to light during the right times the next day.

Tai Chi

*I*t's a raw, cold day in Manhattan, but on the third floor of the New York offices of the international School of Tai Chi Chuan, about 100 tai chi instructors are fine-tuning their teaching techniques. They wear an assortment of comfortable clothing and the Eastern equivalent of ballet shoes—soft, flat black Mary Janes. The mood is warm, mellow, relaxed.

Tai chi is often called a moving meditation. Like all meditation, it mellows you out and calms you. "Tai chi is a very high level meditation. You can't think about anything else or you lose your balance or forget where you are in the sequence of movements," says tai chi instructor Bobbie Fink, who runs the Atlanta branch of the School of Tai Chi Chuan.

Move into Energy

"Tai chi is a nonaggressive self-defense art from Chinese culture," explains Margaret Matsumoto, senior instructor at the Manhattan headquarters of the school. "When the tai chi movements are performed in slow, flowing motion, its benefits for health and relaxation are easily felt. It is also an excellent method for boosting your energy, for giving you sustained energy throughout the day.

"However, learning the sequence of movements is not that hard. Practicing the movements, however, points out where the tension is in your body. In order to make just one step, you have to relax whole groups of muscles that might be tensing up."

Tai chi comes in many forms. The classic type, tai chi chuan, contains more than 100 postures. As you learn the movements, you can go all the way up the ranks until you reach the level of black belt, says tai chi researcher Ralph LaForge, a clinical exercise physiologist at San Diego Cardiac Center Medical Group. There are shorter forms and variations, some adapted for the elderly and other special-interest groups.

"Tai chi is perhaps the best single technique for reducing stress and increasing energy," maintains LaForge. "It very quickly reduces blood pressure. We see remarkable reductions in low to moderate high blood pressure, and it improves your mental acuity."

If you'd like to experience the energy-boosting benefits of tai chi, here's how to get started.

Find a teacher.

Although there are videos devoted to tai chi, the best way to learn is in a class with an instructor. To locate a class, call a martial arts school and inquire about tai chi. Some Ys offer tai chi classes, as do some health clubs, colleges and adult-education programs.

"The best thing is to try a class and see how comfortable you are working with the teacher. Visit a place you are considering and talk with current students," suggests Matsumoto.

Fill the prescription.

"If someone asked me for the ideal exercise prescription for the average man or woman who wants to live a productive life in the fast lane," says LaForge, "I'd say 40 percent of it should consist of aerobic exercise (like walking or running), 20 percent of it should consist of resistance exercise (like weight training) and 40 percent should be relaxation exercise (either a form of tai chi or yoga).

"I know many researchers say that you can show a reduction in anxiety after 25 minutes of aerobic exercise. But tai chi (and also yoga) give a more substantial reduction of anxiety for a longer period of time. The quality is different. Ideally, you need both aerobic and relaxation exercise for stress reduction."

Begin and end the day.

Each course of tai chi is different, but after just a few classes you'll know enough to start experiencing the benefits, says Matsumoto.

"Once you've learned," she says, "the minimum amount of time for doing tai chi is ten minutes in the morning when you get up and ten minutes at night before you go to bed. That will help offset the stresses in your life. In the morning tai chi helps set the body in motion. Before bed the movement is calming and de-stressing."

Touching

*M*others do it to infants, lovers do it to each other, those moved by the spirit do it to whoever needs it. Even animals rely on a touch, a lick or a nuzzle to comfort and connect.

Many kinds of touching—from a friendly squeeze to a brisk massage—can restore energy, both physical and emotional, says Stanley E. Jones, Ph.D., professor of communication at the University of Colorado in Boulder and author of *The Right Touch: Understanding and Using the Language of Physical Contact.*

Certainly, "touch therapies"—massage, acupressure and the like—help to relieve muscle tension, reduce pain and improve blood flow. Research has shown that all those things can boost energy.

And researchers maintain that the ability of touch to comfort, to convey the sense of being loved and cared for, to literally connect, evaporates the biggest energy drain there is—stress.

Touching Goes Deep

Exactly how touch works its magic is under investigation. No doubt it operates in a number of ways, some more mysterious than others. Studies show that a calming touch can reduce stress hormones, strengthen immunity, reduce pain and normalize heart rate and breathing, says Tiffany Field, Ph.D., professor of pediatrics, psychology and psychiatry and director of the Touch Research Institute at the University of Miami School of Medicine.

Studies show that touch is so crucial that if babies don't get it, they may have retarded growth and mental development. In adults certain kinds of touch can confirm and reinforce intimate relationships. That's important because studies show that people who have close personal relationships develop fewer stress-related diseases than those without social ties. "Studies also show that even a casual, friendly touch on the hand, arm or shoulder makes others more open to us and more likely to see us in a friendly light," says Dr. Jones.

Getting and Giving

Still, people in the United States tend not to touch much. "Most people see touch as inherently sexual and are afraid they will be misunderstood if they use it outside the home," Dr. Jones says. Business colleagues, teachers, doctors, nurses, even clergy are concerned that a caring touch will be mistaken for a caress.

So how do we take advantage of all the energy-boosting benefits of touch without raising eyebrows?

Look for opportunities.
Whether it's a caress across a spouse's cheek, a kiss on a baby's bottom or a congratulatory squeeze on a fellow employee's shoulder, countless daily moments provide the chance for a caring touch, especially among family members, Dr. Jones says. "You can learn to see these opportunities."

Know your motives.
"The overriding factor in determining how someone will respond to your touch is your apparent intention," Dr. Jones says. So know what you want to convey.

"You may think you're communicating one thing, but if you have an unconscious desire to flirt or mixed motives, the other person is very likely to pick up on that," he notes. "We are much better at reading other people's messages than we are our own, in many cases."

Your touch should not be aggressive, manipulative or designed to put the person down. "Even an uncomfortable attempt to make contact will usually be appreciated if this rule is followed," Dr. Jones says.

Understand the context.
The meaning of a touch does not come from the type of touch alone, but also from a subtle combination of accompanying behavior and the situation in which the touch occurs, Dr. Jones says. "Get a feel for the total picture to understand what a touch might mean," he says.

Tune in to cultural differences.
Some countries are touchy-feely. In others, touch a person of the opposite sex in the wrong place, and you'll be lucky to return home with both hands.

Mediterranean countries—Greece, Italy and Spain—are big on touch. Israel, France and Brazil also tend to be tactile. To the contrary, you'll definitely want to avoid touching someone of the opposite sex in China and Japan and in Moslem countries. In fact, Moslem countries are a *very* special case because only the right hand is used for touching. The left hand is considered unclean, because it has traditionally been reserved for toilet functions.

"When visiting, take a cue from the people who live in that country," Dr. Jones suggests. "Only do what you see them do."

For an Expert Massage, Call Y-O-U

You might think you died and went to Heaven if you had a personal massage therapist to provide just the right touch whenever you needed it.

But while it's pure luxury to have professional pampering, there's something to be said for doing it yourself. The price is right, it's always instantly available and you never have to say, "Harder, please, and a little farther down to the right." You know exactly what feels good. And what feels good can get you going again if you're sleepy or sluggish.

For an energizing massage concentrate on invigorating strokes—kneading, tapping, pummeling, squeezing, rubbing, even brushing with a rough sponge or hairbrush, suggests Elliot Greene, past president of the American Massage Therapy Association in Evanston, Illinois. "If, on the other hand, you're tired because you're strung out, relaxing strokes may be more restorative," he says.

Here's the lowdown on how to give yourself an energizing massage.

Tap into energy.

Use a tapping touch over your scalp, forehead and upper chest. Keep your wrists loose and tap your fingertips quickly and rhythmically over the area. "Try starting at the back of your head, where it meets your neck, and move forward slowly until you come to your eyebrows," Greene suggests.

Chop out tension.

Use a light chop with the outside edge of your hands to loosen up muscles on your legs, arms and torso. "Spread your fingers out a little bit so your hand is not rigid like a karate chop," Greene says. "Then when you chop, your fingers will collide and open again, diffusing the blow." You can work the same muscles with a slightly cupped hand.

Touch early and often.

It's almost impossible to hold and caress babies too much, Dr. Field says. "Babies that are touched thrive better and score higher on cognitive tests."

The best stroke for an infant is gentle, firm and slow, she says. If the touch is too light, it can overstimulate and even irritate an infant.

Different areas of an infant's body respond differently to touch. To soothe an infant, gently stroke or massage the baby's back and legs. Stroking a baby's face, belly or feet tends to stimulate the infant, says Dr. Field.

Consider roughhousing.

With teenage boys, mock boxing, headlocks and hair tousling may be the only kind of touches you can get in. "Fathers and sons will roughhouse during times

Rub to revive.

To relieve energy-draining tension in your neck, massage below the ridge at the base of your skull where the neck muscles connect. "Put your hands on the back of your head, then move your thumbs down at a right angle and hook them under that ridge," Greene says. "Use your thumbs to massage in tiny circles, working out on both sides from your spine to your ears."

Try foot first-aid.

Foot massage is an excellent way to overcome fatigue and restore vitality. "There are many nerve endings in the feet, so massaging the bottom of the foot stimulates the whole body," Greene says.

Cross one leg over the other so that your right foot is on your left knee. Grasp your elevated foot with both hands and start out by gliding your thumbs in a straight line between your heel and toes. Then make little circles all over sole of your foot with your thumbs.

Pay particular attention to a spot on the sole at the bottom of the ball of your foot, between the bones of the big toe and the second toe. This point, called Bubbling Spring, is a source of energy for the entire body, Greene says. "People can intuitively find these spots, where they'll want to rub a little bit more," he says.

Freshen up with a face "wash."

For a soothing mental pick-me-up, rub your hands together fast to warm them up, move them over your face in a washing motion, then inch your fingertips back through your scalp. To finish, rub your hands together a second time, then cup them over your eyes for 30 seconds or so as you take a few deep breaths.

when a hug would be rejected as too mushy," Dr. Jones says. The only rough-housing rule: Keep it more playful than aggressive.

Know your body parts.

Don't inadvertently escalate intimacy, Dr. Jones warns. "Direct contact to the thighs, buttocks or breasts is clearly a sexual touch."

Touches, according to Dr. Jones, become increasingly intimate in the following order: handshake, hand to arm or shoulder, hand to upper back, arm around shoulders, hand to lower back, kiss on cheek, frontal upper-body hug and frontal full-body hug. (For more information on hugs, see "Hugging" on page 165.)

Because of the intimate nature of touch, touch in the workplace can be dicey in terms of sexual harassment. This is particularly true when a supervisor touches a subordinate, even if the touch is on the less intimate side of the continuum, says Jonathan Segel, a partner at Wolf, Block, Schoor and Solis-Cohen law firm in Philadelphia, and an expert who conducts training for preventing sexual harassment.

Tune in to touch taboos.
Not all unwelcome touches are sexual. Avoid pats to the hand, tickling, picking up the person or interrupting or startling someone with a touch, Dr. Jones says.

Don't be a "glue hand."
The touch that lasts too long is often confusing, suggesting the desire to control, Dr. Jones says. "If you are talking to someone you are touching, take your hand off when you are done talking," he recommends.

Touching a person off and on during a supportive conversation, especially if the person continues to express distress, is more comforting than a continual touch, which can be misconstrued as flirtatious, Dr. Jones says. "Constant contact is considered a togetherness touch."

Practice on a pet.
If you find human contact scarce or uncooperative, find a dog or cat who likes having its head scratched, Dr. Jones suggests. "Petting or cuddling a pet can provide some of the same benefits you'd get from a human."

Talk with your touch.
To make communication crystal clear, say what your touch is meant to convey: "I am really sorry you are having a hard time with this." "That's a great idea!" "Now we're getting somewhere!" The combination of verbal and touch messages underline your support and help to generate energy, Dr. Jones says.

Get feedback.
Look for a response that tells you how your message is received. "If the other person smiles and looks at you, returns the touch, moves toward you or reacts in some other positive way, it's an acceptance," Dr. Jones says.

On the other hand, if the other person looks at your hand, grimaces, scowls—or in extreme cases—says, "What are you doing?" it's a rejection.

"Even if the person simply 'freezes up' physically or doesn't respond in an expected way, it's a rejection," Dr. Jones says. "If people are willing to pay attention, they can almost always tell whether a touch is accepted or rejected. There are few people clever enough to mask their reactions completely to a touch."

Give to receive.
As long as you touch appropriately, the more touches you hand out, the more you'll get back. "If you want to be touched, touch," Dr. Jones says.

Toys

Step on a misplaced Lego while walking barefoot and you'll get a quick boost in energy all right. The problem is that it's usually expressed in language that could make a sailor blush. Or attempt to play Christmas Eve mechanic with those "partial assembly required" playthings and your temper can get hotter than Santa's mug o' chocolate.

Okay, so maybe your experiences with toys aren't all fun and games. They empty your wallet, cover your floors and can even clog your toilet—adding fuel to your parenting or grandparenting ire, a sure energy drainer.

But, hey, that's exactly why *you* need them.

Winning Isn't Everything

"One of the main roles of toys is that they provide an outlet from the stresses of life," says Edward A. Charlesworth, Ph.D., a psychologist in Houston, a recognized expert in the therapeutic use of toys, and author of *Stress Management*. "What toys do is allow us to escape from reality. And that's vitalizing and energizing . . . at any age."

In fact, that's why adults can benefit even more than children from toys—at least when it comes to boosting energy levels. For kids, toys are often used to help them develop and learn new skills. "But for adults, toys provide a recreational outlet for the pressures of life—things that can cause stress and depression and drain energy," says Dr. Charlesworth.

The key to an energizing toy, however, is to choose one that helps you unwind. "The emphasis should be on recreation and fun instead of competition," says Dr. Charlesworth. "Some competition, like that in board games, is fine because it adds to the game. But, unfortunately, too many toys for both children and adults put the emphasis on winning, which only adds to stress and fatigue."

Choosing Your Playthings

Here's what the doctors order when you're looking for amusement, leisure, distractions or any of the other energizing gratifications that grown-up children get from their toys.

Keep it simple.
"If your 'toy' requires too much maintenance, it defeats the purpose," says Dr. Charlesworth. "Many boat owners, for instance, say the best times are when they buy the boat and when they sell it. That's because so many people go into it with all these fantasies, but they don't realize all the upkeep and cost that is involved. Then it becomes more of a hassle than recreation or fun."

The same holds true for complicated machinery or other items. "When choosing a plaything, keep it as simple as possible," he advises.

Do a personality profile.
"It's important that you take a good look at the type of person you are when you're choosing a toy," says Margaret Carlisle Duncan, Ph.D., associate professor of human kinetics at the University of Wisconsin at Milwaukee and president of the North American Society of the Sociology of Sport. "If you're a problem-solver type, then you may find puzzles and other toys that require those skills to be relaxing. But if you're an impulsive, creative type, you might find them too frustrating and will probably enjoy amusing items like wind-up toys better."

Decorate your desk.
Some toys are especially useful in high-stress areas, like your desk at work. "Play is absolutely important at work and other places where fatigue can set in, because these toys help you regress to a childlike phase," says Dr. Charlesworth. "But it's important not to use toys as an ego defense mechanism to lose track of reality." That means that while it's advisable to have wind-up toys, Nerf guns and other knickknacks at work, playing with them too much can take you away from your responsibilities.

"The same holds true for computers and other home toys," says Dr. Charlesworth. "If you're doing nothing but playing with the computer all night, it can go from being a recreational diversion to an obsession and an ego defense mechanism to escape your real responsibilities."

Share the fun.
Toys that have the truest meaning are those that are shared with your family or friends. "I gave my mother a goofy picture frame made of fake fur, and each time she looks at it, it reminds her of me. And each time I see it, I think of her," says Dr. Duncan. "Things like that help us bond with our loved ones, and this social interaction is very good for boosting energy."

Walk down memory lane.

Some experts recommend that you think back to those earlier days when you had fewer responsibilities and stresses and think of the playthings that made you happy—and why. "For me it was cars," says Dr. Charlesworth. "In college I was a car buff, and it wasn't so much the driving that was important but the actual restoration . . . bringing a car back to life. Fixing an old car represents that happy, stress-free time for me, and doing it today gives me energy."

Try hands-on therapy.

Some toys do nothing but occupy your hands. "I often play with a pencil or pen while talking on the phone, because I am a handler," says Dr. Charlesworth. "I used to smoke a pipe for the same reason. It wasn't so much the actual smoking but rather the cleaning and handling of the pipe." If you know you're a handler, have some toys or objects by the phone that you enjoy touching.

Think color when choosing toys.

Studies show that children are more likely to choose and play longer with yellow and red toys over similar items in other colors. Those hues are more energizing, says Harry Wohlfarth, Ph.D., president of the International Academy of Color Sciences at the University of Alberta in Edmonton, Canada. But others find comfort in choosing items in their favorite colors.

"I've always owned blue cars because blue is my favorite color," says Dr. Charlesworth. "I think, given a choice, people should consider color when choosing a toy."

Vacations

Ever come back from a long-needed vacation only to have to spend the next few days—or weeks—recuperating? We've all had vacations in hell—nonstop rain, terminal diarrhea, family feuds, dead cars, leaky tents, tour guides named Adolf...

You get the picture. No wonder you come home feeling as though you need a vacation from your vacation.

You can't completely control a vacation any more than you can control the other events in everyday life. "In fact, a vacation may be even less controllable, since everyday life is pretty much routine and a vacation is never routine," says Brian Baird, Ph.D., professor of psychology at Pacific Lutheran University in Tacoma, Washington, and author of *Are We Having Fun Yet?*

Vacationing for Vitality

If your goal is to take some time off to restore your energy and enthusiasm, you have to know yourself and plan with your needs in mind. Getting energized from your vacation won't happen automatically. You may also need to make some attitude adjustments—maybe even revise your concept of a vacation.

"I found I had to unlearn my idea that a vacation always had to be someplace else," says Ann McGee-Cooper, Ed.D., a creativity consultant in Dallas and author of *You Don't Have to Go Home from Work Exhausted!* and *Time Management for Unmanageable People*. What she gave up, she says, is "spending a lot of money, a lot of packing and a lot of organization." Instead Dr. McGee-Cooper manages to sneak in all sorts of strange and wonderful "sanity breaks" at least twice a month.

Here's what she and other experts in the field of fun recommend for turning your vacations into energizing experiences.

Lighten up.

Do your vacation plans approach the scale and complexity of a military operation? It's time to start taking them less seriously, says Randy Petersen, editor and publisher of *Inside Flyer* magazine and impulse vacation enthusiast. "I suggest you watch one of the National Lampoon vacation movies featuring Chevy Chase," he says. "They are a great way to get some insight on what to do or not to do with vacations."

Find the fun factor.

"Most adults have forgotten how to have fun," says Dr. McGee-Cooper. "While on vacation, they may have changed their clothes but they are still working—trying to get the best deal for their money, shoving the kids in cars, trying to get out ahead of all the other tourists. While you can't avoid all of this hassle, you can be more flexible, make fewer plans, laugh and take time to *be*, not do."

Get your timing right.

Do you feel as if you can never take time off? Lots of people have that feeling, say both Dr. McGee-Cooper and Petersen. The two of them deal with this problem from opposite perspectives, however.

"When you plan your month, plan your fun," Dr. McGee-Cooper suggests. "You need at least two mini-vacations in every month to keep from getting burned out, so decide ahead of time where they will be. After you plan them, they will be set aside as pockets of free time. That's the point."

Petersen prefers a seat-of-the-pants approach (and since he owns his own company, he can get away with this). "The timing is almost never right, so I find the best thing is to go on impulse," he says. "That way, you are not dictated by your work schedule, but by your whims."

Plan ahead.

On a more practical note, major vacations should be planned at least six months in advance to get the best rates, says Petersen. Running around at the last minute can be so depleting that you won't have any energy left to enjoy yourself.

By planning way ahead, you can also take advantage of specials. It's best to travel on the "shoulders" of a vacation season—at the beginning or end, when you'll still get good weather and find open shops but will be able to avoid energy-draining crowds and peak-season prices.

Creative Vacationing

Are you spending every vacation hauling your mother-in-law around Miami when you'd like to be reeling in pike on Lake Kickback in northern Ontario?

While it's realistic to include some family obligations in your vacation plans, that's not all you should be doing, Dr. McGee-Cooper says. Here are some things to consider when putting together a vacation to energize *you*.

Go back in time.

"I ask people, 'What is it that you like to do that you don't get to do?' " says Dr. McGee-Cooper. She suggests that you close your eyes and try to recall the things that were most fun when you were a kid and on vacation. Where did you go and what made it fun? Did you camp out in your backyard? Build a tree house? Go fishing with your dad?

"Getting back to the memories that are filled with joy will help you rediscover the things you love and haven't done in years," she says. You may end up taking vacations that are nothing like the slick, expensive sort we see advertised. "People may visit family members they haven't seen for years, look up old college roommates or go back to that little town they used to live in and find childhood friends," she says.

Explore your dreams.

Another powerful way to come up with unique, fulfilling vacation plans is to recall the dreams you have had that never happened, Dr. McGee-Cooper says.

"When I was a kid, for instance, we didn't have a lot of money, and I longed to be Shirley Temple and have those shiny black tap shoes. As an adult, I bought those shoes and learned to tap dance," she says.

Your dream might be a sailing trip, a week being a cowhand on a working ranch or going to a faraway mountaintop where you can really see the Milky Way.

Consider a solo flight.

You like race-car driving. Your spouse likes antiques. If the two of you have different ideas about what's fun, consider the possibility of separate vacations. Or at least plan some separate activities during the vacation, Dr. Baird says. "If your relationship is secure, this won't be a big deal. This way, you both get to do what you really want, and everyone is happy."

Join a group.

If your family doesn't happen to share your interest in Civil War battlefields, hook up with a tour group of like-minded people. This could be a garden club's tour of British formal gardens, a historic society's trip to castles of the Rhine or a religious organization's talk-with-the-animals tour of the favorite hangouts of St. Francis of Assisi. The choices are truly exciting and endless, and you will have saved yourself lots of exhausting planning and organizing.

Look through special-interest or travel magazines for group trips or ask a travel agent to help you find one to your liking.

Retreat to Revive

You've probably noted that vacations are good for the spirit. Why not take that notion one step further and take a vacation specifically designed for the spirit?

Spiritual retreats let you put aside everyday life, take some time for yourself and create the opportunity for rejuvenation and a fresh perspective, says Stephan Rechtschaffen, M.D., president of the Omega Institute, a retreat center in Rhinebeck, New York.

Most retreats offer natural beauty, peace and quiet and a caring community for self-exploration and growth.

Ask your pastor or rabbi about retreat centers near you. Or, for about $25, you can order a directory of 583 retreats in the United States and Canada from Retreats International, P.O. Box 1067, Notre Dame, IN 46556.

Making Time

Even if you can't quite find room in your schedule for a real vacation, that doesn't mean you have to forgo the energizing benefits of getting away from it all. Here are a few alternatives.

Take mini-vacations.
More frequent three- or four-day weekends are replacing two-week or ten-day vacations for many business people, Petersen says. "And in the long run, they're probably just as invigorating. Depending on how you look at it, there's either less hell to go through or just enough pleasure."

Plan to take Friday off—and leave work an hour or two early on Thursday. By traveling that night to your destination, you avoid some of the major energy drains involved in getting away for the weekend, he says. By beating Friday's crowds you're less likely to get stuck in traffic or lose your baggage on an airline, and it will be easier to get good accommodations. Come back Sunday night or Monday.

"If you plan it right, you're out of the office only a day or two and the time is split between two different weeks, so it's almost like you were never gone at all," says Petersen. "I never feel guilty about leaving work this way."

Work while you play.
With a little forethought, you can combine business and pleasure, says Dr. McGee-Cooper. "I try never to go someplace without taking a vacation while

Get Pampered and Pummeled

Massage and other kinds of bodywork are a regular part of the daily routine at many health spas. If you're looking to de-stress, rejuvenate and energize yourself, a spa vacation is certainly an option to consider.

A visit to a health spa can be especially energizing if you go to one that offers programs that help you break negative health habits such as smoking or overeating. One advantage of a spa is that the environment allows time for you to practice these changes before you have to go home and integrate them into your life.

It's common to think of a spa vacation as the ultimate in self-indulgence. But look at it this way: If you don't take care of yourself, how are you going to be any good to anybody else?

To find the right spa for you, check out *Fodor's Healthy Escapes*, which lists hundreds of spas, fitness resorts and cruises worldwide. Or call Spa-Finders at 1-800-255-7727; in New York call (212) 924-6800. Ask for their catalog, which costs about $8, including postage and handling. The address is Spa-Finders, 91 Fifth Avenue, New York, NY 10003.

I'm there," she says. "It's nothing outrageous. I don't stay any longer. But I'm thinking, 'How can I get out of a rut within the time I have, instead of going back to the hotel and just being tired?' "

She'll ask her host (who may also be her client) about offbeat things to do. On one business trip her host planned part of a meeting, and dinner, on a boat in the nearby bay. "We all got to have fun, not just me," she says.

Don't think you're neglecting your clients if you want to have fun. "Frequently, the people you are visiting will want to do things with you, and you will bond," she adds.

Make part of each weekend into vacation time.
Plan something every weekend that you look forward to doing, Dr. McGee-Cooper recommends. That could be dabbling in some artistic pursuit, gardening, kite flying or a taking long walk. You'll find it energizing during the week to look forward to what you'll be doing, she says.

Be a kid.
Involve your own kids or grandchildren in your weekend "vacation" pursuits if you want, says Dr. McGee-Cooper. But even if you're solo, remember to "play like a kid," she adds. That means no competition or judging whether you're good enough. Just enjoy.

Travel by armchair.

Get your juices flowing with some exotic reading material, Petersen suggests. "I may read about this neat little hotel in the south of France or great new regional park in Queensland, Australia, or an original Japanese teahouse in Osaka, and it is almost as though I've taken a five-minute vacation," he says. Plus, it's a great way to come up with ideas for new places to go.

Take a virtual vacation.

For the price of a local phone call, you can cruise electronically via the World Wide Web, visiting sites around the world. "I am finding that this is one of the more pleasurable things for me now, and it certainly helps trip planning," Petersen says.

Be a tourist in your own backyard.

It's true that New York City natives are the last to see the Statue of Liberty, Dr. McGee-Cooper says. "People take their own environment for granted. They don't realize how much there is to enjoy."

Think about where you'd go if you were showing out-of-town guests around, she suggests. "What things in your locale have you never done that would be fun, that you never seem to have time to do?" What kinds of things would make you feel vital, energized and alive? What about going to an outdoor band concert on a summer night? Spending a weekend at that new bed-and-breakfast spot? Watching bears come eat the garbage at the town dump?

People often ignore great tourist activities simply because they're close to home, Petersen agrees. "I talk with people who want to go to the Australian outback who don't realize that they could see similar terrain in the California or Arizona deserts. Wherever you go around the world, there are still things undiscovered at home."

Getting Away

You've picked your destination and felt that wonderful rush of anticipation. But that doesn't mean you can ignore the details. There are several things you can do to ensure that no matter where you go, your getaway will feed your energy.

Give packing some forethought.

Make up a checklist of the items that you'll need on your trip, Dr. Baird suggests. Then, don't wait until the night before the trip to pack. "That is just a recipe for disaster," he says.

Start a few days early so that you can track down items and buy things you need. Actually check each item off your list as you pack it. Don't take anything back out of your suitcase without noting it on the list, or you may end up having to brush your teeth with your finger all week long or wear a trash bag as a rain poncho.

Go easy on your companions.

You need to adapt your activities to the people accompanying you on your trip. This is especially important if you're a sportsman introducing your family to the great outdoors, Dr. Baird says.

"I could take a 12-mile hike to an alpine lake and impose a forced march on my family," he says. "But how much fun is that going to be? They don't like to hurt themselves the way I do. So why not go on a 2-mile hike to some little pond? Then we'll all have a better time." (What's more, you won't have to listen to all that vitality-depleting whining and complaining.)

Use your experience and judgment to gauge what your family might like, Dr. Baird recommends. "I really mark it down from my own level and consider others' needs. If I know my partner doesn't like to get up at 6:00 A.M. and doesn't like to sleep in the back of a pickup, then why force her to do that? I know she is going to have a better time if we do at least some of the trip her way."

Do regular "fun checks."

What's the ultimate goal of any vacation? To have fun. Find out how your trip is going by periodically taking a break for a fun check, Dr. Baird suggests. "Simply ask each person if he is having fun. If someone is not having fun, find out why."

The idea behind this is to ensure that each person is getting at least some of what they hope for from the trip and that no one is feeling as though his needs or interests are being neglected, he says.

Vacation from your vacation.

Once you're back from your trip, allow a little time for re-entry. You'll have a more leisurely transition back if you give yourself a day at home to decompress after your trip. If you've been camping or canoeing, you'll have time to properly clean and store your expensive gear. Unpack, do laundry, water your plants, read the mail, answer phone calls, pick up Brutus at the kennel and get a good night's sleep in your own bed. You'll have more energy when you head back to work the next day.

Walking

*F*rom lotions to potions there are all sorts of notions about sidestepping fatigue—and it's amazing how quickly some folks will dash off to pursue them. But for a fast, effective and no-cost way to keep one step ahead of the doldrums, all you have to do is stay one step ahead of where you've been.

Walking may indeed be the ultimate energizer—requiring no special talents (chewing gum while doing it is optional, of course), equipment (although proper walking shoes are advised) or environment. And since you've been doing it since those diaper days, there's nothing to learn . . . except maybe exactly how great it can be for your mind and body.

A brisk ten-minute walk can almost immediately raise your energy level and keep it elevated for up to two hours, according to Robert Thayer, Ph.D., professor of psychology at California State University in Long Beach and author of *The Origin of Everyday Moods*.

A Step in the Right Direction

"Even though energy is used during exercise, it creates more," says William J. Evans, Ph.D., professor of applied physiology and nutrition and director of the Noll Physiological Research Center at Pennsylvania State University in University Park. "That's because the muscles and cardiovascular system are like a car engine. Regular exercise can increase the efficiency and horsepower of the engine. Thus, whenever you perform any activity, it feels easier."

While any aerobic exercise is helpful and energizing, walking has an added advantage because it causes less impact on joints than more jarring forms of exercise such as running. And it can be done anytime and anywhere by anyone with two good legs. "For most people walking is the easiest way to get more physical activity into their day," says James Rippe, M.D., associate professor of

(continued on page 238)

Walk All Over Fatigue

On your worst days, do you feel like a lure for listlessness? You can turn the tables on tiredness by taking it in stride—literally. Walking is a great way to dump the doldrums. Even if you can't harvest a couch potato partner to join you in your strolling, it's fun for the mind and body even when done solo. Here's a fatigue-fighting, step-by-step walking program recommended by Mark Bricklin, co-author of *Prevention's Practical Encyclopedia of Walking for Health* to keep you from loafing in your loafers.

Week 1

Day One: Do less than you're able. Take a walk that's comfortable for you, whether it's around the block or two miles—but no more. Concentrate on enjoying it.

Day Two: Evaluate yesterday's walk. If you took our advice, you shouldn't be very sore, if at all. Also check for blisters and other foot problems. If you're able, make today's walk at least as far as yesterday's—maybe a little farther. If you're not up to it, walk less. Just enjoy it!

Day Three: Walk the same distance as yesterday. Again, concentrate on enjoying your walk, not setting a record.

Day Four: Fine-tune your technique. Evaluate your posture and pace. You should walk erect, not hunched over, and you should be able to speak while walking. If you're too short of breath to talk, you're probably going too fast.

Day Five: Increase the distance a bit. If everything's going well, up the ante anywhere from a block to a quarter mile, but no more. If you're sore, take it down a notch from what you did yesterday.

Day Six: Record your strides per minute. Walk the same distance as yesterday if you're up to it, but get a watch and count how many times your right foot hits the ground in one minute. Do this several times, and record the average number in a walking journal. Most people average 60 strides per minute.

Day Seven: Rest. Don't walk today, but if you're curious, drive your walking route to see how far you went. Most people wonder how far they've walked. Also, tune in to your body to see if your walking has made you feel more refreshed and more energetic.

Week 2

Day One: Take your pulse rate on a morning when you wake naturally without an alarm clock, such as a weekend morning. This is what's called your resting pulse rate—in other words, the basic rate of your heartbeat when your body is totally at rest. (It's different with each person.) Take your pulse rate by placing the first two fingers of your left hand on the inside of your right wrist, about an inch above the heel of your hand. Count your pulse for one minute. Record that number in your journal. Later on, you can compare your resting pulse rate to help monitor your fitness.

Also today, walk about the same distance you did two days ago, or two to five minutes longer if you can.

Day Two: Walk the same distance you did yesterday but, again, pay attention to posture and pace.

Day Three: Walk the same distance you did yesterday but now pay attention to your feet. Try to point them straight ahead as you walk. It's good form, but don't be overly concerned if your feet bow out or in a little bit.

Day Four: Increase your walk by another minute or two.

Day Five: Do another foot check. Make sure that you haven't developed blisters or other problems. Walk the same distance as yesterday.

Day Six: Again, walk the same distance as yesterday, but remember posture, pace and pleasure.

Day Seven: Rest. You may think you've been going too slowly, but actually your body's begun to change. You're probably storing more carbohydrate fuel in your leg muscles for energy, and those muscles are probably stronger than they were 14 days ago. Become aware of your energy level. Review the past two weeks. Do you have more stamina? Are you feeling less tired more often?

Week 3

Strategy: Add a few more minutes to your weekly total. You're probably averaging 20 to 40 minutes per day and are ready to increase your time gradually. Remember to take your resting pulse rate at least one morning this week and record it. The more fit you are, the lower your pulse rate will go.

(continued)

Walk All Over Fatigue—Continued

Week 4

By the end of this week, you should have doubled what you walked on your very first day. Measure the distance of your new route again if you're curious. Also, concentrate on your energy levels. You should feel rejuvenated more often. And don't forget to take your weekly resting pulse rate.

Week 5

Keep it steady. Stick with the same distance you walked last week for this entire week. It will give your body a chance to rest. You're now into your second month, and you don't want to burn out early. Don't forget to monitor your resting pulse one morning. And don't forget to give yourself a day of rest.

Week 6

Add up to five minutes to your weekly total. Is your resting pulse showing an improvement? Evaluate your walking program. Is it still fun or does it seem like too much work? Remember to keep it fun.

Week 7

Keep it steady. By now, posture and pace should be second nature. Practice refining your walking skills, but don't increase the distance.

Week 8

You're completing your second month of walking, so evaluate your whole routine. Do you feel less fatigued? Do you have more energy during the day? How is your resting pulse? What about enjoyment—are you still having fun? You should be. If not, is it because you're walking too far, too fast? If so, slow down and enjoy. For this week's walk add a few minutes to your time on alternating days.

medicine at Tufts University School of Medicine in Boston and author of *Dr. James Rippe's Complete Book of Fitness Walking*.

When you walk, you burn about 100 calories per mile—roughly the same as you would burn running (but because runners usually cover more distance, they'll fry more calories). Your heart and lungs work harder, releasing endor-

Week 9

Measure your pace and alternate walks. Take your car and measure a one-mile walk. Walk this course and time your pace. (As you clock your one-mile pace in the future, use this same course.) As for your daily walks, alternate long and short walks, but make sure your "long" walk isn't more than ten minutes longer than your "short" walk.

Week 10

Increase your walk by a few minutes or a quarter mile if you're up to it.

Week 11

Pace yourself on the one-mile course. Include several one-mile walks this week in your daily routine. Again, measure your one-mile pace. Is it about the same each time? If so, good. You've established a steady rhythm.

Week 12

Do two 45-minute walks this week. If you have the time and you're up to it, do the entire 45-minute walk at one clip. If not, break it down into one 30-minute walk and one 15-minute walk. How are your energy levels? Your resting pulse? Enjoyment?

Week 13 and Beyond

You've now completed three months of walking—not bad, since the average person drops out in three weeks. This week, try walking the greatest distance you covered last week—only see if you can do this on three separate days. (But cut your other walks by 10 to 15 minutes to avoid overdoing it.) Tips for the upcoming weeks include gradually increasing your one-mile pace, increasing overall walking time to 45 minutes or more or walking up hills and other challenging courses.

phins—natural hormones that promote a feeling of well-being. Walking has been linked with reducing energy-drainers like stress, anxiety and depression and even heart conditions like high cholesterol and high blood pressure. And if all those benefits aren't enough, it can also boost immunity and even your sex life.

Taking Energy in Stride

Best of all, even a little walking goes a long way. Although experts once believed that, as with other forms of aerobic exercise, you needed to walk for at least 20 continuous minutes (and preferably 30) to reap the benefits, newer research shows that any amount of walking can start this energizing process, says Dr. Thayer. The big benefits begin to kick in at about 10 minutes, and you'll profit even more from walking briskly for longer periods.

Here's what experts suggest to help you get the most from every step.

Start off slowly.

If you're just beginning a walking program, concentrate on form rather than on distance. Walk with your head erect, shoulders back and hips swinging freely to take pressure off your lower back.

"Our first suggestions are always the same: Slow down!" advises David Balboa, who with his wife teaches proper walking form at the Walking Center of New York City. "Remember: form first, speed second. As your heel contacts the ground, feel that connection firmly. Then roll your foot forward toward your toe and allow your foot to press into the ground. The major source of power for moving forward in walking comes from pushing off with the toe and the calf muscles of the trailing leg. Don't bend forward from the waist. The power in your walking gait is directly related to your ability to stretch your trailing leg."

Build gradually.

The American Podiatric Medical Association suggests that you slowly work up to a brisk speed that covers a mile in about 15 minutes—or a four-mile-per-hour pace. Your walks should ideally last at least 20 minutes, and if you're just a beginner, an hour is the max. The goal, say experts, is to try to increase your walking time or mileage by 10 percent each week.

Set a schedule.

If you walk at the same time each day, you'll be less likely to think of it as an expendable activity, says John Duncan, Ph.D., professor of clinical research at the Center on Research for Women's Health at Texas Woman's University in Denton. He advises setting up a firm time—say, from 6:00 to 7:00 P.M., three days per week—to make it part of your routine.

If you can't do that, Dr. Thayer advises going for a walk whenever you need a quick energy boost. For instance, during the midafternoon slump nearly all of us have, go for a stroll instead of a coffee break. Or take a walk just before you eat lunch, since research shows that walking can help decrease your appetite.

Look into shoes.

Although you don't necessarily need walking shoes, most experts agree that they're a good idea. Ill-fitting shoes can lead to blisters, while good shoes can make you feel as if you're walking on air.

Walking shoes have a firm heel that is beveled to keep your foot more stable, says Dr. Duncan. They also have good arches for support and sturdy lacing to keep your foot from sliding. But regular athletic shoes are fine as long as they fit well.

Water

We all know what happens to houseplants when they don't get enough water. They droop, as their cells lose their rigid structure. One look at their flaccid state is enough to remind us that it's time to get out the watering can.

People who don't get enough water don't actually wilt, of course, but they do get a droopy, draggy feeling, with heavy arms and legs and less energy. The problem is that they may not readily connect that droopy feeling with a need for water.

"People are already somewhat dehydrated by the time their body thirst signals kick in," explains Wayne Askew, Ph.D., professor and director in the Division of Foods and Nutrition at the University of Utah in Salt Lake City. Older people have even less sensitive thirst triggers and may be chronically dehydrated if they rely on thirst alone to tell them when to drink.

Water is important for energy production for several reasons, Dr. Askew says. Every cell in your body relies on water to dilute chemicals, vitamins and minerals to just the right concentrations. The body also depends on the bloodstream to transport nutrients and other substances from one part to another. And this, too, depends on optimal fluid concentration. Blood actually thickens when you're dehydrated, which means that the heart has to work harder to supply the oxygen you need.

"Although research has focused on the consequences of severe dehydration, it stands to reason that when vital components are in a less than optimal fluid concentration, cells are handicapped. Fatigue is a very likely consequence," Dr. Askew explains.

Staying Liquid

There are steps you can take to make sure that you get enough water to keep your body running at maximum efficiency. Try some of the following suggestions from Dr. Askew.

Get your eight-a-day.

Even if you're inactive, you should drink the equivalent of eight glasses (8-ounces each) of fluids a day, including water, juice and soup. Watch out for salty soups, though, they'll increase your need for water. You need this much just to replace the fluid lost each day when you're urinating, breathing and sweating normally.

Rise and sip.

When you wake up, you are already pretty dehydrated. So have your first drink of the day while you're still in your jammies.

Get more when you need it.

If you're sweating a lot, taking medications or working in a dry environment, you may need 10 to 20 glasses (8-ounces each) of fluid a day. You'll know you need more water if your urine is dark in color or if you're not urinating much.

Don't wait until you're thirsty to drink.

Your body's thirst mechanism doesn't kick in until you are already pretty well dehydrated. You can, in fact, lose up to 2 percent of your body weight as sweat or urine before you feel really thirsty. For a 150-pound person, that's 3 pounds of fluid!

Fill up before you work out.

To stay hydrated and not feel waterlogged during exercise, drink a large glass of water 30 to 60 minutes before you begin your workout. This gives your body time to absorb it into your bloodstream. Take a few more sips just before you begin.

Sip while you're sweating.

Continue to drink during exertion. Take a few sips every 15 minutes or so. If you wait until you feel really thirsty, you'll already be dehydrated.

Avoid caffeinated drinks.

Coffee, tea and colas can help make you more dehydrated in the long run because they increase urination, resulting in water loss from the body.

If you're sick, juice it.

If you're losing fluid from diarrhea or vomiting, drink diluted fruit juices such as orange or grapefruit juice to replace the potassium you lose.

Don't count beer as a "replacement fluid."

It might go down easy, but if you're really thirsty on a hot summer day, guzzle down a big glass of cold water first, then sip that brew. Alcoholic beverages increase urination, which can lead to dehydration. And even though beer seems like a thirst quencher, its alcohol dries you out.

3

Beating the Energy DEMONS

Aging

You get older with every breath you take. And with age come some inevitable facts of life: Your hair will get grayer and thinner. Your metabolism will slow down. Your reflexes will lose some sharpness. Body parts will show signs of wear and tear. As songwriter Leonard Cohen put it, you'll ache in the places where you used to play.

For the most part, those changes are as inevitable as death and taxes. But a decline in energy is not inevitable. In fact, there are lots of things that you can do to make sure you're raring to go even while you're reeling in the years.

Never Give Up, Never Give In

Older muscles are a bit weaker, and older organs might not function as efficiently, so it can take more energy to do physical activities. But fatigue and lethargy are by no means preordained. Medical experts now know that the energy decline that we associate with age is due to how we think and feel as well as what happens physically.

"We blame a lot of things on aging itself, but we're finding that a lot of what we call aging is due to inactivity," says Ben Douglas, Ph.D., assistant vice-chancellor for graduate studies at the University of Mississippi Medical Center in Jackson and author of *Ageless: Living Younger Longer.*

We tend to be less physically active as we get older. Our concerns change, our time becomes limited, our friends say, "Let's play cards," not "Let's go roller skating." But, says Dr. Douglas, the way to generate energy is by using it.

Here's how to adjust the tempo on the march of time and keep your energy levels up and running.

Check Your Attitude

"The common perception of getting older is, 'When you're 20, you're hot; when you're 40, you're not; when you're 60, you're shot,' " says Stanley Teitelbaum, Ph.D., a clinical psychologist in New York and New Jersey and faculty member and director of supervisory training at the Postgraduate Center for Mental Health in New York City. "This doesn't have to be the reality."

Your age is just a number, he points out. And here's how to keep the number from doing a number on you.

Examine your image of aging.

Do you equate getting older with deterioration? "A lot of our thinking dates back to a time when 50 was considered old," says Ross Goldstein, Ph.D., a psychologist and consultant in San Francisco and author of *fortysomething: Claiming the Power and the Passion of Your Midlife Years.* Question the notion that chronological age determines vitality, he urges: "There have been scientific, nutritional and medical advances that allow us to remain quite energetic, productive and enthusiastic throughout our life span."

You'll find that simply questioning your assumptions is a very energizing thing to do, according to Dr. Goldstein.

Separate the changeable from the inevitable.

The challenge, says Dr. Goldstein, is to accept gracefully the inexorable changes of aging while taking constructive steps to remain youthful. "Develop a realistic, but optimistic awareness of how much control you have," he advises. It would be foolhardy to think that you can avoid all the consequences of aging, but equally foolish to think that you have to cash in your chips ahead of time.

Stay connected.

People tend to narrow their social horizons as they get older, associating only with people like themselves. "Stay exposed to diverse groups of people with diverse opinions and lifestyles," Dr. Goldstein recommends. "The stimulation can be very energizing."

Stay open.

Don't be a fuddy-duddy, passing stiff judgment on new trends and fashions. Instead, try to stay current. "Being open-minded makes available a lot more energy and avoids the drain of negativity," says Dr. Goldstein.

This doesn't mean you have to adopt MTV styles or take up bungee jumping. "It means adopting an attitude of curiosity, asking 'What's this all about?' " he adds.

Hang out with youngsters.

As George Bernard Shaw said, youth is wasted on the young. "Being around young people helps you participate in life in a more youthful way," says Dr. Teitelbaum.

One particularly constructive way to do this is to become a mentor at work or in your community. "The willingness to mentor keeps you connected to younger people and gives you a sense of continuity," says Dr. Goldstein. You might not want a pierced ear and ponytail for yourself, but it's challenging, amusing and energizing to be around kids who are trying out such things.

Cultivate self-acceptance.

"Make a realistic assessment of who you are, what you're about and what matters to you, and accept it," Dr. Goldstein advises. "If you can accept who you are, the energy that used to go into suppression becomes available for constructive purposes." If socializing, taking trips or going to ball games are your preferences, don't fight it. Make the most of those times—and try to get more.

Keep your sense of humor.

In one study Dr. Douglas interviewed a number of people who were over 100. They varied widely in race, religion, national origin, socioeconomic status, educational background and other characteristics. The one thing that they had in common was a great sense of humor.

"Keep laughing," advises Dr. Douglas. "It gives you an internal chemical high. Don't take things or yourself too seriously. And stay around cheerful people—it's catching."

Look at the bright side.

So *what* if you don't look as good in a bathing suit as you did when you were 20? It's energizing to think about what you have going for you, says Dr. Goldstein.

"Consider all the things that you do better now than when you were 20, how much more you know and how much you have going for you as a result of maturity," he says. In other words, focus on the benefits of aging, from senior discounts to permission to be eccentric.

Staying Young in Mind

"Humans are much like bicycles," says Dr. Douglas. "As long as a bicycle is moving forward it does okay. When it slows, it begins to wobble."

Keeping your mind alert and your imagination active will keep you moving forward in an energetic way. Here's how.

Stay productive.

"Doing something meaningful translates into more vitality," says Dr. Teitelbaum. Whether you stay on the job past the usual retirement age or tackle problems in your community, it's energizing to feel useful, he says.

Hang out with the gang.

Studies show that people who are active in society maintain good physical and mental health as they age, says Maria A. Fiatarone, M.D., chief of the physiology

Staying Energized for Sex

One of the more pernicious myths about aging is that you "dry up" and lose your energy for sex. Not so, says Stanley Teitelbaum, Ph.D., a clinical psychologist in New York and New Jersey and faculty member and director of supervisory training at the Postgraduate Center for Mental Health in New York City.

"For physiological reasons we tend to have sex less frequently than we did in our younger years, and it may take longer to get aroused," says Dr. Teitelbaum. "But there is ample research to indicate that people are capable of having sex to a ripe old age."

Older women may need some additional vaginal lubrication, and older men may need some help from their partner to achieve an erection, but such adjustments are easy to make, according to Dr. Teitelbaum. It's worth the effort, too. "Any time you connect sexually, you feel energized," he says.

But isn't sex a drain on your energy? Not if you do it right, says Felice Dunas, Ph.D., a doctor of Chinese medicine in private practice in Los Angeles. "When a man and woman get together in a loving, generous manner, sex can be an energy-generating experience, not an energy-consuming experience," she says. By stimulating blood flow, heart rate, respiration and electrochemical activity in the nervous system, sex can create energy.

Having too many orgasms can be dissipating to your stamina, adds Dr. Dunas, which is why aging couples should not feel compelled to climax every time they have sex. "The ancient Chinese held that conserving sexual energy by not pushing to the finish line is the key to longevity," says Dr. Dunas. "It's called pleasure without pressure. They separate ejaculation from orgasm."

It's a good idea to remember the exquisite, energizing pleasures of affection, touching and foreplay activity, even if it doesn't always culminate in intercourse, advises Dr. Teitelbaum.

---

laboratory at the U.S. Department of Agriculture Human Nutrition Research Center on Aging at Tufts University in Boston. "It doesn't matter what the activities are, whether recreational, volunteer or paid work, as long as it fits your desires and needs," she says.

Think big.

"You have a set of nerve cells with a very large number of connections, and you're endowed with those cells for a lifetime," says Zaven Khachaturian, Ph.D., director of the Ronald and Nancy Reagan Institute for Research of the Alzheimer's Association, which is headquartered in Chicago. "Maintaining them is a critical factor in determining the quality of life."

How can we keep those brain cells ticking along in a healthy, energetic way? An ongoing diet of mental exercises is the way to go, according to Dr. Khachaturian. Do puzzles, for example, or learn a new language. "The brain needs challenges that require concentration, attention, learning and remembering."

Leap into the unknown.

Novelty is important, says Dr. Khachaturian. "Do things that are challenging, new and different." If you have kept house, learn about car engines. If you have worked on car engines your whole life, learn to cook.

Wallow in learning.

"Engage in lifelong learning endeavors," suggests Dr. Goldstein. "Take courses or do self-study, but make sure you're learning something fresh or going deeper into something that you're interested in."

Get into Shape

Using your body is another key to staying energetic as you age. "You have a lot more control than you think," says Dr. Fiatarone. "The things we think have to happen as we get older—losing strength, muscle mass and endurance—can be delayed until very late in life."

It takes only a small amount of time and effort on a regular basis to prevent, or even reverse, a decline in energy, says Dr. Fiatarone. Here's how to stay fit and energetic as you age.

Accept fewer shortcuts.

True, modern conveniences can help you conserve your energy, but they can also encourage laziness. "Labor-saving devices can be counterproductive," says Dr. Fiatarone. "In the long run, you can become functionally impaired and less able to do things." Use the stairs instead of the elevator, she urges. Walk instead of taking a cab. Stand up and change channels instead of using the remote control.

Stretch your exercise plan.

If working out is new to you, consult your doctor or another qualified health care practitioner and design a program that's suitable for your overall condition. A good program might include stretching, strengthening and aerobic exercise, says Dr. Fiatarone. Start slowly and increase the intensity of your workouts gradually. To keep your interest lively, you may want to add variety to the workouts. Make it fun, not drudgery.

Hoof it.

Walking is generally the exercise of choice for older people, according to Dr. Douglas. "It's the best activity because it doesn't cause any joint or leg problems," he says. "It's great for the lower body and also for cardiovascular conditioning." Plus you can do it anywhere, anytime.

Hoist a little weight.

Supplement your aerobic exercise with strength-building activities, says Dr. Fiatarone. "Aerobics don't keep your muscles in shape or keep you from losing muscle mass as you get older," she says. If you do some lifting, your muscles will stay in far better trim. Start with light weights, then gradually increase the weight you're using, she adds.

You're Only As Old As You Eat

With age, the body's metabolism changes. Essentially, your margin of error is reduced. If you eat high-fat, high-calorie, low-nutrition foods, you'll see a more immediate effect. As you age, it's harder to control your weight and keep your energy levels up, says Dr. Goldstein.

With the changes in your body, your nutritional requirements may change also, if, for example, your energy level changes or as your digestive tract ages. The way you respond to nutrients may also change, says Joanne Curran-Celentano, R.D., Ph.D., associate professor of nutritional sciences at the University of New Hampshire in Durham.

It becomes important to have appropriate nutrients at the right time and under the right conditions, Dr. Khachaturian says. Here's how diet can help feed your energy as you age.

Eat less, more often.

It's a good practice to eat smaller meals, more frequently—and earlier, according to Dr. Goldstein. Smaller, more frequent meals keep insulin levels lower and more stable. This may help keep your energy on an even keel. In addition, studies show that the heart pumps more blood after a heavy meal than after a light meal.

Light meals may even help prevent heart attacks. Why? Studies show that cholesterol levels are lower in people who eat mini-meals than in those who eat three square meals a day.

Focus on quality, not quantity.

We tend to eat a lot more than we need, says Dr. Khachaturian. Studies have shown that animals eating fewer calories have less risk of degenerative diseases and live longer. Of course, if you go too far, you can end up malnourished, he notes. "Reduce the total calories you consume, but make sure that you get the appropriate amount of necessary nutrients," he says.

Cut the fat.
Limit foods with high fat content, advises Dr. Douglas. A high-fat diet is a major cause of all kinds of health problems that can slow you down, including cardio-vascular disease, high blood pressure, diabetes, stroke and some types of cancer. A study at the University of Kentucky found that adults ages 30 to 50 with moderately high levels of cholesterol can lower those levels by as much as 9 percent just by trimming their fat intake to 25 percent of total calories.

Limit the simple.
The kind of carbohydrates found in sugar—simple carbohydrates—should be eaten only in moderation, says Dr. Douglas.

"The sugar molecule itself is not dangerous," explains Dr. Douglas, but when you eat sugar, your blood sugar rises. In response your body pours out insulin, which drags the blood sugar way down. This is a normal process within your body, explains Dr. Curran-Celentano. Simple sugars can make blood sugar rise more quickly, which may have a negative effect on your energy level.

Add complex to your diet.
Complex carbohydrates—corn, beans, potatoes, rice, pasta—are high-energy foods, according to Dr. Douglas. "Complex carbs get broken down into simple sugars at a steady pace," he says, "so the blood sugar doesn't bounce up and down and the energy level doesn't wax and wane."

Mind your potassium/sodium ratio.
Getting more potassium than sodium helps you maintain a young cardiovascular system, says Dr. Douglas. "Blood pressure tends to remain lower in some people. It's easier to have a high energy level if you have a healthy cardiovascular system."

So, avoid salty foods and eat more potassium-rich foods. Some of the heavy hitters in the potassium department include raisins, bananas, dates and potatoes baked with the skin on.

Alcohol

You have a couple of drinks, and you start to unwind. The aches and pains that may have slowed you down get numb, your anxieties miraculously disappear and your inhibitions are less inhibiting. Next thing you know you're whirling about like Fred Astaire or Ginger Rogers and flirting like Cary Grant or Mae West. Alcohol lowers your energy? Give me a break.

Sad, but true . . . . Like a pink elephant, the energizing effect of booze is a delusion. Alcohol is a depressant. Like all depressants, it slows down your reflexes, your metabolism and your brain. It's relaxing but actually depletes your energy and reduces your ability to function efficiently.

Over time, many of its effects contribute to chronic energy depletion. It interferes with your sleep. It also damages your internal organs, like the liver, intestines and heart. Alcohol causes blood sugar imbalance, and it adds superfluous calories to your diet, contributing to weight gain. And on top of everything else, it interferes with the absorption of some nutrients and uses up others while it's being metabolized and detoxified.

Daze of Alcohol

If you get really hooked on booze, the energy picture looks even worse. "If you're addicted to something, you expend a lot of energy making sure that you get the substance into your body," says Anne Simons, M.D., assistant clinical professor of family and community medicine at the University of California, San Francisco. "Plus, the physical changes that result from addiction take up a certain amount of energy themselves. The withdrawal symptoms that you experience when you don't drink—tremors, rapid heart rate, elevated temperature—are very taxing to the body."

Need further convincing? Just think how energetic you felt the last time you drank too much. Now think about how you felt the morning after. Did you need a designated driver? How about a designated lover, designated exerciser, designated parent or designated worker?

There's a lot of talk these days about the health benefits of alcohol. It seems that a drink or two a day may lower the risk of heart attacks. Don't let that be an excuse to drink three or four or more, says Dr. Simons. If the juice is draining your juice, here's what to do about it.

Pace yourself.

"Nurse your drinks and take a break between them," advises John Brick, Ph.D., a biological psychologist and executive director of Intoxikon, a forensic and educational consulting firm in alcohol and drug studies, in Yardley, Pennsylvania. After you have a drink, your blood alcohol level rises gradually for as much as 90 minutes, depending on how much alcohol you have consumed and when you last ate. If you drink too rapidly, you might not realize how intoxicated you're going to become and think you can handle even more, says Dr. Brick.

Eat protein.

"Foods high in protein stay in the system longer," says Seymour Diamond, M.D., director of the Diamond Headache Clinic in Chicago and author of *The Hormone Headache*. "This keeps something in the stomach to slow down the absorption of the alcohol." Hors d'oeuvres or other appetizers can do the trick.

Reach for the fruit bowl.

Fructose, a natural sugar, helps the body burn off alcohol, says Dr. Diamond. Nibbling on apples, cherries or grapes may help. Or since honey is high in fructose, you may want to spread it on bread. And some fruit juice the next morning may reduce the impact of any alcohol that lingers in your system.

Drink lots of water.

A glass of water between alcoholic beverages will slow your pace of consumption and reduce your level of dehydration. Liquor inhibits production of a key pituitary hormone, causing more water to leave the body, says Dr. Brick. The result is that brain cells become dehydrated. It's not dangerous, but it does contribute to hangovers and the energy-sapping effects of alcohol. To replenish lost fluid, drink as much water as is comfortable, especially before going to bed.

Take a shot of Gatorade.

With the loss of fluid comes a loss of important minerals and salts, says Dr. Brick. Replenish them with a sports drink after the party or the next morning.

Change drinks.

It's not just how much you drink but what you drink that contributes to the energy-depleting effects of alcohol. People react to beverages in individual ways, but, in general, the darker-colored spirits cause more unpleasant side effects, says Dr. Brick. So vodka and gin may be less depleting than rum and whiskey. And white wine is less likely to cause morning-after discomfort than red.

Do You Have a Drinking Problem?

Most drinkers are not alcohol abusers or alcoholics, says John Brick, Ph.D., a biological psychologist and executive director of Intoxikon, a forensic and educational consulting firm in alcohol and drug studies in Yardley, Pennsylvania. An alcohol abuser engages in unnecessary and dangerous use of alcohol at some legal and social cost, whereas an alcoholic is dependent on alcohol.

No matter what the distinction, here are some questions to ask yourself to determine whether or not you have a problem with alcohol. If you respond positively to two or three of these questions, call your local Alcoholics Anonymous or your county's council on alcohol, suggests Dr. Brick.

1. *How important is it?* One sign of a drinking problem is that you give it too high a priority, says Mark Goulston, M.D., assistant clinical professor of psychiatry at the University of California, Los Angeles, and author of *Get Out of Your Own Way.* Do you look for ways to squeeze it into your daily schedule? Do you sneak drinks? Do you find yourself distracted because you're thinking about when and where you can take the next drink?

2. *How badly do you need it?* Is it difficult to do something unpleasant without the comfort of booze? Do you find the thought of an alcohol-free social event intimidating or boring? Do you ever need an eye-opener first thing in the morning to calm your nerves? Are you ever afraid to not drink (you could be afraid of withdrawal symptoms)?

Stretch it out.
The dehydrating effect of alcohol can prevent the body from effectively moving toxins out of the muscles. "You'll feel more energetic and comfortable if you stretch your whole body for 10 to 15 minutes," suggests Felice Dunas, Ph.D., a doctor of Chinese medicine in private practice in Los Angeles. "It improves circulation and reduces the lactic acid level in the muscles, thereby alleviating muscular aches and pains."

When It's Time to Stop

What if you have done some soul-searching and come to realize that your drinking has become a major-league, energy-consuming problem in your life? Now what do you do?

3. *How's your performance?* Have you ever gotten into trouble at work or school because of alcohol? Has drinking ever led you to neglect your obligations for two or more days in a row? Do you ever cancel meetings because you don't want to be seen intoxicated? Do colleagues avoid you when you have been drinking?

4. *Are you in command?* This is the behavioral acid test, says Dr. Brick. Can you control your drinking? Do you end up drinking more than you intend to? Do you have trouble stopping after a couple of drinks?

5. *What impact does your drinking have on other people?* Have the people closest to you ever expressed concern for your health or safety because of your drinking? Do they nag you to stop? Has alcohol ever cost you a friendship?

6. *Do you have to drink large amounts of alcohol to feel any effect?* This means you have developed more tolerance of alcohol. Having to drink ever greater amounts can lead to greater damage from the toxic effects of alcohol.

7. *What does your intuition tell you?* Do you think you're a problem drinker? Have you ever felt guilty or ashamed about your drinking? Are you hiding it from others? "As a rule of thumb, if you think you might be drinking too much, you probably are," says Anne Simons, M.D., assistant clinical professor of family and community medicine at the University of California, San Francisco.

To begin with, you can congratulate yourself for waking up to the situation. The first and most important step is to recognize that you have a problem and admit to yourself that you need to change, says Dr. Simons. "Once you do that," she says, "it's a lot easier to have the willpower to simply not drink." That doesn't mean that it will be easy. For many people, it's as hard to give up alcohol as it is to quit smoking.

If you simply can't manage to quit on your own, don't hesitate to reach out to others for help. "People won't think worse of you if you solicit help," says Dr. Simons. "More than likely, it's not a big secret and they'll respect you for owning up to the problem."

You can call on friends and family, but don't stop there. Most municipalities have a council on alcoholism that provides information on where to get help. Look for listings under "Alcoholism" in the yellow pages. And, of course, there are support groups, in particular the venerable Alcoholics Anonymous. "Such

Make a Point of Acupuncture

If at first you don't succeed . . . Quitting alcohol, or any other addiction for that matter, is notoriously difficult. Now there's yet another weapon in the anti-addiction arsenal—and it has a sharp point. A number of sharp points, actually.

The ancient Chinese art of acupuncture, which uses needles to stimulate healing responses in the nervous system, has shown some success in the treatment of addiction. "Studies show that acupuncture increases the success rates of addiction programs for all drugs, including alcohol," says Felice Dunas, Ph.D., a doctor of Chinese medicine and licensed acupuncturist in private practice in Los Angeles.

"The physical addiction can be broken quickly with acupuncture. But alcohol leaves systemic imbalances that have to be treated to get the body back to health," says Dr. Dunas. Complete recovery requires a great deal of effort by the body. A few months of weekly or biweekly treatments will help you feel twice as healthy in half the time, she says.

If you're interested in giving this ancient aid to willpower a try, here are several avenues to pursue. Contact addiction clinics—they may be able to refer you to acupuncturists who treat addictions. Speak to physicians who specialize in addiction. Call the National Certification Commission for Acupuncture (NCCA) at (202) 232-1404 or send $3.00 (check or money order) with a written request for a list of certified acupuncturists in your state to NCCA, P.O. Box 97075, Washington, DC 20090-7075.

groups have a twofold benefit," says Mark Goulston, M.D., assistant clinical professor of psychiatry at the University of California, Los Angeles, and author of *Get Out of Your Own Way.* "They help you kick the addiction, and they help you develop ways to be in social situations without resorting to drink."

You can look up Alcoholics Anonymous in your phone directory. It's located just about everywhere, and it has worked for millions of people. "It may not be for everybody," says Dr. Simons, "but I believe that everyone who has a drinking problem or is an alcoholic should give it a try."

Like smokers who are experts in quitting because they have done it so many times, most people who try to stop drinking are not successful at first. If you have a setback, be easy on yourself. "Instead of beating yourself to death for making a mistake," says Dr. Goulston, "convert your self-contempt into self-determination." Ask yourself what you should have done and make a plan of action for the next time the situation arises.

Allergies

Allergies are sly energy robbers. While some allergies knock you out by making you cough, sneeze or itch, others are so well disguised that they slip by almost unnoticed. You feel exhausted, wiped out, without knowing why.

Allergies occur when the immune system overreacts to an otherwise harmless invader, like pollen, peanuts or animal dander. It takes a lot of energy for the body to mount an immune response. What's more, the drugs commonly used to treat allergies can also make you feel tired.

Whether you're allergic to dust or dander, pollen or perfume, experts offer a number of ways to bring your energy levels back to normal.

Create comfortable quarters.
Since you spend a lot of your time at home—and since it's the one environment that you can readily control—it makes sense to begin with an allergy sweep. "Limiting exposure to your allergy trigger should be your first line of defense," says allergist and immunologist Daryl R. Altman, M.D., director of Allergy Information Services in Hewlett, New York. For example:

- Use zippered plastic or vinyl covers on your box spring, mattress and pillows to help reduce exposure to dust mites, a common cause of allergies.
- Substitute hypoallergenic pillows and comforters for feather-stuffed ones.
- Leave floors bare rather than put down carpets or rugs that harbor dust mites.
- Use shades instead of curtains, since shades attract less dust.
- Keep rooms spare, with a minimum of dust-collecting bric-a-brac or clutter.
- Consider installing a high-efficiency air filter to keep the air clean and pure.
- Move your pet out of your bed and into its own.

Investigate medications.
Drugs used to treat allergies are a common cause of fatigue. This is particularly true of older types of antihistamines, like diphenhydramine (Benadryl) or hydroxyzine (Vistaril).

Picture Relief

When it comes to allergies, the mind is a powerful master. Whether you experience minor symptoms or full-blown, energy-sapping attacks, it's ultimately the brain that makes it so.

Just as the brain can knock you down, it can also pick you up again. According to some researchers who study mind-body interactions, people with allergies may unconsciously view allergens—everything from dust to animal dander—as dangerous aliens. By reprogramming your perception of these things, these researchers say, it may be possible to lessen their impact as well.

Using mind power to beat allergies requires a two-pronged attack, consisting of relaxation, followed by visualization, says clinical psychologist Steven Fahrion, Ph.D., director of research at the Life Sciences Institute of Mind-Body Health in Topeka, Kansas. Here's how a one-two punch of biofeedback and visualization can help knock out allergies, according to Dr. Fahrion.

Biofeedback involves using normal body functions, like temperature or heart rate, to help you learn to relax. The idea is that your body will immediately tell you how stressed out you are. "Since stress draws blood away from the hands, warm hands make a good index for relaxation," says Dr. Fahrion.

You can train yourself to warm your hands by placing them together so that the pinkie on each hand rests opposite the index finger of the other hand. Rest both hands on your lap, lightly clasping a cardboard-backed thermometer (available by mail from Echo, P.O. Box 87, Springfield, OH 45501) between your left pinkie and right index finger. (Don't use an oral thermometer; its range is too limited. Instead, use one that registers between 70° and 100°F.)

If you suspect that medications are wiping you out, ask your doctor about the newer, nonsedating antihistamines. Prescription drugs such as astemizole (Hismanal) and terfenadine (Seldane) can relieve most allergy symptoms while causing little or no drowsiness.

Use drugs to your advantage.
Sometimes a drug's side effects can work for you instead of against you. While antihistamines taken during the day can make you uncomfortably drowsy, when taken before you go to bed, they can help you get a good night's sleep, says Dr. Altman. You'll have more energy the next day.

Allow yourself to become aware of any sensations of warmth. Concentrate on letting the sensations get stronger. Over time, you'll find that you can let yourself relax, as measured by warmer hands, just by wishing it so.

"Once you can achieve relaxation with this method, you can start the second step, visualization, to reprogram your body to stop attacking the harmless allergens," says Dr. Fahrion.

Get comfortable, close your eyes and imagine yourself in a perfectly allergy-free room. See yourself standing behind a glass wall, protected from any possible allergens. Then observe yourself sitting there. Relax as you view this scene in detail. To stay relaxed, monitor the warmth in your hands.

While you're in this relaxed state, imagine introducing tiny amounts of something that you're allergic to as you watch yourself sitting there. Tell yourself to stay relaxed as you watch these tiny pieces of allergen drift around the room where you are seated. Monitor the temperature in your hands while you do this to make sure that you stay relaxed. "Over time, imagine yourself with gradually increasing amounts of the allergen in the room," Dr. Fahrion suggests.

By doing this exercise every single day, Dr. Fahrion says, there's a good chance that you'll see substantial improvement in your allergy symptoms in about a month. "Over time, you may even be allergy-free," says Dr. Fahrion.

Don't be surprised, however, if your symptoms temporarily flare up during the first month. Paradoxically, relaxation can temporarily worsen allergy symptoms. This effect usually fades in a matter of weeks, says Dr. Fahrion.

To locate a trained hypnotherapist who can help you learn this technique, write to the American Society of Clinical Hypnosis, 2200 East Devon Avenue, Suite 29, Des Plaines, IL 60018.

Exercise wisely.

Exercise can give you a great energy boost, if you choose your activity wisely and time it well. If you have asthma—which is often triggered by allergies—exposure to cold and dry air can cause an attack, says Richard Podell, M.D., clinical professor in the Department of Family Medicine at Robert Wood Johnson Medical School in New Providence, New Jersey.

Swimming is the best exercise for people with asthma because of the warm, moist environment of the pool. It's best to exercise indoors when it's cold or hot outside, when pollution is high or when it's pollen season, Dr. Podell says.

Timing is also important, Dr. Altman adds. Ragweed pollen counts tend to be highest within three hours of sunrise, so evening is the best time to exercise in late summer. Grass releases pollen around midday, so early morning is the best time to exercise in the spring.

Check your diet.

Many allergists believe that while full-blown food allergies aren't particularly common, many people may experience subclinical reactions. That is, the problem doesn't show up on standard allergy tests but nonetheless may cause a number of uncomfortable reactions, including fatigue.

Wheat and gluten are the biggest offenders that have been documented, Dr. Podell says. "There's a fair amount of evidence that a mild form of celiac disease (damage to the small intestine caused by allergy to gluten, a protein in many grains) can be the culprit in otherwise undiagnosable fatigue. While this is not as common as pollen allergy, it's not so rare that it should be ignored."

If you suspect wheat or gluten in the diet is causing your energy levels to flag, Dr. Podell recommends asking your doctor about going on a special diet. "Have your doctor put you on an elimination diet that also excludes wheat, oats, barley and rye," he says.

Put your mind to work.

Dr. Altman often refers her patients to people specially trained in biofeedback, visualization or other relaxation techniques like yoga. Studies have shown that focusing mind power can decrease the severity of the body's response to allergens, causing it to view them as so many harmless tourists, rather than "dangerous" invaders that need fending off.

Boredom

You would think that boredom was the result of low energy—a shutdown of the imagination caused by a worn-out brain. But in many cases the opposite is true. Boredom *causes* your mental motor to run down.

"It takes a lot of energy to be bored," says Ken Druck, Ph.D., a clinical/consulting psychologist in Del Mar, California. The more bored you are, the less energy you have. The less energy you have, the lower your abilities to get "un-bored."

Most of the time, boredom is a temporary state of affairs: Your life is a little uneventful, for example, or you're just feeling a little under the weather. But in some cases the boredom never seems to go away. "If you're constantly bored, something has dampened your native curiosity," says Neil A. Fiore, Ph.D., a licensed psychologist in Berkeley, California, and author of *The Now Habit*.

Bore through Your Boredom

Whatever the cause of your energy-sapping boredom, the situation is not hopeless. There are ways to stimulate your thinking and rev up your enthusiasm.

Take responsibility.
When you're feeling bored and your energy is low, it's natural to look around to see what's causing it. You could be looking in the wrong direction. "Adolescents say 'B-o-o-r-ing,' meaning something out there isn't entertaining them," says Layne Longfellow, Ph.D., a psychologist in private practice in Prescott, Arizona.

A better tactic is to say to yourself, "*I'm* bored," notes Dr. Longfellow. "That's something you have control over."

Realize that you can change.
People who feel they have little control over their lives are more likely to get bored—and stay bored—than those who are willing to take charge. "You'll stay bored if you feel that you were born with a certain 'you' stamped on your per-

sonality," says Penelope Russianoff, Ph.D., a New York psychologist and author of *When Am I Going to Be Happy?* "You can change. You have ears to hear, eyes to look, a body that moves. Entertain yourself."

Diversify.

Just as diversifying investments can increase your assets, spreading out your interests can improve your energy. "People who are prone to boredom are often not well-rounded," says Mark Goulston, M.D., assistant clinical professor of psychiatry at the University of California, Los Angeles, and author of *Get Out of Your Own Way.*

Put some of your eggs in new baskets, he advises. That way, if one area of your life is somewhat underwhelming, others will be full and exciting.

Practice excitement.

When we're stuck in the doldrums, we often say we're in a rut. That's another way of saying that everything, including bad things, get more automatic the longer we do them. People who are often bored, says Dr. Russianoff, are practiced at being bored. "You won't get un-bored unless you practice being the person you want to be," she adds.

Ask yourself, "What do I really want to do? What am I really interested in?" At the same time you need to let go of all your self-defeating thoughts, like "It's not me" or "I don't think I can do it." Remember, there is no such thing as a single, unchangeable you, says Dr. Russianoff. You can reinvent yourself as often as you want.

Whatever your new interest, just go for it. "Think about it, write notes about it and then say, 'I'm going to try it,' " says Dr. Russianoff, who practices what she preaches. At age 69 she bought herself a set of drums and learned to play jazz.

Take stock of where you are.

If you're spending a lot of time in one activity or you have had a sudden change in lifestyle, it might be time to take a fresh look at what interests you. "You may not have taken inventory of what is truly interesting to you in 10 to 20 years," Dr. Druck points out. What's thrilling at 20 is unlikely to be quite as stimulating at 30 or 40.

Even if you're not sure of what direction you'd like to be moving in, take some time to explore various options. For example, peruse the offerings at a local university or community college. Subjects that you may have found dull in the past—like photography or philosophy or calligraphy—may be just what you're looking for now.

Take one step at a time.

Sometimes we avoid new things because they seem overwhelming, says Dr. Fiore. New challenges always appear more manageable if you break them down into small, easy-to-achieve increments, he says. For example, don't put off writing until you become a famous writer. Start out by writing letters. Keep a journal. Write notes to the mail carrier. Write anything. As your confidence rises, so will your enthusiasm. "Taking success-assured steps allows what I call the shy tendrils of the self to move out into life gradually," says Dr. Fiore.

Take a breather.
It's natural for new experiences to cause tension and anxiety, which in turn can result in fatigue. When stress levels rise, Dr. Fiore says, pause for some deep, relaxing breaths. He recommends taking deep breaths and holding them for a couple of seconds before exhaling. "Do it for a minute or so," he says.

Stop obsessing.
People who say they're bored often spend their time obsessing about one particular thing, says Dr. Russianoff. They burn up so much energy worrying about work, for example, or problems at home that they don't have the necessary drive to tackle more exciting things.

It's almost impossible not to think about obsessions (that's why they're called obsessions). What you can do, however, is limit their influence. Dr. Russianoff recommends putting aside 15 minutes in the morning and evening to do nothing else but think about the subjects that are worrying you. "Don't do anything else during that time," she says. "The idea is to get it out of your system." If you stick to it, eventually you'll find you have more mental energy for other, less-fatiguing ideas.

Stay fit.
"Your mind may feel like it needs a rest, but your body needs to be used," says Dr. Druck. In fact, people who exercise regularly have more energy than those who don't. "By doing something physical, you might take care of the mental exhaustion and become more alert," he says.

Stretch it out.
Dr. Russianoff recommends stretching exercises, like yoga. "If your body is alert and flexible," she says, "there's a better chance your mind will be, too."

Coping with the Nine-to-Five

Boredom is not in your job description—but somehow over the years it has seeped its way into your workspace like recycled air. You used to be excited and invigorated in the morning; now you can barely drag yourself out of bed.

"There's no such thing as a boring job, just an individual who is forced to continue an activity for which he's reached the satiation point," notes Arthur

Just Do It!

When you're sick, you call a doctor. When the car breaks down, you call a mechanic. When you're bored, you call . . . The Boring Institute.

"There's no excuse for being bored," says Alan Caruba, founder of the Maplewood, New Jersey, organization that has dedicated itself to banishing the blahs and boredom. "There are countless things you can do." Suggestions from his list include:

- Read a book.
- Take up photography.
- Bake cookies.
- Write a letter.
- Visit a comedy club.
- Dine at a new restaurant.
- Join a rescue squad.
- Become a volunteer firefighter.
- Coach a Little League team.
- Be a tutor.
- Throw a party.
- Get a pet.
- Visit a museum.
- Visit a zoo.

- Shoot billiards.
- Collect stamps, coins or antiques.
- Make Christmas decorations.
- Learn to knit.
- Attend a play or concert.
- Climb a mountain.
- Become a hospital volunteer.
- Trace your family history.
- Learn to square dance.
- Learn carpentry.
- Go to a ball game.
- Go dancing.
- Take up bird-watching.

It really doesn't matter what you do, says Caruba. Just do it!

Witkin, Ph.D., professor of industrial psychology at Queens College in Flushing, New York. In other words, the longer you do something, the more likely you are to find your energy flagging.

To keep your job exciting and your spirits high, here's what experts advise.

Follow your bliss.

The most exciting job in the world will quickly become a yawn if it's not in an area that interests you. To stay energized year after year, it's critical that your job and your interests coincide. "If you're not sure of your interests, you can have them measured by a psychologist who specializes in career counseling," adds Dr. Witkin.

Even if you can't do exactly what you want—be a professional dancer, for example—there are other ways to combine your livelihood with your loves. "If you love dance but lack the ability to earn a living as a dancer, you can do public relations for a dance troupe or make costumes for a ballet company," says Sarah Edwards, a Los Angeles psychotherapist and co-author of *Working from Home* and *The Secrets of Self-Employment*.

Turn to your colleagues.

Going to work involves more than just a paycheck. Whether you work for a small retail shop or a giant corporation, you spend hours every day with co-workers—more than you spend with your spouse or children. Having a good social life at work, far from detracting from the bottom line, makes you more productive and energized. Be part of the group, Dr. Witkin advises. Talk to your colleagues. Join sports teams. Organize outings. "People forget about boredom if they enjoy their fellow workers," he says.

Enrich your job description.

One of the best ways to stay energized is to always be pushing yourself to try new and different things. Let it be known that you're ready to take on new jobs and responsibilities, advises Dr. Witkin. "It will push back the point of satiation because the new work won't be boring," he says.

Take five.

Even the best day has moments of boredom—mental downtime when you'd like nothing better than to take a two-hour lunch break followed by a three-month vacation. When work is starting to seem too much, well, like work, take a break, advises Dr. Witkin. Take a walk outside. Get something to eat. Read the newspaper. Even a brief respite from work will help you feel refreshed and energized when you start again.

Get a Helping Hand

Although boredom usually fades on its own, sometimes it never seems to go away. If days, weeks or months go by and your enthusiasm for life seems to be at a permanent ebb, it's probably time to get professional help.

Start with an exam.

Illness can masquerade as long-term boredom, says Dr. Druck. People with sleep disorders, for example, may have a terrible time feeling motivated. "You might be physically depleted by something like chronic fatigue," he adds. In fact, any physical problem can cause your energy to take a dive.

Ask about depression.

Caused both by physical and emotional problems, depression can leave you feeling profoundly bored, says Dr. Fiore. Don't be surprised if your doctor asks

Ennui to Energy

Although boredom is often a result of not having enough interesting things to do, it can also be the mind's natural reaction to overload. "As a society, we've become habituated to increasing levels of stimulation," says Layne Longfellow, Ph.D., a psychologist in private practice in Prescott, Arizona. "We've raised the critical mass at which we get stimulated. We can't tolerate quiet."

Driven, ambitious, hardworking people—the very ones you'd think would never get bored—often get restless the minute there's a lull in their hectic pace.

Does this sound like you? Don't fight the feelings, says Dr. Longfellow. Instead, try to savor them. Let yourself be bored for a bit. "When you've been on a treadmill for a long time, what seems like boredom can be a blessing and a freedom. Go further into it until it becomes relaxation."

Dr. Longfellow recommends taking regular time-outs every day. Call them boring, if you like, but do them anyway. "Set aside time to walk on the beach or listen to music or meditate," he says. Eventually, you'll learn to appreciate the quiet time—and you won't believe you ever got by without it.

questions about your mental and emotional health. (If the doctor doesn't bring it up, you should.) Are you feeling sad lately? How are things at work? Is your marriage okay? Just talking about problems can help bring them to the surface so that you can deal with them. In addition, there are a number of drugs that can relieve depression and help keep your energy high.

Consider therapy.
For many people boredom is a direct result of being afraid. "They can't immerse themselves in things that keep them alert and alive because they're thinking, 'I wouldn't be good enough at it' or 'They won't like me,' " says Dr. Longfellow. The mind, not surprisingly, responds to these fears by taking the path of least resistance—zoning out in front of the TV, for example, or staying home rather than socializing with friends.

There are many types of therapy that you may want to explore, ranging from the traditional (and often lengthy) psychotherapy to more-modern approaches like cognitive therapy. Ask your doctor which approach might be best for you. Although counselors or therapists can't prescribe drugs unless they are M.D.'s, they can refer you to a doctor if they think therapy should be combined with medication.

Burnout

*I*f you put a frog in a stew pot and light a fire under it, the heat increases so gradually that the frog doesn't notice. It stays in the pot even when the water starts to boil.

Burnout is like that, says Perry W. Buffington, Ph.D., a psychologist, lecturer and radio talk-show host on Amelia Island, Florida. The stress builds up, the pressure gets more intense, the joy of living fades, but you shrug it off, hardly even noticing that your energy is oozing out of you like a slow leak. "You go from stress to stressed out to burnout to burned up," says Dr. Buffington.

Burnout is not the result of mere overwork. Working too long and too hard can certainly drain your energy. But five minutes of overtime might be too much for one person, while others might work 16-hour days and love it so much that they gain energy. Besides, for most of us, overwork is a temporary nuisance—we don't like it and we can't wait to stop. Once we do, our bodies tend to recover quickly.

Face Up to Activity Addiction

Workaholism is another story. "Workaholics are addicted to incessant activity," says Diane Fassel, Ph.D., an organizational consultant in Boulder, Colorado, and author of *Working Ourselves to Death*. They need the adrenaline fix that work provides and get depressed without it. They keep pushing themselves until one day their nervous systems and endocrine systems shut down, and they just can't crank themselves up anymore.

Beyond workaholism, the chief cause of burnout is feeling powerless, says Beverly A. Potter, Ph.D., a psychologist in Berkeley, California, and author of *Beating Job Burnout* and *Finding a Path with a Heart*. "When people feel trapped, without control over what they do, they go from anger to anxiety to apathy." And once their motivation is sapped, their physical energy follows. It becomes harder and harder to get moving.

If your stew pot is heating up, the best thing to do is hop out before it's too late. Meanwhile, there are a number of things that you can do to cool things down and make yourself burnout-proof.

Recognize the Signs

As with heart disease or cancer, spotting the warning signs of burnout is a crucial prevention measure. Here are some tips from expert fire-spotters.

Look for the common signals.
Dr. Potter lists six categories of burnout symptoms.

Negative emotions. Anger, frustration, anxiety and depression crop up more and more often.

Interpersonal problems. Communicating with friends, family and colleagues is a strain. You overreact, get into conflicts, feel like withdrawing.

Health problems. You're tired, run-down, beset by minor ailments like colds, headaches and insomnia. Sex doesn't seem worth the effort.

Below-par performance. You're losing interest, unable to concentrate, forgetting things. Your productivity and efficiency are declining.

Substance abuse. You're drinking and smoking more, relying on caffeine. Maybe you're using medications inappropriately.

Feelings of meaninglessness. Work seems pointless. You find yourself thinking, "Why bother?" Your enthusiasm is being replaced by cynicism.

Monitor your friends' and co-workers' comments.
Sometimes the people around you notice signs of burnout before you do, says Dr. Buffington. They'll remark on little things—frowns, for example, or forgetfulness or a slumping posture. They'll say things like, "Are you okay?" or "Do you feel all right?" or "You don't seem yourself."

Look for danger signs at work.
Demoralizing job conditions are major contributors to burnout, says Dr. Potter. If you're beset by any of the following, you're a candidate.

A critical boss. Is he impossible to please, no matter how hard you try?

Lack of recognition. Do your contributions go unnoticed? Are you inadequately compensated or stuck at a level beneath your talent and aspirations?

Ambiguity. Is it hard to figure out what's expected of you? Do you lack the information to get your job done? Are the goals of your organization or department unclear?

Overload. Is your "in" basket always overflowing? Is your "to do" list always off the page? Do you have too many things to do and too little time to do them in?

No-win situations. Are the various demands of your job incompatible? Are you expected to do your tasks quickly and be thorough at the same time? Do your work needs conflict with the needs of your family?

Lack of control. Are you unable to influence the decisions that affect you? Do you feel helpless? Are you in danger of being laid off with no recourse?

"The essential component of burnout is a feeling of loss of control," explains Dr. Potter. So it's important to build a sense of control, even if it's by becoming a better manager of just yourself. Other ways to build feelings of control are to practice stress-management techniques, build strong social support, change your job to fit you better, adopt an attitude of "detached concern" without becoming cynical or analyze your job for its good points as well as its bad points, suggests Dr. Potter.

There are a number of other things that you can do to deal with burnout.

Check Excess Baggage

One of the key steps to regaining the energy that you have lost to burnout is to prioritize and cut back in the least important areas. Here's how to do it.

Just say no.

It might be time to give up some obligations. "The problem is, people who are burning out are prone to anxiety," says Mark Goulston, M.D., assistant clinical professor of psychiatry at the University of California, Los Angeles, and author of *Get Out of Your Own Way.* "They can't say no without fear or guilt, and they can't say yes without resentment." The key is to realize that saying nothing will be taken as a yes. "If you act with honesty and integrity, you should be able to set boundaries without being unfair or unreasonable," he says.

Make others feel important.

For busy people, trying to juggle every role—parent, spouse, child, sibling, boss, subordinate, co-worker, friend—can be a major energy drain. "If you spread yourself too thin, you not only risk burnout but also the scorn of people who expect you to be there for them," says Dr. Goulston. With everyone competing for your time, the key is to make each person feel important. That means showing them, not just telling them. "If you convince people they're important to you, they won't feel deprived of your time," he says.

To help you do this, use Dr. Goulston's three Cs: concern, curiosity and confidence. To show concern, hear your friend or family member out, listen. To show curiosity, be specific, even if they are not having problems. Ask, "How was that meeting?" instead of "How was your day?" When another person shares a problem with you, show confidence by helping him brainstorm a solution and show support for his final decision.

"Following the three Cs may be simple, but it's not easy," warns Dr. Goulston. But it is worth making the effort. Even if you don't have time now, the three Cs will give you more time in the future because the other person will be more self-reliant, he says.

Take Care of Body and Soul

One reason overextended people burn out is that they're too busy to take good care of themselves. Developing and maintaining good, sensible, healthy habits will keep you "un-fried" and help restore your energy if you start burning out. Here's what to do.

Get appropriate exercise.
Keeping your body fit is crucial, but the wrong regimen can backfire. "It should be pleasant, and it should be appropriate for your age, shape and ability," says Rob Krakovitz, M.D., a medical doctor in private practice in Aspen, who specializes in alternative medicine and is the author of *High Energy*. "If you're pushing yourself to do it, it's not an asset. Working out should not be one more have-to on your list."

Eat right.
People in a burnout situation tend to grab whatever's available and eat on the run, says Brian Rees, M.D., medical director of the Maharishi Ayurveda Medical Center in Pacific Palisades, California. "That inhibits good digestion, promotes the formation of toxic by-products and makes you feel heavy, dull and fatigued," he explains.

It doesn't take long to eat a nutritious meal without rushing, Dr. Rees points out. He recommends a moment of silence before eating and another moment when you're done. "Sit quietly and comfortably for five minutes to let the digestive process switch over to automatic pilot," he advises.

Don't be a junk-food junky.
Burnout victims have a penchant for on-the-run infusions of sugar, fat and salt. But that practice is counterproductive, says Ann McGee-Cooper, Ed.D., a business consultant in Dallas and author of *You Don't Have to Go Home from Work Exhausted!* and *Time Management for Unmanageable People*. A healthy diet includes a wide variety of foods and foods rich in fiber.

Snack for energy, she advises. Fresh fruit, vegetables and whole-grain crackers will take you a lot further than high-fat or high-sugar foods. "Learn how to enjoy strawberries instead of a candy bar," advises Dr. McGee-Cooper.

Take your vitamins.

To maintain energy, Dr. Krakovitz recommends taking a daily multivitamin/mineral supplement to provide the essential nutrients that you may not be getting enough of in your diet.

Get some friendly fat.

"Fat has become a dirty word," notes Dr. Krakovitz, "but you can shortchange yourself if you don't get the essential fatty acids." Essential fatty acids are a beneficial type of oil especially abundant in fish.

Drink up.

Your body needs lots of water to flush toxins out of your system and for your brain to think clearly, says Dr. McGee-Cooper.

"Plain water is best because other liquids tend to carry additional calories or substances that should be limited, such as caffeine and aspartame," says Joanne Curran-Celentano, R.D., Ph.D., associate professor of nutritional sciences at the University of New Hampshire in Durham.

Don't leave the rest behind.

"Rest is the absolute key to avoiding burnout," states Dr. Krakovitz. "You need a day or a couple of afternoons a week to commune with your spirit, where there are no have-tos and you can be with your family, or by yourself, in a quality way."

Take a break.

Workaholics sometimes hesitate to take breaks, thinking that it will make them less productive, adds Dr. Fassel. "It's a myth that the way to get ahead is to work longer and longer and more and more. Workaholics get less rest than they need and consequently make more mistakes and are not as creative. The harder they work, the harder they have to work to get results."

Frequent brief respites can be as beneficial as one or two longer ones, says Harold H. Bloomfield, M.D., a psychiatrist in Del Mar, California, and co-author of *The Power of 5: Hundreds of 5-Second to 5-Minute Scientific Shortcuts to Ignite Your Energy, Burn Fat, Stop Aging and Revitalize Your Love Life*. "Introducing short breaks into your routine actually speeds up work. You accomplish more, with less distress and loss of energy."

Take a breather.

One particularly helpful way to use your break time is doing deep breathing, says Dr. Bloomfield. "It's one of the most powerful ways to activate your energy and alertness."

When your body says, "Gimme a break," try Dr. Bloomfield's one-breath meditation.

1. Inhale naturally, without forcing it.
2. Relax your shoulders, straighten your back and let the air open your chest.
3. Imagine that you're drawing vitality and strength into every cell of your body as you inhale.
4. Hold the breath for a few moments.
5. As you exhale, let your attention sink into the center of your chest, releasing the darkness from your thoughts and tension from your muscles.

Take time to meditate.
Setting aside regular periods of solitude is a great way to prevent burnout or to recover from it. There are dozens of ways to relax or meditate, with books, tapes and instructors galore.

One method is transcendental meditation (TM), a natural technique that does not require concentration and is practiced 20 minutes, twice a day. "A number of studies have shown that TM is about 2½ times more efficacious in reducing anxiety and lowering blood pressure than other relaxation methods," according to Dr. Rees. He notes that meditating can help with another key factor in burnout, control. "Tests indicate that meditators become more inner-directed, so they're less battered about by forces out of their control," he says. To learn more about TM, call the Transcendental Meditation Program in Fairfield, Iowa, at 1-800-888-5797.

Reach Out and Touch Someone

"People who burn out often think, 'I can handle this. I can do it myself,'" says Dr. Fassel. "They have to learn that they can't handle everything by themselves." If you could, you wouldn't be reading about burnout. Here's how to recruit others to help banish burnout.

Find others like you.
Talk to other people who are experiencing burnout, suggests Dr. Fassel, or join a support group. "Workaholics Anonymous (WA) is a good first line of defense. You learn things about workaholism and burnout, and you see what others are doing to address the problem." To locate a WA group near you, call (510) 273-9253.

Encourage feedback.
"Teach people to let you know where you stand, so you don't have to guess," advises Dr. McGee-Cooper. It might seem risky to ask how you're doing, but when you seek feedback, it usually gets expressed in a more positive way. "Think of it as an opportunity to learn," she adds. "It will energize you."

See a professional.
Often, people who are prone to burnout don't even feel that they have the time to see a health care provider. "Have a thorough physical exam to see how you

have been affected by all the stress," Dr. Fassel suggests.

It can also pay to see a therapist, especially if you're having a hard time dealing with the problem on your own. "You might want to deal with some fundamental questions," says Dr. Fassel, "such as 'Why am I doing this to myself? Am I keeping constantly busy to avoid something that I don't want to face or feelings that I don't want to feel?' "

Create a Sanctuary

Home should be a place where you go to recover from the forces that lead to burnout, a place to recharge your creative energies. But for many people the atmosphere at home adds to the chaos that leads to burnout, according to Mortimer R. Feinberg, Ph.D., chairman of BFS Psychological Associates in New York City and author of *Why Smart People Do Dumb Things*. Here are several suggestions from the experts for correcting that situation.

Plan on some home repairs.
Don't avoid domestic problems, but don't think you have to solve them all at once, says Dr. Feinberg. Sit down with your spouse and try to reach agreement on those that need immediate attention, even if it means putting off the other problems.

Be home at critical times.
You can't always be available, but be there when your kids need someone to talk to and on important family occasions like birthdays, the school play and the big game, suggests Dr. Feinberg.

Develop some allies.
Let your family know about your work. Explain what you do, advises Dr. Feinberg, the pressures you're under and the importance of your job to their livelihood.

Use modern technology.
Phones, beepers, fax machines and e-mail can help you and your family stay in touch, says Dr. Feinberg.

Create a buffer zone.
Greeting your family with a rundown of your day can be a formula for resentment, says Dr. Bloomfield. For a more peaceful, energizing transition, keep your initial comments brief and warm, as in "What a hectic day. It's great to be home." Save the details for later. "Use the interlude to exercise, shower or change clothes," suggests Dr. Bloomfield. "Or do something with your partner—take a walk, give each other a back rub, listen to music."

Child Rearing

When Linda Keys became a mother, she did it in a big way. She gave birth to quadruplets—three girls and a boy. "The hardest thing in those early years was that somebody needed me all the time," she says. "I don't know how I would have done it without help."

Energy draining? Of course. But Linda learned a few survival tricks that she still practices today.

"If you're organized, that's half the battle," says this Philadelphia mom who also works part-time as a hairdresser. "In my house, lunches are made the night before school and the clothes are laid out. That way we're not running around in the morning looking for somebody's sneakers because it's gym day."

Linda also accepts help when it's offered. "Even if somebody just does a load of wash, it can be a big help. A good mother-in-law really saves your life!"

Superwoman Is a Fictional Character

Forget what the magazines say about having it all. Nobody can do it all, so don't even try. "As parents we've become more de-energized than ever before because our world is less forgiving of not getting enough done," says C. Wayne Jones, Ph.D., a child and family psychologist at the Philadelphia Child Guidance Center. "We're supposed to be outstanding parents, professionals and employees. There is not a lot of support for letting go of anything."

The trick, whether you're rearing one child or an entire brood, is finding shortcuts that can make your daily tasks go a little bit easier. Here's what experts advise.

Welcome catnaps.

For new mothers, perhaps the biggest energy drain is providing constant attention to a baby while getting little sleep in the bargain. After you have a baby, it may be months before you get another full night's sleep, so you have to catch winks when you can.

"When your child is resting, give yourself time to rest," suggests Joan Test, Ed.D., adjunct professor of education and director of the nursery school at Washington University in St. Louis.

It's tempting to try to catch up on other household tasks while your baby is sleeping, but sometimes taking a little downtime is the more efficient strategy. "Try not to feel like you have to catch up on everything," says Dr. Test. "In the long run you'll come back faster."

Have an open house.

Once your child (or children) are old enough, having one or more of their friends over will keep them occupied so you have at least a few moments to yourself in which to catch up, says Dr. Test.

Develop routines.

If your children know what it is they're supposed to do and when they're supposed to do it, you can save a ton of energy. One routine that many parents find to be effective, for example, is having the child bathe every night and lay out his school clothes before he goes to bed. Once he is accustomed to doing this, it will become routine. He'll be less likely to slack off, even when you're not around to supervise him. "Get children to do as much as they can themselves without being asked," suggests Barry G. Ginsberg, Ph.D., a child and family psychologist and director of Ginsberg Associates and Center of Relationship Enhancement, both located in Doylestown, Pennsylvania.

Have the routine go with the flow.

Rather than trying to carefully structure your family life, be flexible, says Dr. Ginsberg. "If you grew up having a special meal every day, you may think that's important. Yet, it may not be realistic today."

Dr. Ginsberg suggests designating certain days as "flex" days, when dinner is something you make speedily—peanut butter and jelly, for example, or tuna fish or cold cuts. Just as important as keeping the meal simple is stepping back, not taking charge. What's your most hectic night of the week? If the children are old enough, let them grab their own dinner on that night each week. Having this type of "routine flexibility" will open up free time in your schedule so you can get other things done—or simply relax by taking some time for yourself.

Be a team leader.

Family members of all ages should work as a team to accomplish what needs to be done around the house. Otherwise, you're doing it all yourself or wearing yourself out trying to get everyone else to do their part.

Rather than simply giving commands that generally require lots of energy to enforce, encourage the family to come up with their own solutions. If laundry is building up, try asking various family members what they feel is the most efficient way to take care of it.

"Call a family meeting and turn over the problem to other family members to solve. Let them brainstorm what chores have to be done," says B. Kaye Olson, R.N., an instructor and adviser in stress management at Lansing Community College in Lansing, Michigan. She has worked with parents for 30 years and is author of *Energy Secrets for Tired Mothers on the Run.* "Rotate the chores. Cooperation in the family goes up 100 percent when involvement takes place."

Accept the job done.

It's a fact of life that other people may not perform tasks the way you would if you did them yourself. When you delegate responsibility, you simply have to learn to back off, to let others solve problems in their own ways. "Let go of perfectionism," says Olson. At the end of the day, when you've actually had a few relaxing moments to yourself, you'll be glad you did.

Share the shopping.

No one can clean out a pantry or refrigerator faster than a teenager. To prevent the never-ending shopping from wearing you down, let the older children do some of it. Not only will this save extra trips to the store but also it will give the kids experience learning about prices and shopping for quality and good deals, Olson says.

Double your time estimates.

It's frustrating to plan your day only to find out later that the time you allotted for individual tasks was way too short. Trying to meet unrealistic deadlines can be extremely stressful and draining, particularly when you look back and realize how little you got done.

It's true that most tasks take a lot longer than anyone anticipates, says Olson. Her solution: Figure how much time you're going to need for a task, then double it. By the time you allow for interruptions, stops and starts and the snags and snafus that invariably crop up, it's probably going to be a lot more realistic than the original estimate.

Make lists.

Make a note of everything you need to do, then cross off each item the instant it's done. "Keeping lists helps relieve stress by keeping things from whirring around in our minds," Olson says. There's something about writing things down that makes them tangible and—equally important for keeping your stress levels down and energy levels high—achievable.

Take advantage of TV.
Given the poor programming that is a staple of today's television industry, it's not surprising that many people have opted simply to turn the thing off. But TV can provide some valuable time out—not only for children but for exhausted parents as well, says Cynthia Whitham, a staff therapist at the University of California, Los Angeles, Parent Training and Children's Social Skills Programs. She is also the author of *The Answer Is NO*.

She recommends using TV time as a reward: turn it on after the children have eaten breakfast, brushed their teeth *and* packed their book bags. At night it can go on after homework and chores are done. By using television as a reward, it can actually save you a bundle of supervision, while relieving you long enough to relax and recuperate.

Make Time for Fun Times

When the bills are due, the house is a wreck and the children are throwing tantrums for who knows what reasons, it's hard to remember that fun is what good memories are all about.

But fun doesn't just happen, experts remind us. Sometimes you have to give it more than a little nudge. Once you start smiling, the surge of energy can last you all day.

Start off on the right foot.
How often do you come home at the end of the day only to swap one set of tasks for another? Next time, before opening the mail, before starting dinner and before returning phone calls, take a few minutes just to play. "Playing with children first, before you do anything else, makes them easier to manage," Dr. Jones says. You'll get an emotional lift (and so will they) that translates into a healthy shot of energy that can last until bedtime. "We get big gains out of just a little play with our kids," he says.

Plan ahead.
We like to think that quality time is something that just happens, but today's busy parents may find it helpful to block out specific periods of time just to have fun. "When I plan that time and carry it out, I feel successful and energized, not drained," Dr. Jones says.

Allow for improvisation.
While it's helpful to set aside some time for play, you don't want to go overboard and create an entire social calendar. Sometimes we get so busy driving our children from one "fun" activity to another that we find ourselves even

more exhausted than when we began, notes Dr. Jones.

We would all do ourselves a favor by remembering that the word *recreation* means re-*create*. Creating fun—like creating a painting, sand castle or a snappy tune—is among the most energizing things you can do. Children are great at improvising, which is why they can make toys out of sticks, pebbles or anything else that comes to hand. All you have to do is set aside the time to let it happen. Then stand back and watch the fun begin.

Share your joys.
When you and your children have similar interests—walking in the park or building model planes—that means you spend less "extra" time trying to keep them entertained. "Children learn to like what they see their parents enjoy," says Marilyn M. Segal, Ph.D., dean of the Family and School Center at Nova Southeastern University in Fort Lauderdale, Florida.

Your children won't be enamored of all your activities, of course, but every interest that you share translates into quality time together—and that makes you and the child both more energetic. "It makes child rearing so much fun," says Dr. Segal.

Create your own space.
Parents who try to be everything for their kids—social director, partygoer and head joke-meister—typically find themselves so exhausted at the end of the day that their batteries never have time to recharge.

To keep yourself energized, it's critical to cultivate interests that have nothing to do with the children, says Dr. Test. Parents need time away from kids, both physically and mentally. Try to get out of the house on a regular basis. Go to the library. Spend an hour at the gym. Take yourself out to lunch. Allowing yourself to have regular adult fun means you'll have more energy to spend on your family later on.

It can be difficult, of course, for parents to get out of the house, particularly when the children are young. Perhaps the best solution is to trade off babysitting time with a neighbor or a friend, Whitham suggests.

Know when it's quitting time.
There's simply no way you can keep the children entertained all day without taking care of yourself. Downtime is more than a luxury; it's absolutely essential to keep yourself fresh and your energy levels high, says Whitham.

Many parents simply tell the children that certain hours—say, after eight or nine o'clock at night—are "parent time" when the parents are "off duty." Ideally, that means children should be in bed with quiet activities such as reading. For parents that means no getting drinks of water or night snacks or refereeing squabbles. The point is to create an opportunity for quiet time that will give your energy a chance to bounce back.

Do's and Don'ts of Discipline

Disciplining children can be one of the most difficult and energy-demanding tasks of parenthood. To keep your children on the right track without derailing yourself in the process, here's what experts suggest.

Ask once.

Never more. "It's exhausting to have to ask a child three times to do something," says Dr. Segal. Here's how she suggests you get a child of any age to respond the first time you ask.

"If the child doesn't respond the first time, say in a very low voice, 'I asked you because I wanted you to do it; I don't want to ever ask you more than once.' If the child still doesn't do it, say, 'I'm not going to ask you again.' Then call a family conference with the child and your spouse to discuss this behavior."

Don't reward persistence.

"Another thing that exhausts parents," says Dr. Segal, "is when children say, 'I want. I want. I want.' Don't reward them for whining long enough and loud enough. Decide immediately if you will stand your ground or give in.

"If you're going to give in, do it right away. If you're going to say no, offer an explanation. Then, if the child asks again, say, 'The answer is the same as it was before, and I don't like being asked the same question more than once.' "

Discipline with humor.

Dr. Segal says humor works well with all ages and helps you avoid energy-draining arguments. With a young child who doesn't want to get dressed, for example, say, "Here are your socks. Put one on each ear." The child will have fun getting dressed, and you'll avoid an argument. For an older child, instead of threatening punishment or raising your voice, explain that if he doesn't clean up his room, the garbage truck will be arriving in the morning. The point is to always enforce behavior without having energy-draining emotions run high.

Be ready to talk.

A lot of misbehavior occurs because children are unhappy and aren't quite able to express themselves. Don't hesitate to ask what's bothering them, says Dr. Segal. If your child doesn't want to talk, say, "That's fine, but I'm here if you change your mind." Simply asking about the problem shows that you care, which can help prevent the child from getting into a negative or uncooperative mood that will sap energy from the whole family.

Take a united stand.

"Be sure to include your spouse in decision making as well as in caring for your children. Even if one parent is the primary disciplinarian, it's important that there be consistent communication to the children that this is a rule or decision both parents agree upon," says Dr. Ginsberg.

Take a deep breath.

"It's the quickest, most powerful tool we can use," says Olson. Simply take a breath through your nose and hold it for four seconds. Then pucker your lips and slowly release the breath over six seconds. Breathe normally four or five times and then take a second deep breath. Deep breathing is a quick fix for frustration, stress and anger. It stops your mind from spinning and allows you to concentrate again.

Performing deep-breathing exercises over a period of several minutes lowers your pulse and heart rates, helping prevent a moment's stress from taking over and wearing you down.

Chronic Disease

Prolonged illness can drain your energy. Whether it's arthritis, colitis, diabetes, heart disease or Lyme disease, one symptom seems to be a given: fatigue.

Why is that?

The answer seems to vary with the disease. Doctors know that some conditions tax your immune system with infection. Other conditions pull the plug on your energy stores by creating constant pain. Still others wreak havoc on your body's chemistry, preventing you from converting the food you eat into a reliable energy source.

Making the Mind-Body Connection

Doctors know one more very important thing when it comes to dealing with the fatigue brought on by chronic disease. Feeling tired when you're sick or in pain is not entirely physical, according to David Spiegel, M.D., professor of psychiatry and behavioral sciences and director of the psychosocial treatment laboratory at Stanford University School of Medicine. It seems that thoughts, emotions and behavior play important roles, too.

People who are very sick go through the same emotional stages that researcher Elizabeth Kubler-Ross, M.D., identified in people who are dying, says psychologist Robert H. Phillips, Ph.D., director of the Center for Coping in Hicksville, New York. "Once they go through shock, denial and anger, they may become depressed and grieve for the way they lived before the illness," he explains. "Such negativity is draining—it makes you feel more fatigued."

Most medical treatments for chronic disease focus mainly on the physical, and many of these treatments will make a difference in your energy level, says Dr. Phillips. You don't have to stop there, however. In addition, you can do a great deal to boost your energy by taking control of how you think and feel, he says.

"It's not the medical problem that determines how well you cope, it's your thinking, attitude and perspective that counts. How you think is far more important than what you do," says Dr. Phillips. "One of the best ways to boost energy is to reduce stress, to think more positively and to empower yourself to live life more successfully."

Here are some positive steps that you can take to re-energize your life.

Think small.

When you're feeling down and depleted, you can improve the way you perceive your energy level by focusing on small accomplishments, according to Dr. Phillips.

On days when you feel as if you can hardly lift a finger, try to concentrate on activities that are still within your reach, he advises. He suggests asking yourself, "What activities have I put off doing because other things were more important?"

Low-energy days are a good time to catch up on activities that aren't very physically demanding, like making phone calls or writing letters.

Think positive.

"Changing negative thinking requires a huge mental effort, but it's worth it," says Dr. Phillips. With practice, it is possible to identify the negative thoughts that contribute to your feelings of being overwhelmed. When you catch yourself thinking these kinds of things, the trick is to reword them realistically and positively.

How does this work in practice? You may catch yourself thinking something like, "I can't do what I used to do" or "I'm no good for anything anymore." As soon as you become aware of such thoughts, advises Dr. Phillips, stop and say firmly to yourself, "I can handle this" or "There are still things I can do."

Learn how to communicate.

If you don't feel understood or have difficulty making yourself understood to your doctor, your family and your friends, you'll experience energy-draining stress in your relationships, says Dr. Phillips.

"People can't see pain or fatigue," he says. "They may not understand why you need a lot of rest. If your family accuses you of shirking your chores, for example, you may challenge them by saying, 'Do you really think I enjoy feeling so weak or sore that I can't do what I want?' "

Speak softly.

"If you can't see eye-to-eye with friends and family, try discussing your differences in a whisper," suggests Dr. Phillips. "Whispering eliminates the negative tone of voice that can bog down understanding and forces both parties to listen harder." Getting your feelings out in the open will also help eliminate energy-draining stress, he explains.

Seek support.

Your friends and family may listen well and offer sympathy, but, let's face it, they probably don't understand what you're really going through. They can't; they don't have the disease. That's why medical experts advise joining a support group composed of people who have the chronic illness that you're facing.

Giving and receiving emotional support and expressing your innermost feelings and fears in an atmosphere of acceptance can go a long way toward relieving stress, according to Dr. Spiegel.

To find a support group near you, ask your doctor for a referral. You may also try calling hospitals and clinics in your area.

De-stress with biofeedback.

Many doctors recommend biofeedback because the procedure enables you to relax, enhances your body's healing abilities and lowers energy-depleting stress, says Angele McGrady, Ph.D., professor of psychiatry at Medical College of Ohio in Toledo. "Some people with diabetes and some people with high blood pressure can reduce their blood-glucose levels and blood pressure with biofeedback therapy." But, initially, it's not something that you can do on your own. Biofeedback is a technique whereby a person learns to be aware of, and control, a physiological process. Biofeedback is often coupled with relaxation therapy.

A trained specialist will use equipment to monitor the physiological response, such as muscle tension or heart rate, and help you learn how to control that response. After a while, with practice and coaching, you'll be able to do this without the device. If biofeedback is appropriate for you, your doctor will be able to recommend a qualified practitioner in your area or you can call the Association for Applied Psychophysiology and Biofeedback at 1-800-477-8892 for a referral in your region.

Banishing the Pain

One of the most energy-depleting aspects of many chronic illnesses is dealing with the pain. If medications and other treatments from your doctor just aren't providing the relief you need, there are other options to consider.

Get needled.

A number of medical researchers believe that acupuncture needles may stimulate the release of the body's natural pain relievers—endorphins and enkephalins. The acupuncture procedure may block the pain pathways to the brain, says Bruce Pomeranz, M.D., Ph.D., a neurophysiologist who has studied acupuncture extensively at the University of Toronto.

Studies suggest that in some people, acupuncture may help ease pain—including musculoskeletal, angina, arthritis and dental—in a host of chronic conditions.

In one study done at the University of Maryland, for example, 40 people with osteoarthritis of the knee received eight acupuncture treatments every other week for eight weeks in addition to treatment with painkillers and anti-inflammatory drugs. Preliminary results on 19 of these study participants showed significant improvement in levels of pain and knee function compared to those of a group who received only the painkillers and anti-inflammatory drugs.

So if you think acupuncture may help, ask your doctor if it may be appropriate for you, especially for treatment of chronic or serious illness. Your doctor may be able to recommend a qualified acupuncturist in your area.

For referrals to physicians who do acupuncture, you can call the American Academy of Medical Acupuncture referral line at 1-800-521-2262 to have a list of physicians in your state sent to you. The organization is based at 5820 Wilshire Boulevard, Suite 500, Los Angeles, CA 90036.

Call in the heavy hitters.
Sometimes pain resists even the best medical efforts to relieve it. In such a case, pain-management experts advise having a customized pain-relief program to address your individual problem on all fronts.

To find an accredited pain-management program in your area, send a self-addressed envelope with double postage to CARF, The Rehabilitation Accreditation Commission, 4891 East Grant Road, Tucson, AZ 85712.

Chronic Fatigue Syndrome

*T*ired. You wish you were *just* tired. Garden-variety tired—too tired to do the dishes, maybe, or to read the newspaper.

What you're experiencing is something else entirely. You're so tired you stay in bed and think about taking a shower for three days before you can actually do it. So tired you can't add three sevens in your head, much less go to your job. So tired you can't remember a phrase like "chronic fatigue," even though the two words describe exactly how you feel.

That's how tired people with chronic fatigue syndrome (CFS) feel in the earliest stage of their illness. But there are other symptoms as well. Their muscles ache. And their joints hurt. They either can't sleep or they sleep too much. Whenever they work out, they are sick for days. What kind of nasty bug is this sickness that never goes away?

Nobody knows for sure yet. In the field of public health, chronic fatigue syndrome is a presence without a face. Doctors do not have any lab test that helps them readily identify CFS. It has no known cause and no reliable cure. In fact, it isn't even a formal disease—just a constellation of symptoms called a syndrome.

Lowdown on the Slowdown

But there is a ray of light in this dimness: Even though CFS can't be cured by writing a prescription or specifying a certain therapy, the symptoms can be treated. And with treatment many people who have it may regain some of their former energy. "The natural course of CFS in many people is one of gradual recovery," says Mark A. Demitrack, M.D., assistant professor of psychiatry at the University of Michigan Medical School in Ann Arbor and director of its chronic fatigue syndrome clinic.

Chronic fatigue syndrome usually starts with something severe and infectious that feels like a very bad flu—such as fever, sore throat and tender or aching joints. Like those with the flu, people who have CFS may also have tender lymph glands—areas around the jaw, armpits and groin that ache when there's a problem with the lymphatic system. While those symptoms may let up, they can return with any kind of exertion—or even with none at all.

Along with these symptoms comes steady fatigue, the kind that settles in, hangs its hat and calls your body home—for six months, at least, and often for long years. About 25 percent of the people who have chronic fatigue syndrome have to stay out of work, and another 33 percent can only maintain part-time jobs.

The collection of symptoms that we now know as CFS made its first big public splash in 1984 in the small resort town of Incline Village, near Lake Tahoe, Nevada. Doctors began reporting cases of what looked like mononucleosis, but no one was getting better and a virtual epidemic had broken out, which was unheard of for mononucleosis.

Those who had the symptoms included about 200 teachers and students in two local high schools. The outbreak was large enough and unusual enough to attract the attention of investigators from the Centers for Disease Control and Prevention (CDC) in Atlanta, the nation's prevention agency responsible for gathering information and researching diseases in the United States. They began gathering statistics and evidence about the newly identified health problem.

Since then, the CDC has been conducting an ongoing surveillance study of CFS, and results indicate that the chances of your having it are extremely low—less than 1 in 10,000. Women account for 81 percent of the total. The CDC found that the age range for most people with chronic fatigue syndrome is from 25 to 45.

What bothers people with CFS as much as their fatigue and pain, researchers discovered, are the strange cognitive problems that come with it, including memory loss, concentration lapses and a kind of "mind fog." Doctors say chronic fatigue syndrome affects both the body and the mind, disturbing both the immune system and the central nervous system. More than half of the people with the condition, according to researchers, also wrestle with symptoms of depression.

One of the big problems with diagnosing CFS is that it has many of the symptoms of unrelated illnesses like Lyme disease (carried by deer ticks), fibromyalgia (aching joints) and dozens of others. So diagnosis of CFS involves eliminating all other possible diseases through lab tests and physical examination.

Finding the Answers

Despite all the research on CFS, some people still doubt the existence of chronic fatigue syndrome—including many doctors.

"One of the worst things is not the illness itself but the ignorance about it. The mainstream medical community minimizes the importance of CFS in part because people don't die from it and because the majority do get better," says Dr. Demitrack.

So if you suspect you have this problem, the process of seeking medical help is really in your own hands. Here's how to go about it.

Seek a savvy doctor.
Suppose you've been feeling sick, tired and exhausted for more than six months. You're not sure exactly why you feel so bad, but you have many of the symptoms that are associated with CFS (see "The Symptoms of CFS" on page 290). The problem now: What kind of a doctor to call?

Doctors at the CDC suggest that you start with a call to a university medical center. A teaching hospital can put you in touch with doctors who keep abreast of current research and who are adept at hard calls like CFS.

Keep a health diary.
Since symptoms of CFS mimic other problems, you'll help yourself and your doctor if you keep a running daily health journal of your symptoms and activities. Reviewing the journal can reveal patterns that show whether you have the condition or one of the look-alikes.

"If you feel exhausted and miserable, you can see why it happened. Maybe you have these symptoms because you've been pushing yourself for a month," says Meredith A. Titus, Ph.D., a senior psychologist at the Menninger Clinic in Topeka, Kansas. The journal should include notes on your energy highs and lows as well as symptoms during different times of the day.

Getting Geared Up When You're Worn Out

If you're diagnosed with CFS, it's likely that the doctor will prescribe a number of medications that may help ease some of the related symptoms, ranging from soreness and inflammation to allergies and depression. But here are some other things doctors recommend for those who have it.

Exercise caution.
If you're the kind of person who's been used to the sporting life or getting regular workouts, the slowdown that comes with CFS may be a real shock. People

The Symptoms of CFS

In 1988 the Centers for Disease Control and Prevention (CDC) in Atlanta published the definitive list of symptoms of chronic fatigue syndrome (CFS). It was a tricky feat because CFS is an easily misdiagnosed syndrome with shifting shape and many disguises. So, in order to study the disease and the people who have it, the CDC developed a "case definition"—a diagnostic map. This is a modified version.

Two Top Diagnostic Tools

- Identifying debilitating fatigue that continues for six months or more, reducing your normal activity by at least 50 percent.
- Eliminating the probability of other diseases through doctors' examinations and lab tests.

Three Symptoms to Measure

These three symptoms are the ones the doctor can measure, observe or test. People with CFS generally have at least two.
- Mild fever (between 99° and 101°F)
- Inflamed throat
- Tender glands (the lymph glands) in the neck or armpit

A CFS Checklist

These are the symptoms that accompany CFS fatigue, but many of them can't be measured. People with CFS usually come down with about eight of them.
- Chills or mild fever
- Sore throat
- Painful or swollen lymph glands
- Muscle discomfort
- Fatigue for at least 24 hours after regular exercise
- Unusually severe headache
- Joint pain without swelling or redness
- Concentration and memory problems, irritability, confusion, depression
- Disturbed sleep
- Unexplained general muscle weakness
- A quick onset of symptoms within a few hours or days

with the condition tend to overdo, doctors note. It may be hard to accept the fact that you can't be a regular visitor to your favorite health club anymore. "Health clubs are largely for healthy people," notes Phillip Peterson, M.D., an infectious-disease specialist at the Hennepin County Medical Center in Minneapolis.

"People with CFS have to get their physical activity under control," says Burke A. Cunha, M.D., director of the Chronic Fatigue Syndrome Center and chief of the Infectious Disease Division at Winthrop–University Hospital in Mineola, New York. "That doesn't mean sitting in a room and not moving. It means a walk around the block in the evening instead of a hike. If they overdo it, they'll relapse. Instead of one bad day a week, they may have five or six."

When muscles are in poor condition, they start to lose tone rapidly—after just two weeks of inactivity. Even the muscles in your heart aren't exempt. If you don't get some sort of mild aerobic exercise, your heart will pump more weakly. Then the blood circulates less efficiently, and you end up tiring even faster. That's why CFS specialists recommend small amounts of carefully graded mild exercise, especially walking or water exercise.

Play games.
Just as muscle grows slack without use, so can the mind, says Stephen E. Straus, M.D., a virologist at the National Institutes of Health in Bethesda, Maryland. And using the mind when you have CFS is no simple matter, since loss of memory and trouble with concentration are two main symptoms of the syndrome.

"The memory thing really drove my morale down. I couldn't even remember how to take shorthand—which I'd done all my life," says Shirley Mynatt of Gladstone, Missouri, who has CFS. "But you have to accept that part of the disease. It doesn't mean you're crazy."

Television or board games can give the brain a needed workout. Some days, for instance, Mynatt exercises her mind by playing along with the TV game show *Jeopardy*, or playing Trivial Pursuit with friends or booting up a solitaire card game on her home computer.

Learn new ways of reading.
"I can't read for long periods of time. So I've quit trying to read long, thick novels," says Mynatt. But since she loves reading, she didn't want to give it up. "So I read short articles in magazines instead. And I have rediscovered the joys of short stories," she says. Short stories are easy to consume at one sitting. And people with memory problems don't have to worry about retaining complex plots.

Books on tape were attorney Brian Lutterman's coping tool for dealing with his CFS problem. "I have trouble sleeping. But I also have to spend a fair

The Help Hotline

A telephone rings on the second floor of an office building at 3521 Broadway in Kansas City, Missouri. A person with chronic fatigue syndrome (CFS) answers. A person with CFS speaks.

It's the hotline of the National Chronic Fatigue Syndrome and Fibromyalgia Association. And it rings anywhere from 25 to 100 times a day.

"Most people want to know three things: 'Is it fatal? Am I contagious? How long will I be sick?' " says Orvalene Prewitt, co-founder and president of the association.

Prewitt tells the callers no one has died from CFS. She tells them contagion is unlikely and has never been proved. Even in the same family, she points out, it's rare for more than one person to have the condition. "And we tell them we don't know how long CFS lasts. There are no good studies on it. But we tell them what we know based on the people we've talked to." People with CFS are so glad to have someone who understands the "mystery syndrome" that they sometimes talk for an hour.

The telephone at headquarters is at the heart of a network of more than 400 support groups and phone contacts located throughout the country and abroad. "We can also give people the name and number of a local support group they can go to or just someone nearby to talk to," says Prewitt.

The chronic fatigue syndrome (CFS) hotline operates 24 hours a day. Write to them at National Chronic Fatigue Syndrome and Fibromyalgia Association, 3521 Broadway, Suite 222, Kansas City, MO 64111 or call (816) 931-4777.

More Helpful Numbers

The Centers for Disease Control and Prevention in Atlanta has a hotline with the latest recorded information on CFS diagnosis, causes, treatments and support groups. Call (404) 332-4555.

The Consumer Health Information Research Institute operates a hotline in Kansas City, Missouri, where you can get information on any CFS treatment or remedy you hear about. Call (816) 228-4595.

amount of time resting. That's so boring that I don't rest as much as I should. But I look forward to listening to these books. They're a help, really a godsend," says Lutterman.

Most libraries have audio books that you can borrow with a library card—sometimes with a minimal rental fee. Check your local library to find out about the availability and selection.

Energy Management

For people with CFS, clouds of fatigue don't always shift according to patterns. That's where your health diary can come in handy—telling you whether you tend to feel better in the mornings or in the afternoons.

You can take advantage of any upsurge in energy if you know exactly what you want to do at different times of the day. Here's how to plan.

Rank activities and projects.
Suppose you've let your phone calls lapse since you've been sick, and that report you meant to write is still in files on your desk. As for the laundry, it's rising faster than bread dough on a summer's day. You're feeling well enough to tackle one of those chores right now, but not all three. "You have to figure out what's most important for you to do with the energy you have," says Mynatt.

Friends wound up at the top of Mynatt's list of priorities. She says, "I was involved in many activities and organizations. Every time a door opened, I was there. But I couldn't continue to do everything. So I chose getting together with my friends on the good days that I had."

For someone with CFS, energy is precious—and needs to be spent carefully. To help you keep the books on your energy budget, list the activities you want to do on a piece of scrap paper. Then rank them in another section of your home health diary in the order of their importance, says Dr. Titus.

Don't do it all.
Mynatt describes folks with CFS this way: "They were used to bringing home the bacon. And then frying it up." Experts on the condition remark on their hard-driving, take-charge nature, too.

But people with CFS can't handle the bacon anymore. Instead, they have to learn how to direct others. "You have to revise your expectations of what needs to be done and how much you have to do yourself," says Dr. Titus. Instead of doing the laundry yourself, for instance, have your spouse do it—or send it to a laundry service or the cleaner.

Wherever possible, find shortcuts. Instead of preparing dinner from lengthy recipes, for example, "cook something simple," Dr. Titus suggests. "Or ask people to bring something. Or get some gourmet take-out food."

Building a Bounce-Back Strategy

Former administrative assistant Shirley Mynatt, 50, of Gladstone, Missouri, has been living with chronic fatigue syndrome (CFS) for 2 years. Former attorney Brian Lutterman, 37, of Minneapolis is into his sixth year of living with CFS. And former math teacher Judy Basso, 47, also of Minneapolis, has experienced chronic fatigue syndrome for 11 years. All three adapted creatively to the intrusion, either through trial and error, help from support groups or occasional counseling.

This is what happened and how they have coped with CFS.

An Administrative Assistant on Overload

Mynatt was working many 12-hour days, managing an understaffed office while also attending school. On average she was sleeping five hours every night, and she had so little time for meals that she was fueling up on fast food. Then both her sons decided to get married within six months of one another—and her already overloaded schedule went into hyperdrive.

CFS struck. Mynatt came down with a bout of what felt like extreme influenza or some other virus. She partially recovered, then had another bout of the same. After the third, she went to a doctor. Several months later, when chronic fatigue syndrome was diagnosed, she attended her first support-group meeting. "I found people there who had had CFS a long time and who had found ways to cope," she says.

Mynatt found ways to cope, too.

- The moment I feel the extra fatigue coming on, I stop whatever I'm doing. I had to learn that I couldn't go beyond that or my symptoms would flare.
- I use the answering machine so I can return calls when I feel at my best—usually in the afternoons.
- I use a temporary handicapped sticker when I don't have enough energy to go to the store *and* do the extra walking in the parking lot.
- I read funny things and rent funny videos. My friends and family have helped me keep a sense of humor.

Safe Swimming

Ironically enough, getting some exercise is particularly helpful when you have CFS. "We recommend exercise for everyone with chronic fatigue syndrome, no matter what condition they're in," says physical therapist Barbara D.

A Lawyer's Lows

Like many others, Lutterman can date his CFS siege to a case of acute mononucleosis. Instead of shaking his case of mono after six weeks, the usual duration, Lutterman found that his symptoms hung on. He plugged away at his law work anyway—until 18 months later, when he collapsed.

Lutterman summarizes all the tough lessons he's learned since then: "The single most important thing for me was attitude adjustment, mainly being realistic in my expectations. I can't predict what's going to happen with CFS. I could start to get better. I don't think I'll get worse; that's not the usual course. So I try to plan for the short term and assume I'll have CFS indefinitely. I live in the present as much as possible. And take pleasure in what I can right now, especially our ten-month-old baby."

Small Steps for a Long-Distance Runner

Basso thought she was just getting a cold after she ran a six-mile race in the rain. But when the cold worsened and she saw the doctor, she learned that she had developed acute mononucleosis. Then CFS moved in.

As a way of coping with CFS herself, Basso organized a support group in Minneapolis and wrote a brochure on the subject for the National Chronic Fatigue Syndrome and Fibromyalgia Association. Among her suggestions:

- When something important comes up, I clear my calendar, rest up beforehand and allow downtime afterward, so I have the energy and then the recovery time.
- I try to schedule only two major things a week.
- I don't stand in the kitchen. I use a kitchen stool.
- I buy vegetables and fruits that are already cut up, and I have my groceries delivered.
- I focus on what I can do, not what I can't. For instance, I don't think I'll ever do long-distance running again. But I hope that eventually I'll be well enough to play golf.

Alexander, supervisor of adult rehabilitation at the National Jewish Center for Immunology and Respiratory Medicine in Denver. "And, for anyone with muscle or joint pain, exercise in water—especially warm water—is the most comfortable."

Recreation centers, Y's and even some hospitals offer water exercise classes for the elderly or for people with arthritis. Those classes are generally safe enough for people with CFS. But if you want to start water exercise on your own, here's what you need to do, according to Alexander.

- Pick the time of day when you're most energetic.
- Exercise two to four days a week.
- Exercise for 8 to 10 minutes and stop before you feel like you're so worn out that you have to stop.
- Increase your exercise time by no more than 2 minutes a week until you reach 20 to 30 consecutive minutes.
- Exercise at a moderate or comfortable pace.
- Warm up and cool down your muscles by doing the same water exercises at a slower pace.
- Don't give up too quickly. It's only natural to feel a little tired for two to three weeks. Then you'll start to feel the benefits—more energy and better sleep.

You can get a sufficient workout by walking, marching or jogging in the water for eight to ten minutes. But if you want to try something more structured, here are three water exercises.

The March. Stand sideways to the edge of the pool in chest-high water. Lightly hold on to the side of the pool. March in the water by bending each knee and lifting each leg to hip height if you can. Go at your own pace and use smooth, slow and controlled movements.

Arm sweeps. Stand shoulder deep in the water with your back to the side of the pool. Under the water, push your arms straight out in front of you. Then sweep them widely—out to each side. Bend your elbows and bring your hands toward your shoulders as you drop your elbows. Push your arms out in front of you and make the wide sweep to the sides again. Do ten repetitions.

Leg swings. Stand in chest-high water, turned sideways, with your left forearm resting comfortably on the side of the pool. Swing your right leg straight out to your right side. Then lower the right leg while swinging it across your left leg. Do ten repetitions. Switch sides and work the left leg ten times in the same manner.

The CFS Stroll

Many doctors also advise mild walking for people with CFS as the most convenient form of safe exercise. The following "start-walking" program for someone with the condition is recommended by researcher James F. Jones,

M.D., who has been studying exercise and CFS at the National Jewish Center for Immunology and Respiratory Medicine in Denver.

Start slowly.
Pick a reasonable length of time to walk—ten minutes, for instance.

Take it easy.
Whatever length of time you choose, only walk to the point of exhilaration. Then stop, while you still feel good.

Turn up the effort.
Increase your walking time very gradually, by no more than five minutes once a week. "Eventually, people with CFS will regain pretty good physical function," says Dr. Jones.

Here's the sample program:

Week	Time Limit (minutes)	How Often (times per week)
1	10	2–4
2	15	2–4
3	20	2–4
4	25	2–4
5	30	2–4

Colds
and Flu

For an organism that's a fraction of the size of one cell in your body, a virus packs a mighty punch. It's bad enough that it makes you sneeze and cough and blow your nose all day, but does it also have to make you feel as though your flesh has turned to heavy rubber?

Catching a cold or the flu saps your energy because it forces your body's defense system to mobilize in order to fight the foreign invader. This effort requires energy.

"Being tired is a natural response," says Thomas A. Gossel, R.Ph., Ph.D., dean of the College of Pharmacy at Ohio Northern University in Ada. "It's the body's way of assuring that we slow down and let our natural defenses fight back."

Little Bug, Big Impact

Because colds and flu affect your airways, you also have to work harder to breathe, and that takes energy, too.

As for the flu bug, it's even more pugnacious than the viruses that cause the common cold, and it doesn't stay localized in the upper respiratory tract. Rather, it spreads throughout the body, causing fever, muscle aches and so much energy drain that you can barely get out of bed.

"The fever itself will increase your metabolism and therefore lower your total amount of energy," says Jeffrey Jahre, M.D., clinical associate professor of medicine at Temple University School of Medicine in Philadelphia and chief of infectious diseases at St. Luke's Hospital in Bethlehem, Pennsylvania.

On top of the enervating effects of the illness, many of us compound the energy loss by taking medicines with sedating ingredients, like antihistamines and cough preparations containing codeine.

Coping Mechanisms

Unfortunately, there are no quick and easy cures for colds and flu. The best advice that doctors can offer is that you just have to muddle through, doing what you can to alleviate the symptoms and speed your recovery. Here's how to function while keeping your energy loss to a minimum.

Listen to your body.
"You'll get your energy back faster if you follow the impulse that nature is trying to communicate to you," says John Hibbs, a doctor of naturopathy, associate clinical professor of naturopathic medicine at Bastyr University in Seattle. "The impulse to slow down is natural, and it might be the most important thing you can do."

You should rest as soon as you feel the first hint of symptoms, he states. Don't wait until you're very sick. "Stay home, take a long nap, go to bed early," he advises. "The whole thing will be dramatically shortened and might even blow over."

Make rest stops.
Take the time to rest frequently, advises Dr. Gossel. "This doesn't necessarily mean that you have to sleep a lot. Take naps or just relax, even if it's for ten minutes to read or listen to music or take a hot bath."

Each person has different requirements, he adds. Try to design your schedule so that you can get the relaxation periods you need.

Don't interfere with sleep.
If ordinary rest is important, then deep, natural sleep is even more so.

"The body's immune function can diminish with a lack of sleep," says Dr. Jahre. Try not to use cold remedies that might disturb your sleep. "Oral decongestants, which can stimulate your nervous system, should be avoided at night. The use of a nasal decongestant spray is usually preferred since most of the drug can then be isolated to one area of your body instead of being fully released into your bloodstream," he explains. If you find that you need medication for more than three days, see a doctor, he advises. People who have high blood pressure or heart disease should consult a doctor before taking any of these medications.

Drink lots of fluids.
"Drink a minimum of eight to ten glasses a day, preferably of clear liquids, and more if you can handle it," recommends Dr. Gossel.

Drinking plenty of liquids is one way of helping to eliminate harmful substances that your body produces as it's battling the virus. "If they're not eliminated, they stay in the blood longer, and that leads to more tiredness and lethargy and energy loss," explains Dr. Gossel. And by keeping your system properly hydrated, you'll also help the mucous membranes get rid of foreign invaders.

Watch your diet.
Eating complex carbohydrates like pasta is preferable to focusing on sugar, according to Dr. Gossel. "Sugar will give you an immediate energy boost, but after an hour or so it will make you feel more tired. There's an influx of insulin that follows a sugar load, which lowers your blood sugar, which makes you feel tired."

Reduce your fat intake.
It's important to keep your diet balanced, says Dr. Gossel. So, if you increase your carbohydrates, give up something else so that you don't just add to your total calories. The best place to cut is in the fat department. "If you're going to have pasta, have it with tomato sauce, not with a heavy meat sauce," he advises.

Keep a sunny outlook.
"A positive attitude can help the way you respond to illness," says Dr. Gossel. "If you have the attitude that you don't have to lose all your energy, that you're going to take care of yourself and get over it quickly, you'll feel better." But don't let your upbeat attitude carry you to the never-never land of denial. "Don't fool yourself into thinking that you can do whatever you want as if there were no symptoms," he cautions.

Reduce stress.
"Studies show that a person can become infected with a virus and not get cold symptoms," says Dr. Jahre. One of the influencing factors is stress. "The more stressors you have experienced in the recent past, the more likely you are to become ill."

A Panoply of Remedies

Want your energy back? Take steps quickly to alleviate debilitating symptoms and keep the virus from making things worse. Here's how.

Get a dose of relief.
Take a pain reliever if you have the flu, says Frederick Ruben, M.D., professor of medicine at the University of Pittsburgh. Acetaminophen or aspirin can reduce the fever and combat aches and pains, according to Dr. Ruben.

Shake a Leg to Shake a Cold?

You're feeling under the weather but not quite so laid out that you feel as though you need to stay in bed. In fact, you suspect that a bit of exercise may make you feel better. Should you indulge? The answer is: It depends.

If you have a cold, researchers have found that a brief walk in fresh air keeps your blood moving. The exercise helps your body heal and enhances your energy level.

Studies show that being infected by the rhinovirus, the one that causes most common colds, does not seriously impair your ability to exercise, according to David C. Nieman, Dr.P.H., professor of health and exercise science at Appalachian State University in Boone, North Carolina. Nor does exercise make the symptoms caused by the cold virus any worse. It may even help to relieve them.

If you have the flu virus, however, it's a different story. "It's a systemic virus," says Dr. Nieman. "It diminishes performance capability. And exercising when you have the flu can make the symptoms worse."

In fact, exerting yourself when you have the flu can lead to something called post-viral fatigue syndrome. "You're not actually sick," observes Dr. Nieman, "but you don't feel quite right. You fatigue easily and get lethargic."

What if you're not really sure what you have and you feel as though a little exercise may do you some good?

Dr. Nieman advocates the neck rule: "If the symptoms are from the neck up, it's usually okay, and perhaps beneficial, to exercise moderately. If the symptoms are below the neck, it's better to rest and wait for the symptoms to go away before getting back to exercise, especially if you have a fever."

Try vitamin C.

Taking vitamin C as a cold remedy is controversial, and the jury is still out on whether it can actually prevent colds. But there seems to be solid evidence that it can hasten recovery. In one study done by Elliot Dick, Ph.D., professor of preventive medicine at the University of Wisconsin Medical School in Madison, researchers found that taking 2,000 milligrams of vitamin C every day "greatly moderated people's colds."

Taking that amount in doses of 1,000 milligrams, two times a day, is helpful as a basic preventive measure, according to Dr. Dick. "If you start to notice cold symptoms, increase the dosage sharply." He suggests taking 1,000 or 2,000 milligrams immediately, then 1,000 milligrams every hour or so for a few hours. While a few thousand milligrams a day is considered safe, tolerance for vitamin C varies, says Dr. Dick. As little as 1,200 milligrams a day can cause diarrhea in some people. You should discuss this therapy with your doctor before trying it.

Think zinc.

Studies on zinc gluconate as a cold remedy have yielded conflicting results, according to Melvyn Werbach, M.D., a Los Angeles physician and author of *Healing with Food*: "Some studies find that sucking on zinc lozenges reduces by more than half the number of days it takes a cold sufferer to recover. Others have found no evidence that it's effective."

Use zinc at the first sign of cold symptoms, advises Dr. Werbach. Suck one lozenge every two hours. He recommends using 180-milligram zinc gluconate lozenges containing 23 milligrams of elemental zinc. This therapy far exceeds the Daily Value of 15 milligrams, but taking extra zinc on a short-term basis is generally safe. It is a good idea to take it along with 2 milligrams of copper, as zinc depresses copper levels, he adds. He suggests trying it for a week to see if it works for you.

Try some echinacea.

A number of herbs have been found to stimulate the immune system, making white blood cells more aggressive in attacking viruses, says Dr. Hibbs.

"The first line of defense against colds and flu is echinacea," he says. "It's a very safe herb. Start taking it at the first sign of feeling run down or achy." He recommends taking freeze-dried preparations compacted into pills or capsules in doses of 300 to 800 milligrams, three times a day. If you take it in tincture form, a liquid extract that contains the therapeutic ingredients from fresh or dried herbs, he notes, you have to take more of it, and it ends up being more expensive.

Give licorice a try.

Licorice root is another good antivirus herb and can be taken as an alternative to other cold remedies, according to Dr. Hibbs. Though it can be brewed into a good-tasting tea, it's not strong enough in that form. It's more effective as a pill or tincture, he says. Take one or two capsules, two times a day, or a half-teaspoon, three times a day in tincture form, he suggests. One note of caution: In these large doses licorice root can raise blood pressure. If you have high blood pressure, you should avoid this remedy altogether, says Dr. Hibbs.

Eat garlic.

Vampires are not the only creatures who hate garlic; viruses don't like them, either. "Garlic is a great antiviral," says Dr. Hibbs. You can eat some raw, brew it in tea or, of course, cook with it. Don't fret if your sweetheart doesn't particularly enjoy the smell, he says. You can take garlic capsules that don't leave an odor on your breath. If you want to take it raw, he suggests two to six cloves a day. If not, two to four garlic capsules a day does the job just as well, he says.

Ask Mom for chicken soup.
Sometimes, old folk remedies have validity. "There is scientific evidence that chicken soup may be helpful with respiratory illness," says Dr. Jahre. Its healing power might not come from the chicken, though, but from the fact that it's a hot liquid. It may be that the warm vapors help the nose to produce mucus flow, which in turn clears the cold viruses out of your body, he adds.

What Not to Do

Some people take steps to cure colds and flu that actually make their problem worse. The trouble with these quick fixes is that you may end up prolonging your illness and sapping your energy even further. To avoid that, here are some words from the wise.

Limit your coffee.
Don't increase your caffeine consumption in an effort to boost your energy, warns Dr. Gossel. "If you try to stimulate yourself past a certain point, you'll end up more tired. Caffeine stimulates the cells to increase their metabolism, and that requires a great expenditure of energy."

Drink decaf or herbal tea, he suggests. And go easy on chocolate, since that contains caffeine, too.

Don't drink alcohol.
A hot toddy can feel great going down, and it may soothe your throat and ease your pain temporarily. But, says Dr. Gossel, "it won't be long before you really slow down."

It's especially important to stay away from beer, wine and liquor if you're taking medicine that can interact with alcohol to depress the central nervous system. Read the labels on any medicines that you're taking before you drink so much as a sip of wine, says Dr. Gossel.

Don't take antihistamines.
Medicines that contain antihistamines aren't effective for viruses, says Dr. Ruben. "If they work, you don't have a cold, you have an allergy."

In general, over-the-counter remedies are a waste of money if you have the flu, he adds. They'll only make you sleepier.

Don't smoke.

Quitting is important under any conditions, but especially when you're sick. "Smoking makes you more susceptible to disease," says Dr. Jahre. It also reduces lung capacity, lowers the oxygen capacity of your blood and disturbs sleep. Put all of these things together, and they add up to major energy drain.

Don't try for a quick comeback.

If you're physically active and then become sedentary even for a brief period of time, your energy level and your capacity for exertion can be substantially reduced. Take that into account when you restart your activity after a cold, says Dr. Jahre. If you try to start up where you left off, you may quickly wear yourself out. "Ease back into it and gradually build back up to your norm."

Commuting

Do you have a tough drive to work every morning? If you do, that old energy slayer, stress, probably hovers over your head like a vulture over roadkill.

Nobody has measured the amount of energy that commuting costs the 84 million workers across the nation who drive alone to work. But Raymond Novaco, Ph.D., professor of psychology and social behavior at the school of social ecology at University of California, Irvine, has been tracking the traffic issue for more than 15 years. It's clear that long-distance commuting takes a major toll on health, he says.

"The longer the distance, the higher the blood pressure," he says. Not only that, but the cumulative effect of those bad trips spills over into your life at work and at home. Your frustration level at work rises, your brainpower falters and your mood at home sours. You have no energy left for enjoying life.

Don't Let Commuting Take a Toll

"The best way to deal with commuting is not to do it," says Robert Ostroff, M.D., associate professor of psychiatry at Yale University School of Medicine. "You're better off walking to work or riding in a car pool. But most people don't have that option, so you have to find a way to reduce the stress of being in the car for a long period of time."

There are lots of ways to shoo off the energy vultures, however. Here's how to thrive while you drive.

Juggle your work hours.
If you have ever driven your daily journey early in the morning or late at night, you know that there's nothing actually evil about your route. It's the chokehold of 23 million cars on America's highways at 9:00 A.M. and 5:00 P.M. that clogs our pikes and expressways—and seems to gang up on you to block your way. Avoiding peak commuting hours is an obvious solution to spending time in traffic congestion.

Depending on your company's work policy, you can try a ten-to-six or an eight-to-four shift to lighten your highway woes. But if you don't have that kind of flexibility, just leave for work earlier so that you miss the worst traffic, suggests Dr. Novaco.

Work out after work.
The evening rush is worse than the morning one because stress is compounded by fatigue from the workday, notes Dr. Novaco. So it's a good idea to wait out that traffic.

Instead of getting worked up, work out at a gym near your job, he suggests. Taking a yoga class is a great way to relax. If you plan to go to dinner, see a movie or go shopping, try to do these things near work, delaying your departure enough to miss the worst of the traffic.

Share your ride.
It may be a hassle to coordinate your arrival and departure schedules with another person or two, but carpooling is worth it. Studies show that ride-sharing lowers commuter stress significantly, says Dr. Novaco.

Cocooning in Your Car

Folks tend to regard their cars as extensions of themselves, says Dr. Ostroff. So it's a good idea to outfit your auto as comfortably as you dress yourself. Here's how to make a simpatico nest that will help you get rid of energy-depleting stress during long commutes.

Widen your listening horizons.
"The main way to reduce the stress of being in your car for long periods of time is to do other things," says Dr. Ostroff. Of course, you can always listen to the radio or to music tapes, but there's so much more. Consider learning a foreign language with the use of audiotapes, he suggests. And if you like to read but commuting has stolen all your reading time, check out books on cassette at your local library. You can find novels, dramas, biographies, history books—whatever suits your taste—and many libraries have full-length books on tape as well as abridged versions.

There's even an exercise tape called Karkicks, which has exercises that you can do in your car, according to Jane Sullivan-Durand, M.D., a physician in private practice in Contoocook, New Hampshire, who specializes in behavioral medicine. It combines gentle movements that help you stay awake and relieve stress—shoulder rolls, neck extensions, tummy tucks—with safe-driving messages. You can order the tape by calling 1-800-666-2230.

Pillow your back.

When you're standing, the lower portion of your spine (the lumbar section) normally curves inward, toward your abdomen. When you're sitting, however, it tends to slump outward. That squeezes your spinal disks, puts stress on them and cuts off their supply of nutritious fluid, says back expert Malcolm Pope, Ph.D., director of the Iowa Spine Research Center at the University of Iowa in Iowa City.

It helps to support your back on long drives, says Dr. Pope. He suggests tucking a rolled towel or a pillow in that lumbar curve. Or you can get back pillows that are designed specifically for this purpose at bed-and-bath stores and medical supply stores.

Fidget and squirm.

Even if you have a back pillow, sitting in one position for longer than 15 minutes will start to stiffen you, says David Viano, Ph.D., principal research investigator at General Motors in Warren, Michigan. "Our bodies are designed for movement."

You can't move much while you're driving, but you can make adjustments that will help you ride in comfort so that you don't feel totally depleted by the end of the trip, says Dr. Viano. Put most of your weight on one buttock and then the other. Shift the position of your seat or your buttocks slightly. Slide down in your seat a hair and then sit up. If your car has cruise control, use it on the open stretches—and while your legs are free, flex your knees and wiggle your feet, he says. (Just remember to keep your eyes on the road and your feet away from the gas and brake pedals.)

Depression

In the latter years of the nineteenth century and into the first decade of the twentieth, Harvard professor William James was a pioneer in the fields of philosophy and psychology. William James also was plagued with depression for many years.

His *Principles of Psychology* is included in the Great Books of the Western world, alongside volumes by Freud and Marx. His *Varieties of Religious Experience* remains a highly acclaimed work on the subject of religion.

And in 1907 James published a short essay titled *The Energies of Men*. Its point is that each of us has the capacity to reach down and find more energy for our lives. Each of us, he insists, can catch a second wind. Deep within us all, we can find untapped resources to energize our lives, James asserts.

The Energies of Men reads like a very personal essay. As William James wrestled with depression, perhaps researching this book was his attempt to find answers many of us are still seeking.

Nearly a century later, depression is a serious problem. It affects approximately 17.6 million Americans each year, and women are about twice as likely as men to be depressed.

You can even be depressed and not know it. Doctors use the term "depression" to cover a wide range of less-than-chipper mood states, from the occasional blues to a chronic, disabling and possibly even suicidal condition.

There's no doubt, however, that for most people energy and depression are linked—that day-to-day feeling of being wiped out, spent, washed up and drained can leave you with hardly a memory of what it was like to have energy in your life. What can you do about it?

Getting Help

The introduction of psychotherapies and antidepressant drugs such as Prozac has meant the difference between hopeless despair and a renewed outlook on life for many people who are depressed. In fact, one notable effect of the new medications seems to be a new vitality, a new energy for life.

"Despite some controversy surrounding the new antidepressant drugs, they have an excellent track record for restoring energy and improving the overall quality of life in people who are depressed," says David Allen, M.D., clinical professor of psychiatry at Georgetown University School of Medicine in Washington, D.C.

Still, doctors believe that most depression goes both undiagnosed and untreated. Whether you are being treated by a doctor or not, there are things you can do to have more energy in the midst of depression, if you're simply having a down-in-the-dumps day or even if you're going through a very long, dark, hopeless season in life.

Studies on coping with depression suggest that dwelling on symptoms of depression (for example, fatigue or lack of motivation) or responding in passive ways may make you feel worse. On the other hand, distractions, particularly active and rewarding ones, may help even the most down-spirited person feel more upbeat.

Dr. Allen has assembled a list of possible "distractions" to boost your energy if you're depressed.

Put your shoes on.
Aerobic exercise has been shown to be the single most effective treatment for depression. "Its energizing effects are nearly immediate," he says. "A brisk walk, or a jog if you can manage it, is sure to lift your energy level."

Breathe deeply.
Deep breathing, like exercise, increases the flow of oxygen, expands and stretches your weary body and can have a nearly instantaneous effect on your sense of well-being.

Bring music to your ears.
Forget those sad country music songs about the woes of life. Both relaxing and up-tempo music can have a dramatic effect on the energy level of someone who is depressed. The Muzak folks have mastered the art of changing mood to get us to shop more, shop longer, shop with more energy—shop until we drop. Take a lesson from them. "Listen to music that refreshes you and peps you up," Dr. Allen says.

Focus on inspiring affirmations.
More and more research has shown the value of spirituality for emotional and physical health. "I often have my patients memorize the 23rd Psalm," Dr. Allen says. Its hope-filled message inspires people and urges them on, he insists. Dr. Allen also encourages his patients to read, memorize and reflect on brief, af-

firming passages from inspiring writings such as the Bible and to make an effort to read uplifting writers such as Henri Nouwen, author of *Lifesigns* and *Road to Daybreak*.

Get away.
A change of scenery, especially going outdoors, seems to have a positive effect on those who suffer from depression. The seashore is Dr. Allen's favorite destination. "There is something soothing and healing about it," he asserts. "The rhythm of the waves washing on the sand has a cleansing and stimulating effect."

Lend a helping hand.
Doing kind deeds seems to have a double benefit. Besides helping the individual on the receiving end, it lifts the spirits of the doer as well. "I try to get people to help others who are less fortunate than they are," says Dr. Allen. "If you are depressed, you may think you are at the bottom of a pit alone. It is important for people suffering from depression to see that there are others who are suffering who may be worse off." He encourages people to get involved with the poor, the homeless or those in recovery and treatment centers.

Taking Stock

When you're depressed, it's all too easy to let feelings of uselessness creep into your life and take over, according to Robert D. Kerns, Ph.D., associate professor of psychiatry, neurology and psychology at Yale University School of Medicine and chief of the psychology service at the Veterans Administration Connecticut Health Care System in West Haven. Your dark mood casts a gray shadow over your life, making you feel like you're going nowhere fast.

In fact, Dr. Kerns asserts, you probably fail to appreciate how much you actually accomplish. Simply knowing that you are getting more done than you think can be energizing. Therefore, he recommends a technique for taking stock of your accomplishments. Make a list of what you get done. Or keep a diary so you can go back and see all the activities of your day-to-day life as concrete accomplishments. You may feel that you don't have the energy to log your day, but at least try to.

Dr. Kerns also recommends making a pleasures list to help keep you motivated. There are three categories to include in your list.

1. *Things you used to do and liked but have stopped doing.* Identify the things you have enjoyed over the course of your life. Some, if not many, of

these things may be long lost. Then ask yourself whether you can get them back into your life. Perhaps it was a form of recreation or a commitment to something you believe in. Returning to it may pick you up and energize your life.

2. *Things you have enjoyed and still do but have cut back on.* Perhaps increasing your participation in the activity or your level of commitment to it, or changing how you do it, will work as an energizer.

3. *Things you have never done but have always wanted to do.* You may have unfulfilled goals and dreams. They seem far away, even lost, but they may be possible. After you've made your list, ask yourself if each one is feasible. Forget the easy "no" answer. Give each item serious reconsideration.

If you take on your unfulfilled dreams, you may find the second wind you need that lifts you up to soar above the low-hanging cloud of depression.

Difficult People

Whether they're dominators or doormats, windbags or whiners, users or victims, difficult people are little less than energy vampires. They suck your life force, making you weaker even as they themselves get stronger—and more difficult.

Their behaviors may run the gamut from sweet to obnoxious, but what they actually do or say is less important than their impact on you. If you find that you constantly feel drained, challenged, defensive or simply irritable around someone—well, *that's* a difficult person. Never mind what other people say about him. If you have a problem with that person, then something needs to be done before you pour too much energy into damage control.

"They're often such strong personalities that they control you whether they're present or not," says William J. Kreidler, senior conflict resolution specialist at Educators for Social Responsibility in Cambridge, Massachusetts. "You put a lot of energy into wishing they would change and into fantasizing about revenge."

Expecting a difficult person to change is like waiting for a leopard to shed its spots. "You can't fix them," says Mark Goulston, M.D., assistant clinical professor of psychiatry at the University of California, Los Angeles, and author of *Get Out of Your Own Way.* "If you try to fix someone who's not fixable, it drains your energy."

Kreidler agrees, "Difficult people behave the way they do because it meets their needs. They have very little motivation to change."

Since there's no way to stay away from difficult people entirely, it's up to you to learn strategies for managing them—and yourself—to minimize the damage before you wear yourself out with your efforts to fix them.

Building Mental Strength

When dealing with difficult people, remember that their behaviors and the negative messages that come your way are not aimed at you specifically. To prevent them from wearing you down, you have to put their behaviors in perspective.

Five Makers of Trouble

Difficult people come in all shapes and sizes. Which one is pushing your buttons? William J. Kreidler, senior conflict resolution specialist at Educators for Social Responsibility in Cambridge, Massachusetts, has identified five main types, along with a few tips for handling them.

1. **The Tank.** These are extremely aggressive people who roll over everyone who gets in their way. "Their goals are all that matters," says Kreidler. "They see life as a power struggle."

Strategy: Don't engage them. "People like this are always in a tug-of-war with others. But if you won't pick up the other end of the rope, they can't play the game."

2. **The Doormat**. These are very passive types who always abdicate responsibility. "The catch is that they often get their revenge in subtle ways, and they're aggravating. They drain your energy because they won't take responsibility, so you have to take over."

Strategy: Wait them out. "They want someone else to pick up the ball, so let the ball lie there. Eventually, they have to respond in some way."

3. **The Complainer.** Kvetch, kvetch, kvetch.

Strategy: "If something's annoying, don't engage them," says Kreidler. "Just say that you don't want to talk about that."

4. **The Hot-Air Balloon.** They always claim to know the right answer, but usually they don't have a clue. "They're relatively harmless until they start passing false information," says Kreidler.

Strategy: Correct their misinformation gently, without attacking them personally.

5. **The Know-It-All.** Unlike the Hot-Air Balloon, Know-It-Alls do know what they're talking about, but they're nasty when someone disagrees or makes a mistake. "They tend to be black-and-white thinkers who can't accept that someone with a different opinion may also be right, and they're very defensive when challenged."

Strategy: Don't tell them they're wrong. Instead, try to use phrases like "You're right but . . . "

Don't take it personally.
"We have a tendency to think that people are being especially difficult with us, but typically they're difficult with others as well," says Frank M. Dattilio, Ph.D., clinical associate professor at the University of Pennsylvania School of Medicine in Philadelphia.

If someone's giving you fits because he's critical or what he says is even insulting, taking it personally may cause you to get angry or defensive. But what good does it do to snipe back? This in turn tends to escalate the situation, which ultimately wears you down even more.

"Step back and realize that you're probably dealing with someone who's that way with everyone," advises Dr. Dattilio. "That doesn't diminish the unpleasantness, but it helps you think through your methods of responding."

Welcome some helplessness.

When dealing with difficult people, you tend to focus on their behaviors. "Then you feel helpless because you can't change them," says Robert Strock, a psychotherapist in private practice in Santa Monica, California. But if you just give up trying to change that person, you'll probably feel a sense of relief.

Speak your convictions.

When dealing with people who are truly difficult, sometimes it takes the patience of a saint not to explode. But while venting anger can make you feel better in the short run, you often risk saying or doing something that you'll later regret.

The way to keep your temper in check is to find out what bothers you by thinking about what has been said or done. "Ask yourself what made you angry," advises Dr. Goulston. "Then identify the principles that have been violated and put your conviction into words. Whenever you can rise above the personal offense and stand up for your values instead, you gain clarity, strength and the courage of conviction."

Let your feelings out.

Although it's generally not a good idea to vent your feelings in the heat of the moment, it can be very soothing and energizing to let them out in other ways. After any difficult encounter, says Strock, take a few minutes to release all the negative feelings. He suggests writing down your feelings—but just for yourself, not in an angry letter. Or talk into a tape recorder. Or "express your feelings creatively in art or music," he advises.

Once you get the feelings out, take a moment to evaluate what you said. Maybe your feelings are so strong that it would be best to keep them to yourself. On the other hand, you may feel that you've just had an excellent rehearsal session and that it may be time to confront the person directly.

If you decide to go public, you'll probably want to understate the truth a bit. "Depending on the sensitivity of the situation and the individual, understatement can be safer and more sensible than the truth in its raw form," says Strock.

Heal it with humor.

It's not always easy to see the lighter side of things, but infusing difficult situations with humor will go a long way toward keeping your own energy levels high.

"Find something to laugh about, either in the situation itself or outside of it," says Rick Brinkman, a naturopathic physician in Portland, Oregon, and co-author of *Dealing with People You Can't Stand*. "Make it absurd and funny," he adds. "You can't laugh and hate people at the same time."

Taking Control

If you can't beat them, join them. While experts don't recommend coping with difficult people by becoming difficult yourself, there are ways to preempt their behaviors with some cagey tactics of your own. The more you put yourself in control of the situation, the less they'll be able to wear you down. Here are a few things you may want to try.

Be unpredictable.
The next time you're face-to-face with the person who's driving you nuts, make a conscious decision to act in a totally different way than you usually do. If you're usually silent, talk up a storm. Argue instead of agreeing. Change the subject rather than staying on course.

"They expect you to react in predictable ways that they know how to manage," says Kreidler. "They've been in training since childhood, and they're used to their difficult behaviors bringing them what they want." If you defy their expectations, he says, it disorients them. Eventually, they may find it easier simply to leave you alone—which means you have more energy for the things that matter in your life.

Round out the relationship.
Particularly in the workplace, we often find ourselves re-creating over and over again the very situations that bring out the worst in people. Rather than waiting for difficult people to do "the usual," why not change the rules? Have a meeting over lunch instead of in the boardroom. Call them on the phone rather than dropping into their offices. Do anything you can to engage them in situations that are less likely to bring out their worst qualities, Kreidler advises.

"No one is difficult all the time," he says. "There are other aspects to them that you can try to bring out and develop. It won't necessarily change them, but it might soften their overall behaviors."

Kill them with kindness.
Some difficult people become downright impossible when they're confronted aggressively or put on the defensive. "Don't challenge them," Dr. Dattilio advises. "Defuse the situation by keeping your cool and by not being difficult back. If you absorb what they dish out without letting it get to you, it disarms them and tells them you're not a threat."

Draw a line.

"Sometimes you have to be firm and define your boundaries," Dr. Dattilio says. "Let them know what you will and will not tolerate." Make clear the reasons for your stand, he adds, and acknowledge that while you know it might upset them, your position is firm.

Show them you understand.

Difficult people are often convinced that they're misunderstood—that the world is simply too slow, too disorganized or too stupid to get what they're trying to say. One of the best things you can do, says Dr. Brinkman, is make it very clear that you understand what they're trying to say. "Once people feel understood, the doors to their minds open," he says.

Experts have defined four listening techniques that help give the message "I'm listening." Here are some modes of communication.

• Give meaningful looks (or, if you're on the phone, make meaningful sounds). This is a way of letting the difficult person know that you're hearing what is being said. You aren't necessarily agreeing with every word, but you're not interfering with the message, either.

• Backtrack. Every so often, summarize in a few words what you've just been told: "If I understand you correctly, what you're saying is . . ." This is an easy way of letting the person know that you're listening and digesting what is being said, says Dr. Brinkman.

• Clarify. Everyone appreciates being asked questions. It shows that you not only hear the person but are interested enough to want to get it right.

• Summarize. Periodically in the conversation, you should go over everything that you've discussed and ask if there's anything more that the person wants to say. This will result in fewer misunderstandings later on. In addition, the difficult person will be less likely to get angry, because he was allowed to get in the last word.

Each of these listening techniques can be used with all kinds of difficult people, says Dr. Brinkman. "With a know-it-all, for example, you want to ask fewer questions and do more backtracking. With a whiner, you want to do more clarifying."

Entertaining

You can bet that anyone who sings the praises of parties hasn't thrown one of her own lately. If she had, she'd be way too pooped to sing.

Cleaning floors. Vacuuming drapes. Making a dozen trips to the store. Sending out invitations. Putting up decorations. Cooking. Straightening. Organizing. The very idea of having a party can be so exhausting that you want to climb into bed for a week.

There's no question that giving a party is hard work. But don't let it get you down. With careful planning and by deciding in advance what you can do yourself and how you can get some extra help, you can have a great bash and still have enough energy left over to enjoy it.

According to Brett Frechette, chef at Wellesley College in Massachusetts, the trick is not letting yourself be overwhelmed by the sheer enormity of all the tasks that need to be done. After all, every big event is made up of many smaller, more manageable jobs. "Break your tasks down into doable portions," Frechette advises. "That will help you avoid that frenzied feeling, and you'll always be in control."

Staying in Control

Acting on impulse can be fun. Invigorating. Risky.

Not to disparage spontaneity, but to have a bash on the spur of the moment is to invite disaster. Even professional chefs and caterers make it a point always to prepare a point-by-point plan before putting on a party.

"Plan your menu at least a few days before the party," advises John Nihoff, an instructor at the Culinary Institute of America in Hyde Park, New York. "Make a day-by-day list of what you need to do. Think of it as a countdown to the shuttle launch."

As your party approaches takeoff, here's what you can do to keep everything on schedule and ready to fly.

Start with a list.

Things that don't get written down have a way of not getting done—or of getting done only at the last minute, with a lot of exhausting, last-minute rushing around. "Plan it on paper first," advises Nancy Grigor, owner of Hamptons Locations, a company that handles catering and other details for film and photo crews in New York City. "If you can visualize the party in your mind and make notes, you could save energy by knowing exactly what you need to buy. You'll have to make only one shopping trip."

Stick to the list.

When shopping for a party, it's easy to get distracted by exotic (and usually expensive) trifles you don't need. Things like smoked squid. Rose-flavored candy. Chocolate truffles. "Don't deviate from the list," cautions Pina Manzone, part-owner of a special events consulting firm in Westport, Connecticut. "That's what drives people crazy. They think, 'I'll make this, too,' and they run back to the supermarket to get it."

Follow a theme.

One way to keep your party simple is to organize it around a central theme. Have steak and potatoes on Western Night or use red linens and hearts for Valentine's Day. "Having a theme helps keep you focused," says Manzone. The less work you spend ahead of time, the more energy you'll have for your guests on the night of the party.

Decorate simply.

You don't have to spend hours racing around town trying to find the perfect decorations. Simple set-ups are often the most elegant. In the autumn a pumpkin and some leaves make an attractive centerpiece, says Grigor. Lighting candles adds ambiance, as does a nice fire burning in the fireplace or a bouquet of fresh flowers.

Stick to the tried-and-true.

The night you're having guests is not the time to try out that extravagant new dish you read about. "Stick with the dishes you do best," says Grigor. Remember, the idea is to have a good time with your guests, not to wear yourself out before the party even begins.

Keep the cooking simple.

As host you have to mingle, which means you don't want to be chained to the stove all night. "I try to make something that doesn't take a lot of stove time, such as Bavarian pot roast," says Grigor. Lasagna is also good, particularly since you can assemble it the day before, then pop it in the oven the evening of the party.

Don't squeeze 'em in.

Even if you're planning an outdoor party, don't invite more guests than your home can comfortably hold, Grigor says. Your yard may have room for 50, but bad weather may send everyone indoors.

In addition, when planning a dinner party, don't try to squeeze 12 or 14 people around a dining room table meant for 10, Grigor adds.

The close quarters will make everyone uncomfortable, which will cramp after-dinner conversation—the most important part of the party. "You spend 25 percent of your time eating and 75 percent of the time socializing and conversing," Nihoff observes.

Share the cooking.

One of the easiest ways to keep a party from wearing you down is to have a potluck. "Have your friends bring their favorite dishes," says Laurie H. Meyer, president of Programs Plus International in New York City. "Just be sure to specify whether you want them to bring an entree, appetizer or dessert."

Work ahead.

No matter how well-organized you are, the day of the party is going to be a busy one. To lighten the exhaustion factor, do as much of the cooking ahead of time as you can. Many appetizers, like dips, crudites and deviled eggs, can usually be made one (or more) days in advance. So can most desserts, cakes, sorbets and pies. Even main courses, like stews, can often be made ahead of time.

Not everything has to be homemade, Meyer adds. Don't hesitate to stop at the supermarket or gourmet store to pick up things you need. The less time you spend cooking, the more time you have for entertaining guests.

Hiring Help

No matter how talented or hardworking you are, some affairs are too large or too important to take on by yourself. You'll probably feel more energetic and in control if you hire help. Here's what the experts advise.

Call a caterer.

Perhaps the easiest way to entertain with flair and grace is to have a professional help you out. Depending on your needs, caterers will handle everything from food preparation and service to decorations. The more work they do, the more time and energy you have to spend with your guests.

"It's probably not a good idea to trust the cool caterer-of-the-month that you've only recently heard about," adds Frechette. "Choose someone you already know or who has been recommended by someone you know."

When using a caterer, always be clear in advance about exactly what they're responsible for. (If it's not in the contract, you can assume it won't be done.) By knowing in advance who's doing what, you'll be able to avoid those frantic, last-minute problems that can transform a party to be remembered into an event that's best forgotten.

Hire a babysitter.
If you have young children or are inviting guests with young children, hiring a babysitter for the evening makes it a lot easier for everyone to have a great time, says Frechette. The children will be entertained, and the adults can relax without worrying what the young ones are up to.

Bring on the entertainment.
Depending on your budget, one way to keep a party rolling is to bring in professional talent—a stand-up comedy team, for example, or a quartet of musicians from a local college. You can even rent karaoke equipment for the evening. High-energy parlor games will help relieve you of nonstop entertaining, while at the same time guaranteeing that everyone has a great time.

Party Time

Have you ever looked back on the evening and realized that you didn't have a complete conversation with even one guest? From cooking, bringing food and clearing places to chopping ice and filling punch bowls, you never even had time to sit down. You went to bed exhausted—and determined never to do it again.

In order for your guests to have a great time, however, *you* have to have a good time. Here are a few ways to have a wonderful party without wearing yourself out in the process.

Accept extra help.
Hosts are often reluctant to accept help from friends, because a guest's job is to relax. Don't be so quick to turn them down. "If friends offer to do something for you, accept their offer," says Frechette. "It gives other people a little investment in your party. Support is a great way to relieve stress."

Establish no-enter zones.
By restricting the party only to certain rooms, you can reduce the amount of cleanup that has to be done before or after the party. Particularly when young children will be attending, "you may not want your entire house to be open," says Frechette. Simply keeping doors closed will let people know which areas are part of the party and which are out-of-bounds.

Let the dishes pile up.
Even if you hate having a sinkful of dishes, the party is your chance to catch up with friends, and they with you. You can always clean up the mess later on, says Frechette.

Take some quiet time.
A half-hour before guests arrive, sit down and enjoy a glass of wine. Or just relax for a few minutes, says Manzone. "I need that half-hour to pull myself together so that when my guests come, I'm totally relaxed."

Don't sweat the details.
Your friends don't care if every dish is placed exactly so or if there's a speck of dust on the living room floor. Don't wear yourself out making the house absolutely perfect, advises Meyer.

Stretch to de-stress.
Kitchen work can be extremely strenuous for your hand and arm muscles, says Nihoff. To stay alert and refreshed, here is a stretch that he recommends.

Hold your left arm straight out in front of you. With your right hand gently bend back the four fingers of the left hand until you feel a good stretch. Hold for a count of five and relax. Repeat with the other hand.

Touch your temples.
Need an instant relaxer? "When you can't find the cream, and the guests are due in ten minutes, and you sent your spouse to the store, it's time for this exercise," Nihoff says. "Put your thumbs on your temples with light pressure and rotate them." Breathe deeply for a few moments. You'll feel refreshed fast and be ready to start the party.

Getting Up
in the Morning

Do you hate the sound of the alarm? Do you cringe away from those first rays of morning light as they pierce through your bedroom window? Do you feel as though you simply can't muster up the energy to roll out of bed in the morning?

Don't let the fact that you resist leaping out of the sack get you down. There is good reason for you to want to stay snug in your bed.

"You're taking your body from a complete resting state into an active one," says Art Mollen, D.O., medical director of the Southwest Health Institute in Phoenix. "Physiologically, it's hard to kick up the metabolism from the nice, comfortable sleep and resting state we enjoy. It's a drastic change, so it has an effect on your mind and your mood.

"Right after you wake up, your body's just not flexible enough. Your blood sugar is low and your muscles are still cold," says Dr. Mollen.

A Little Upstart

While there's a good reason for wanting to stay put, the fact remains that you have to get up. How can you get yourself in gear right from the start and call up the kind of energy you need to face the day?

Here are a few tips from the wake-up experts.

Relish your routine.
One common reason that people struggle with getting up in the morning is that they fail to keep a regular sleeping and rising schedule, says health and fitness consultant Robert K. Cooper, Ph.D., co-author of *The Power of 5: Hundreds of 5-Second to 5-Minute Scientific Shortcuts to Ignite Your Energy, Burn Fat, Stop Aging and Revitalize Your Love Life.*

"Sleeping in on weekends actually confuses your body's clock and tends to lower your energy level rather than raise it," he says. You're better off getting up at your usual hour and taking a nap later in the day. And if you do sleep in, Dr. Cooper says, don't stay in bed more than an hour or so past your usual wake-up time.

Shed light on things.
Once you're awake, turn on the lights right away or open the curtains to expose yourself to daylight, says Dr. Cooper. If you can, take a walk in sunlight or sit near a bright window. These actions help stabilize your sleep/wake rhythm.

Moving into Daytime

If you can't get up the gumption to get yourself up, then exercising may be the furthest thing from your mind. But a number of experts suggest doing a few easy movements before you swing your feet to the floor to help you rev up your energy level.

Don't bolt out of bed like a soldier at boot camp, Dr. Mollen says. Instead, stay in bed another ten minutes or so and gradually exercise your way into the day. Here are several exercises suggested by Dr. Mollen to get you going.

Pull your knees.
This exercise stretches your lower back and your buttocks. With your back flat on the bed, arms at your sides, bend your left knee toward your chest. Then grab your left leg behind the knee with both hands. Slowly pull the knee toward your chest as far as it is comfortable. Hold for ten seconds, then release slowly. Repeat with your right leg.

Do the twist.
Torso twists loosen up your waist, back and shoulders. Lie on your back with knees bent and your feet flat on the mattress. Clasp your hands together, with fingers interlocked, and extend your arms straight up toward the ceiling. Keeping your arms straight and perpendicular to your chest, slowly lower them to your left, allowing your right shoulder to rise up off the mattress. Hold this position for a second. Then repeat the twist to the right side. Do 10 twists to each side, 20 in all.

Try some crunches.
These will get you going and also help tone the tummy—a get-up bonus. Lie on your back with both feet flat on the mattress. Lift your left leg and place your left ankle against your right knee. Place your hands lightly behind your head and slowly lift and twist your torso to the left. Twist as far as you can without

pain, hold for a second, then return to the starting position. Do this ten times, then switch, putting your right ankle against your left knee and twisting to the right.

Make like a cobra.
This movement limbers your spine and strengthens your back muscles. Lie on your stomach with your feet together. Put your hands flat under your shoulders, as if you were about to do a push-up. Using your neck and back muscles, raise your head, then chest, then stomach. Hold for five seconds, then slowly lower yourself—stomach, chest and finally your head. Don't strain yourself, only lift your body as far as you are able. Repeat three times.

Lift your legs.
This movement helps develop the thighs and buttocks. Lying on your left side, let your left arm stretch out comfortably above you on the mattress and rest your head on your left shoulder. Place your right hand on the mattress in front of your chest. Bend your left knee so that your left foot extends behind you (this keeps you from rolling backward). Extend your right leg and lift it off the bed as much as a 45-degree angle. Hold it for a second, then lower it. Do ten of these, then switch sides.

Row, row, row your back.
This movement will loosen muscles in your shoulders and chest, helping to relax you even as it feeds you energy. Sit on the edge of the bed with your feet dangling over the side. Extend your arms straight out in front of you and make a fist with each hand. Pull your arms back slowly as you lean back, as if rowing a boat. With your elbows as far back as comfortable, hold the position for five seconds. Relax your arms, return to the starting position and repeat five times.

Gentle Movements for a Gentle Start

If all those in-bed exercises don't appeal to you, there are also a number of less vigorous movements that help you get off to a good start even before you clamber out of bed. These come from Michael Reed Gach, Ph.D., founder and director of the Acupressure Institute in Berkeley, California, and author of *Greater Energy at Your Fingertips*. The exercises he recommends are particularly gentle, but also stimulating.

Make like a windshield wiper.
Lie on your back with your legs straight and your heels on the bed. Turn your feet in and out, making semicircles with your toes like a windshield wiper. As you swivel your feet, take deep breaths. Repeat the exercise until your legs feel

energized. It will take several minutes until your legs feel stimulated, but continue seven more times even after your leg muscles start to ache. Before jumping out of bed, close your eyes for several minutes and experience the benefits.

Roll your head.
Lie on your back with your arms and legs comfortably relaxed. Gently roll your head from side to side. Close your eyes, notice your neck relax as your head slowly moves and take long, deep breaths. Continue the exercise until your neck is completely relaxed. Complete the movement with your head straight in line with your spinal column.

Breathe and stretch.
Breathe slowly and deeply in and out through your nostrils. After several long, slow breaths, gently stretch your arms and legs. Stretch your whole body. Move and extend your limbs and back in whatever ways make you feel good. Continue to breathe deeply as you slowly rise to a sitting, then standing position.

"No matter what exercises you do, you can boost your energy by doing deep breathing as well as the exercises," Dr. Gach stresses. "Slow, deep breaths may be the single best thing you can do to increase your energy level."

Sing yourself awake.
From your first waking moments, positive thinking can raise your energy level, says Dr. Gach. How you look at the day ahead, even before you get up, can color your whole day.

"To get out of bed, try singing, 'Oh, what a beautiful morning, oh, what a beautiful day . . . ' " Dr. Gach recommends. The combination of a positive attitude with the use of your lungs and vocal chords is bound to launch your day with a burst of energy.

Trick yourself.
As a last resort, you can always put the alarm clock across the room, or even in the next room, so that you can hear it but not reach it. It may not give you more energy, but with the alarm blaring, at least you'll have to get up. Then you can turn on the lights and head for a bracing shower.

Grief

Emotional loss is a lot like a physical wound. Whether you've experienced the breakup of a relationship, a death in the family or simply a failed project or dream, the pain can be excruciating. And like a physical injury, grief can be so energy-depleting that often you don't know how to get started again.

Healing begins almost immediately, but that in itself requires a great deal of strength. "Grief takes time and a lot of physical energy," says Daniel Dworkin, Ph.D., affiliate professor of psychology at Colorado State University in Fort Collins and co-author of *Helping the Bereaved.*

Those suffering grief often feel lethargic, depressed and disinterested in life. On top of this is the energy-sapping need to take care of business— money matters, paperwork and helping loved ones—along with the wrenching emotional issues stirred up by having to adjust to a world turned topsy-turvy.

"Some people throw themselves into their work, or they eat, shop or have sex a lot, or they wallow in fantasy with books or movies," says Russell Friedman, executive director of the Grief Recovery Institute in Beverly Hills. This type of behavior, while usually short-lived, can overload your entire system, causing it to shut down from exhaustion.

Whatever the cause of your grief, it's important to remember that it's never bottomless. Human beings are resilient. What you're feeling will eventually ease and pass. That's something we probably all recognize, but when you're in the midst of grieving, it's not so easy to keep in mind.

Understanding the Process

Unlike anger, fear or other everyday emotions, grief is something we experience only rarely. Most of us have little practice coping with its painful effects. To blunt the ache, experts say, you have to know what to expect and what you can do.

Accept the pain.

This doesn't mean dwelling on painful events or assuming that grief must somehow be good for you. It means that whatever you're feeling, whether it's a mild sense of loss or a prolonged sense of devastation, is a natural process.

"Many people are surprised by the profoundness of their reactions during grief," says James R. Averill, Ph.D., professor of psychology at the University of Massachusetts at Amherst. But grief and grieving are normal reactions to loss, so give yourself the freedom to let those feelings out.

Be prepared.

The one thing that's certain about grief is that it's entirely unpredictable. "Pain, sadness and depression are obvious reactions to loss, but they're not the only ones," says Harold H. Bloomfield, M.D., a psychiatrist in Del Mar, California, and co-author of *How to Survive the Loss of a Love.* You may feel helpless, fearful, empty, despairing, disappointed, irritable, angry, guilty, restless, hopeless or regretful. You may start feeling better right away, or the pain may persist for weeks or even months. Every person is different, so be prepared for a wide variety of feelings.

Follow your own path.

"There is a tremendous amount of misinformation about dealing with grief," says Friedman. "You're told to put it behind you, to bury your losses, to be strong. But you want to be human, not strong.

"You're told to put your grief on hold, but you can't because it's happening, and if you try to stop it, your grief will suck the energy out of you. You're told to keep busy, but you can stay busy all day long and when you go to bed at night there's still this big hole in your heart," he says.

Letting It Out

Left to fester inside, the intense emotions of grief can sap your energy, weaken your motivation and make your whole life seem hopeless and gray. Here's what experts advise for getting those feelings out.

Find a good listener.

"Having the horror heard helps to heal the hurt," says Mark Goulston, M.D., assistant clinical professor of psychiatry at the University of California, Los Angeles, and author of *Get Out of Your Own Way.* At the same time, having someone to talk to eases the intense loneliness that often accompanies a loss.

Therapists and grief counselors are trained to be good listeners, but an empathic friend or relative can also be a great source of comfort, says Dr. Goul-

Finding Comfort

Many people can overcome grief on their own or with the help of family and friends, but others may need extra help. The Grief Recovery Institute, based in Beverly Hills, California, helps people work through painful losses.

"It's that unfinished business that keeps the arrow in your heart and drains your energy," says executive director Russell Friedman.

To help people nationwide cope with grief, the institute operates the Grief Recovery Helpline. Staffed by trained counselors, the Helpline is a free service for people who need additional comfort as well as practical advice for getting on with the business of living.

To talk to someone at the Helpline, call 1-800-445-4808. Or write to the Grief Recovery Institute, 8306 Wilshire Boulevard, Suite 21-A, Beverly Hills, CA 90211.

ston. "Find someone who will listen closely without imposing time restraints and who will accept your feelings without judging, questioning or commenting."

Join a support group.
The best listeners are often those who have experienced similar losses. Finding a support group in your area can be the first step toward long-term healing. "Such people are in the best position to say convincingly, 'I understand' or 'You're not alone,' " says Dr. Goulston.

Hospitals and newspapers often have listings of support groups. Or you can ask your doctor or therapist to recommend a group in your area.

Be your own best friend.
You don't necessarily need company to get your feelings out. "It's nice to have a listener, but if you don't have one, you can do it for yourself," says Judy Tatelbaum, a grief therapist in Carmel, California, and author of *The Courage to Grieve* and *You Don't Have to Suffer*.

Take a few moments to get comfortable. Imagine that you're facing the object of your grief—a spouse who has died, for example, or a best friend who's moved away. Speaking aloud, complete one (or more) of the following sentences.

"I'm sad . . ."

"I long for . . ."

"I'm angry . . ."

"I resent . . ."

"I'm sorry that . . ."

"Speak until you feel empty of feelings," says Tatelbaum. "End each session with 'I forgive you. I forgive me. Good-bye.' "

Write your feelings.

An alternative to speaking aloud, says Tatelbaum, is to express yourself in writing. "Write as if you were composing a letter to the person you've lost," she suggests. Or write your letter to God or whatever higher power you believe in. There can be great comfort in letting your feelings out and knowing that you have been heard.

Let it out.

Whatever method you use to vent your emotions, allow yourself to express what you truly feel. "Don't hold it in because it feels silly or useless," says Dr. Dworkin. "People often think they're not supposed to feel certain emotions, but the grief process generates a full range of feelings, many of which are not necessarily tied to logic."

Getting On with Life

Grief is such an overwhelming emotion that fulfilling even the basic necessities of life, like eating well, taking care of children and so forth, can seem excruciatingly difficult. Yet taking care of yourself, both physically and mentally, is key to the healing process. Here are a few ways to manage your life and your grief.

Turn to tradition.

Experts have found that people who go through traditional mourning practices—viewing the body, for example, or visiting the cemetery—fare better than those who do not. "There's a tendency to look at certain practices as silly or old-fashioned or macabre, but they can be a great source of comfort," says Dr. Averill.

Put yourself in control.

"Nothing inhibits your energy or sense of power more than thinking you're a victim," says Tatelbaum. "Instead, shift to the idea of yourself as a survivor."

It may be helpful, for example, to think of all the people in the world who have undergone similar losses and who were strong and resilient enough to survive and even thrive. Ask yourself, "What can I learn from this?" she suggests. "It's a way of empowering and re-energizing yourself. Painful experiences are the things that help us grow the most."

Keep up with basics.

In times of grief, we have a tendency to neglect our basic needs. "Some people will eat too much, some won't eat at all," says Dr. Dworkin.

Good nutrition is critical for helping the healing process, adds Dr. Bloomfield. He advises getting plenty of protein, cutting back on sweets and junk food (which can sap your energy) and perhaps taking a multivitamin/mineral supplement as well.

Try to get moving.
It's natural to withdraw in response to grief, even to the extent of not getting out of the house or walking to the mailbox. The lack of exercise saps your energy, Dr. Dworkin says, which in turn makes you even more vulnerable to the painful emotions of grief.

At the very least, you should try to get out for walks once or twice a day. As you gradually feel stronger physically, you'll also find that you're feeling stronger emotionally.

While some exercise is always good, be careful not to overdo it, Tatelbaum says. If you use exercise as a way to avoid feelings of grief, the entire process may take much longer to resolve. "You may be trying to work your feelings out of your system so that you don't have to deal with them, but you can never skip the emotional part."

Give in to rest.
Don't consider weariness and fatigue as a sign of weakness, advises Dr. Dworkin. "It's your body telling you it needs time to regenerate."

Allowing yourself ample rest entails more than getting enough sleep at night, adds Dr. Bloomfield. "You may want to get help with ongoing tasks, avoid rushing around too much and schedule times for naps or meditation."

Start making new memories.
While experts advise against making major decisions in the turbulent early stages of grief, eventually the time will come when you've sorted out the loss and you're ready to reconnect with the world again. Don't put it off for too long, says Dr. Goulston.

"People say they can't move on until they get over their loss, but the reality is just the opposite: unless you go on with your life, you can't get over the loss," he says. "New memories dilute the intensity of the painful ones." The sooner you start living fully again, the sooner you'll begin feeling rejuvenated and excited by life.

Give it time.
"Grief is a process that evolves over time," says Dr. Dworkin. "Take it day to day and don't beat yourself up if it doesn't seem like it's going fast enough." Don't be surprised if thoughts and feelings you thought you had seen the last of come back at unexpected times, he adds. Like any biological and emotional process, it has its own schedule. Eventually, you'll find you're feeling energized and ready to begin life anew.

Headaches

There's no doubt about it: The steady pounding pain of a headache can drain your energy. While intense migraines tend to be the most draining kind, even garden-variety tension headaches can tire you out.

"Headaches wear people down physically and psychologically," says Fred D. Sheftell, M.D., co-director and founder of the New England Center for Headache in Stamford, Connecticut, and president of the American Council for Headache Education (ACHE). "The more severe or frequent the pain, the more tired you're likely to feel. But the biochemical events that cause headaches can also cause fatigue. While no one knows exactly what the link is between headaches and fatigue, we have some interesting leads."

Pain Means Drain

Research suggests that some people's brains are genetically programmed to translate physical and emotional stress into headaches. How does this work? Researchers have found that stress triggers biochemical and electrical changes in your brain. These changes in turn irritate your nerves and adjacent blood vessels. The irritated blood vessels open wide and become inflamed, creating the flood of blood that you experience as pounding, throbbing headache pain.

So far, so bad. But where does fatigue fit in? It could be related to biochemical messengers that reach the brain—most likely, serotonin, which is a messenger molecule that has been associated with many kinds of mood reactions. "One theory," says Dr. Sheftell, "holds that disturbances in the way your brain uses serotonin and other biochemical messengers in the central nervous system can cause headaches, depression and fatigue. The pain may also be related to depleted levels of endorphins, the body's natural painkillers."

Migraines can affect every waking moment, and sleep problems caused by headaches may also zap your pep, notes Dr. Sheftell. If you get a migraine while you're sleeping—as sometimes happens—the pain can wake you. But even if it doesn't, the headache can prevent you from getting restful sleep. A vicious circle begins: The headaches wear you out, and the fatigue can make you more vulnerable to headaches.

Stress and anxiety contribute to both fatigue and headaches, says Dr. Sheftell. And changes in sleep patterns, shift work, jet lag and other schedule glitches that cause fatigue can also trigger headaches.

But that doesn't mean that headaches need not get the best of you. With a number of tried-and-true approaches recommended by experts, you can reclaim the energy that your headaches take away.

Make Medications Work for You

Though most of us reach for aspirin, acetaminophen or ibuprofen when headaches start, the painkillers that you use to deal with headaches can actually work against you rather than for you. Overuse can actually cause headaches and fatigue, and so can going off the medication, according to Paul Duckro, Ph.D., professor in the Department of Community and Family Medicine at St. Louis University Health Sciences Center, clinical director of the Chronic Headache Program at the St. Louis Behavioral Medicine Institute and co-author of *Taking Control of Your Headaches*.

"Some headache sufferers find they're trading debilitating pain for debilitating fatigue," says Dr. Sheftell. It's easy to get caught up in a rebound effect in which the medication you take to kill the pain actually makes it bounce back even more strongly, he explains.

Even taking as little as two to four aspirin or acetaminophen a day can bring on rebound headaches. If the medication itself doesn't make you drowsy, the perpetual rebound headaches will, says Dr. Sheftell. Here's how to deal with the problem.

Examine your headache pattern.
Dr. Duckro lists five signs indicating that you may have medication-induced headaches.
1. You have headaches 15 or more days per month.
2. The medication you use doesn't seem to help or, when it does, the benefit wears off quickly.
3. You require higher dosages of your medication to get the same effect.
4. You begin to use medications to head off headaches before you even get them.
5. Your doctor tells you that you may be relying too heavily on medication.
If any of these items describes your situation, consult with your doctor.

You'll need to make some changes in the way you use medications if you're going to put an end to this cycle, says Dr. Duckro.

Recruit your doctor to help you.

Taking the maximum dosage of over-the-counter pain relievers like plain aspirin or acetaminophen twice a week is generally safe, but be sure to tell your doctor about all the medications you take. With your doctor's advice you can find alternative ways to cope with your pain that can help keep drug use to a minimum, says Dr. Sheftell.

Seek help from a specialist.

"If your doctor can't get you off the offending medication in one or two tries and your headaches have become chronic, daily affairs, it's time to seek more specialized care," says Dr. Sheftell. "Family doctors—and even some neurologists—often can't give the kind of care you'll get from a headache specialist."

If your doctor can't refer you to a headache specialist, try calling a university-affiliated medical center in your area to find one.

Dropping the Caffeine Lift

Along with the rush it provides, caffeine can help relieve headaches—or cause them. This druglike stimulant jogs your adrenal glands into action, which in turn constricts your blood vessels. Once this effect wears off, your blood vessels can dilate, resulting in a pounding headache. If you seem to be sensitive to this effect, here's how to deal with the problem.

Say no to seconds.

It's a good idea to limit yourself to a five-ounce cup (not mug) of brewed American coffee or tea per day, says Dr. Sheftell.

Cut off your chocolate supply.

Coffee isn't the only caffeine carrier. "Cocoa and chocolate don't contain a lot of caffeine, but eating and drinking various caffeine sources can add up," says Dr. Sheftell. If you must have your hot cocoa, which contains small amounts of caffeine, he suggests limiting it to an eight-ounce cup a day provided that chocolate doesn't trigger your headaches. If you get frequent headaches or migraines caused by a reaction to chocolate, he recommends staying away from it all together.

Can the colas.

Don't think that you can switch from drinking coffee to colas, either. Not only do colas contain caffeine, diet colas contain potentially problematic artificial sweeteners, according to Dr. Sheftell.

People who ingested aspartame (NutraSweet) as part of a study conducted at the University of Washington in Seattle reported a higher incidence of headaches than those who took a placebo. Dr. Sheftell recommends avoiding all sodas that contain either sugar or aspartame, because of their headache-triggering qualities. If you can't do without them, limit your intake to one can a day. Better yet, "try switching to plain seltzer flavored with lemon or lime instead," he says.

Working with Your Body

Watching what you eat and monitoring the medications you take are only the tip of the iceberg when it comes to preventing energy-depleting headaches. Exercise can also play an important role in keeping you headache-free.

Aerobic exercise will energize and relax you *and* help you deal with your headaches, says Seymour Solomon, M.D., professor of neurology at Albert Einstein College of Medicine and director of the Headache Unit at Montefiore Medical Center, both in New York City.

Regular exercise not only can ease headache pain but also can reduce headache frequency, too, by easing the physical and psychological tension that can trigger headaches, according to Dr. Solomon. Regular exercise also increases the body's production of two substances that are natural painkillers, endorphins and enkephalins. If all that weren't enough, exercise also reduces depression and anxiety and promotes restful sleep, he says.

One caution: While exercise may relieve a tension headache, it may make a migraine worse. So consult your doctor about the proper way to exercise for pain relief.

Here's how to use exercise and body awareness to boost your energy level while promoting headache relief.

Focus on aerobics.
Regular, noncompetitive exercise such as walking briskly or swimming is particularly helpful, says Dr. Duckro. The treadmill or cross-country skiing machine is good, too, if you don't push too hard.

Be selective about your exercises, however. Some types of aerobic exercise can actually contribute to the headache problem, according to Dr. Duckro. The worst offenders are jogging, high-impact aerobics and cycling on bikes with downturned handlebars, which strain your neck.

Ease away from pain.
Also pay attention to stretching, which keeps upper-body muscles relaxed, says Dr. Duckro.

Here's a tension-relieving exercise from Dr. Sheftell: Do ten slow, gentle neck stretches to each side. Lean your head to the left and hold for five seconds.

Then slowly lean your head to the right and hold for five seconds. You should sense a slight stretching in your neck as you do this. With each stretch, inhale and exhale deeply as you count.

Do a body scan.
"Muscle tension can be both cause and effect in headache pain," explains Dr. Sheftell. "Tense muscles can bring on a headache, but the muscles clench against pain, too."

He recommends lying on your back with your feet flat on the floor and knees bent. Breathe so that your stomach (not your chest) rises and falls. Now, conduct a body scan, checking every body part to see where you hold tension. Systematically tense then release each body part as you check from head to toe.

By doing this regularly, you'll locate the places where you're holding tension in your body and release it, says Dr. Sheftell.

Massage away pain.
"Massages relax the muscles of the head and neck," says Dr. Sheftell. To perform a headache-relieving massage on yourself, "Try placing a partly inflated beach ball between your forehead and a wall," he says. "As you stand facing the wall, gently rotate your forehead against the ball. This creates a gentle forehead massage while stretching tight neck muscles."

Use a mental eraser against pain.
You can recruit your imagination to help you deal with pain, according to Dr. Sheftell. He invites his patients to visualize their tensed forehead muscles as a series of crisscrossed lines. "I tell people to even out those lines so that they become parallel," he says. "The act of imagining this is naturally relaxing."

Supplement Your Relief Efforts

In some cases, herbs and vitamins offer natural alternatives to drugs without harmful side effects, according to Dr. Solomon. Not only can they reduce your dependency on drugs, natural pain relievers may also eliminate the problem of rebound headaches. Certain nutrients and herbs may also boost energy while relieving pain. Before trying natural remedies, check with your doctor.

If you're headache-prone, you might require additional B vitamins, according to Dr. Sheftell. B vitamins help the body cope with stress, assimilate nutrients and regulate metabolism. Specifically, riboflavin and vitamin B_6 have been found helpful to people who suffer from frequent headaches, says Dr. Sheftell. Most B-complex formulations don't contain enough of these, however. To get the B vitamins you need, along with other nutrients that might help, here's what experts recommend.

Beef up your riboflavin.

The important vitamin riboflavin actually stimulates energy production in the mitochondria—your cells' power packs. The Daily Value for riboflavin is 1.7 milligrams, but you need much more than that to take advantage of its anti-headache, energy-producing potential, according to Dr. Sheftell. He recommends starting with 100 milligrams a day of riboflavin and increasing the daily dosage every three to four days by 50 milligrams until you're taking 400 milligrams a day. While taking this much riboflavin is safe, it will turn your urine fluorescent yellow, according to Dr. Sheftell. And since the doses are hundreds of times above the Daily Value for this nutrient, make sure you discuss it with your doctor.

Consider B_6.

Vitamin B_6 can also prove helpful to some people, according to Dr. Sheftell. He suggests taking 50 to 100 milligrams a day. Don't exceed 100 milligrams a day, he cautions, since that can cause nerve disorders. And be sure to discuss this high dose with your doctor before trying it.

Look into magnesium and vitamin E.

Some people find that taking daily supplements of magnesium and vitamin E helps reduce the frequency and intensity of headaches, according to Dr. Sheftell. He recommends taking 300 milligrams of magnesium a day. He also suggests taking 800 international units of vitamin E daily, dividing the dosage into 400 international units in the morning and another 400 at night.

The Daily Value for magnesium is 400 milligrams a day. The Daily Value for vitamin E, however, is only 30 international units, so this therapy should also be discussed with your doctor before you try it on your own.

Try a little ginger power.

Ginger capsules may reduce the frequency of migraines along with the nausea that often accompanies them, says Dr. Sheftell. He recommends taking 400 milligrams in capsule form two to three times a day as a preventive. You can buy ginger capsules at most health food stores and some drugstores.

Give feverfew a try.

Feverfew can be an effective headache medicine, notes Dr. Solomon. "While some European studies have found it effective, there are no long-term studies of toxicity," he says.

Feverfew comes in various forms, including loose tea, capsules and tinctures. You can find these at health food stores. Whatever way you take it, Dr. Solomon advises using feverfew with care—cutting back or discontinuing use if you experience any stomach irritation or other discomfort. "The trickiest thing is knowing how much you're getting," he says. "Since this herb is unregulated, there is no guarantee that the product contains its advertised dosage."

Holidays

For children, Christmas is all about fun and eager anticipation. From the first glimpses of lights and decorations in late November to the final dash for presents Christmas morning, the excitement rarely dips below the bubbling point.

For adults, however, sustaining Christmas cheer isn't so easy. For one thing, the season seems to get longer every year. These days it seems to begin right after Halloween. Add to that the never-ending rounds of shopping, baking, wrapping presents and visiting friends, and the traditional "Season's Greetings!" starts feeling more like season's groanings.

"We are on the go constantly," says Elaine Masto Copeland, a national fitness training specialist in Flagstaff, Arizona. The holidays, for many of us, start feeling more like a full-time job than a time of joy.

To enjoy the holidays, you have to use your energy wisely. "Look for ways to simplify," says Copeland. The trick, she says, is learning how to be together with family and friends without doing too much.

Even if you don't observe Christmas as a religious holiday, you're likely to find that the time of year is jam-packed with social obligations. Escaping the stress of this allegedly all-joyous season is often easier said than done. But if you plan carefully, shop wisely and do your best to take good care of yourself, you can enjoy this holiday season and still get everything done that needs doing.

Planning Ahead

All holidays are a time of celebration, of enjoying family rituals. Yet they can also be incredibly stressful and exhausting—in large part because we have such high expectations of how we want everything to be.

But of all the seasonal celebrations that place demands on energy, Christmas takes the cake. The house must be decorated and always clean in case unexpected visitors drop by. The tree should look just so. There should be fresh cookies and mulled cider and candles in every window.

Lovely images, indeed, but not always realistic. Here are some ways to make the season more enjoyable and less energy-draining.

Remember what it's all about.

"Set reasonable expectations," advises Deborah Swiss, Ed.D., of Lexington, Massachusetts, a consultant for gender equity and work/family issues and author of *Women Breaking Through*. You'll be a lot less stressed and more energetic if, rather than micromanaging every holiday detail, you just sort of let things happen. The point of the holidays is being with family, renewing ties, enjoying traditions. Does it really matter if the house is immaculate?

Check your list twice.

Take a lesson from Santa: You need a list, and you need to review it more than once. To keep holiday plans from wearing you down, advance planning is critical, says Judy Kern, M.D., a psychiatrist in private practice in Chicago. Discuss in advance with your partner what sorts of things you want to achieve—and what you can do without. Maybe that "perfect" gift for your spouse, which will require about three trips to the mall, isn't something your partner even wants. Home-cooked meals are nice, but maybe you'd both prefer an elegant carryout. "Work with each other's expectations," says Dr. Kern. The only rule is to enjoy the holidays. Anything that takes away from your enjoyment is an energy drain—and should be jettisoned.

Don't plan on everything.

Cross every third item off your list, suggests Theresa Farrow, M.D., a psychiatrist in private practice in Tulsa, Oklahoma. Most of us do way too much for the holidays. Reducing your workload is the surest way to stop fatigue from setting in. "What's important is that we concentrate on the meaning of the season and sharing and giving instead of accomplishing a whole bunch of tasks," she says.

Don't sweat the details.

Do you want to invite friends over, but the whole house is a mess? Remember that your friends aren't going to see the whole house. So prepare only those rooms that they're actually going to see. By setting reasonable expectations you'll keep energy levels high, says Dr. Swiss.

Be flexible.

Every family celebrates the holidays differently, so perhaps it's not surprising that the one tradition more common than Christmas lights is fighting about whose holiday tradition to enjoy. This is particularly true in young families that haven't been together long enough to feel secure in their own traditions.

To avoid the drawn-out, exhausting battle of dueling traditions, discuss in advance with your partner how he celebrated the holidays as a child. Understand what was most meaningful in your partner's past—and what you can do to incorporate some of those things in your family today.

"Don't say things like, 'I can't believe you only got one present' or 'I can't believe you didn't have a tree,' " says Bob Lewis, Ph.D., a clinical program supervisor in the Department of Psychology at Washington University in St. Louis. Be supportive, understanding and creative. Look for ways to combine both of your pasts into a holiday tradition that's uniquely your own.

Take the initiative.
Even though it's important to respect each other's traditions, there's no reason to follow them by rote—particularly those that are causing you stress. Spending Christmas at your in-laws may be a tradition, for example, but look at what that means. Every year you may feel totally worn out even before you leave your own house to embark on that obligatory mission.

Why do something that you don't want to do? This year, for a change, maybe you would like to invite the in-laws to join in your celebrations, says Dr. Lewis. There's nothing more energizing than doing things that you genuinely want to do, he notes. Trying to live up to someone else's expectations can sap all the holiday enthusiasm right out of you.

Create new rituals.
One surefire way to excite the family and help energize the entire holiday season is to start your own family rituals. These don't have to be elaborate. Go to a tree farm and chop down your own tree. Shop for new ornaments. Bake a special dessert on Christmas Day. Then stand back and watch the excitement grow. Not only will you have a great time this year, but the whole family will enjoy the fun of doing it again next year.

Make reservations early.
As any travel agent can tell you, the holidays are when families come together, so those days are the busiest travel times of the year. Not making travel plans until the last minute is guaranteed to leave you wiped out and drained—particularly when you're stuck at the airport for eight hours trying to snag a standby flight.

Always make travel plans well in advance, advises Judi Galst, general manager of marketing for Rosenbluth Vacations, headquartered in Newtown Square, Pennsylvania. "To get preferred dates, times, destinations and accommodations—and the best price—plan as far ahead as possible."

Back to Basics

Every year the holidays get a little more commercialized. The message on television, in magazines and even from family and friends seems to be: If you aren't spending a lot of money, you don't deserve to be happy. As a result, we usually spend more time (and money) shopping than we planned to. And shopping for the holidays can be a major drain on your energy resources.

It doesn't have to be this way. To get through the season and the mall with your energy intact, here's what experts advise.

Make a budget.

Most people begin the holidays with good intentions, but gift lists have a way of growing. The resulting strain on your budget can be extremely stressful and draining—not just during the holidays but for months to come.

It's important to decide in advance who you're going to buy presents for and how much you're going to spend, says psychiatrist Paul J. Rosch, M.D., clinical professor of medicine and psychiatry at New York Medical College in Valhalla, New York, and president of the American Institute of Stress. Once you know exactly what your limits are, you'll find it easier to prevent the traditional shopping frenzy from spinning out of control.

Be firm.

It's not surprising that most of us feel a little, well, guilty during the holidays. We get more invitations than we can accept; we receive gifts from people we didn't shop for; the children want more than we're offering. The pressure to always be doing more is exhausting.

A good solution is to do what you want but find a kind way to do it, advises Daniel Kegan, Ph.D., a lawyer in private practice in Chicago and an organizational psychologist at Elan Associates, also in Chicago. "You don't have to participate in somebody else's game," he says. "Just say no."

This applies not only to gift giving but to all the festivities associated with the holidays. If you don't want to go to an office party, you can graciously decline. "A lot of people fall into patterns out of habit rather than choice," says Dr. Kegan. "Just explain that this year you want to spend some quiet time at home." The downtime may help you feel more relaxed and energetic for the things that you really want to do.

Set some rules.

As every parent knows, shopping for children can be exhausting. Shopping with children ("Mom, can I have another cookie, please?") can become even worse.

To keep the I-wants from wearing you out, plan ahead. "Before you go into a store with your child, talk about what you are going to buy," says Joan Test, Ed.D., adjunct professor of education at Washington University in St. Louis. "This helps them be prepared to resist all the items that they will see on the shelves."

Your Personal Best

Have you ever noticed how short the days seem to get around the holidays? Not because it gets dark so much earlier, but because there's so much to do. Shopping. Wrapping Presents. Baking. School concerts. Getting clothes ready. The work never seems to end. As you rush around trying to accomplish your long list of tasks, it's easy to forget the basics, like eating well or taking a little time out for exercise.

To keep your energy high, experts advise that you take care of yourself. Here's how.

Listen to your instincts.
Due to the stress of the holidays, it's natural to eat more than you usually do. Don't fight it. "If your body tells you it needs food, take the time to eat," says Debra Waterhouse, R.D., a dietitian in Oakland, California, and author of *Outsmarting the Female Fat Cell*.

It's important, however, to be aware of when you give in to the craving for sweets because taking in too much sugar will cause your energy levels to plunge. A better choice is to snack on complex carbohydrates like bread, Waterhouse says. This will stabilize sugars in the bloodstream and help prevent the highs and lows that can leave you feeling drained.

Catch some rays.
Sunshine can be in short supply during the winter months, but you need all you can get to keep your energy levels high. "I recommend getting 15 minutes of sunlight during the day as another way to boost your energy and lower your stress level," says Waterhouse.

Keep a pleasure diary.
It's a way of keeping life simple and focused during the hustle and bustle, says Copeland. Take a few moments to enjoy a hot cup of tea or the peace and quiet of reading a newspaper. Reflect for a moment on how good it feels to relax. Then record the moment. This will help you stay focused on what's really special about the holidays.

Keep up with exercise.
Even when you're dedicated to your workouts, it can be tough to maintain an exercise schedule when every minute of your time is precious. Here's an easy way to stay in shape without taking extra time. When you're at the mall, park the car in Siberia, in the lot farthest from the store. Walking quickly to and from the store will get your heart rate up, boost your supply of oxygen and help keep you feeling fresh even on days when you don't have time to exercise.

Feel deeply.

It's extremely common to feel a vague sense of uneasiness during the holidays, says Robert Oresick, Ph.D., a psychologist and assistant dean at Boston University. "It's a time when people notice the passage of time. They are reminded of things that happened in the past—of sad times or times of loss and disappointment. A lot of energy is tied up coping with negative emotions."

To overcome these feelings and keep your energy high, Dr. Oresick recommends allowing yourself to feel them. "Then you can release energy, and it flows and begins to transform," he explains. "Anger transforms to forgiveness, grief changes to acceptance and disappointment is replaced with optimism. But you have to go through the feelings."

Reward yourself.

No matter how busy things get, experts say, always take a little time for pleasure. Go to a movie. Read the paper. Take a nap. It's these little quiet moments that make the holidays special. Go ahead and enjoy them—you'll be glad that you did.

Housecleaning

*D*oes the top of the range have little chunks of baked-on food? Are you confronted with greenish mold around the corners every time you step in the shower? Or how about the sticky floors and smudged drinking glasses?

If the thought of cleaning it all zaps your zip, take some cues from the experts. There are many ways that you can make housework easier, faster and even pleasurable, they say.

But before you begin, maybe you need to have a look at the goods that you're keeping and consider which things can go.

De-junk Your Home

Junk is not only a burden but also one of the major contributors to unnecessary housework. Everything stashed away in your house is also stashed away in your mind and is draining your mental energy, says Don Aslett of Pocatello, Idaho, author of 25 books on housework.

Here's how to pare down what you own, simplify your cleaning requirements and have energy left over for what *you* want to do.

Lighten your load.
"Junk requires maintenance and takes up so much time in your life that it frequently leads to stress," says Barbara Kramer, an organizational consultant in Orefield, Pennsylvania. "You become a slave to what you own. So only save what you need."

To identify what you really should keep, Kramer suggests asking yourself these questions.

Why do I need this?

What does it do for me?

Do I have some place to store it?

Is it always around and in the way?

"If you don't have a place to store something, ask yourself if you should even have it," says Kramer. "If you should have it, then find it a home."

Just say no.

People who have a difficult time throwing away what they don't need often try to find another home for it. "It helps alleviate their guilt about throwing it away," says Kramer. "But if you take it, you end up with more garbage." When someone offers you something you don't really want or need, all you have to do is decline it.

Impose a strict time limit.

Don't save things because you may have a use for them someday. "If you haven't worn an item of clothing in the last three years, you're not going to wear it in the next three years," says Eugenia Chapman, a professional house-keeper for 42 years and author of *Clean Your House and Everything in It*. Similarly, she advises going through your mail as soon as it comes in and tossing what's junk in the trash.

Give 'em two weeks.

No matter how good you are at ridding yourself of clutter, if your family doesn't do the same, you'll be wasting energy when you clean. Chapman, who has 11 children and 54 grandchildren, imposes junk time limits on everyone in the house.

"I give everybody two weeks. If they haven't gotten rid of junk, then in the garbage it goes," she says. "When they get married or move away from home, I give them two months to get their stuff out of the house."

Raid the attic.

"It's so easy to just open the door and throw things in the attic," says Kramer. To counteract that automatic buildup, "go through the attic every spring and fall. Get rid of what you don't use. If you get something new, throw out something to make room for it or create a place to store it."

Tear up your magazines.

A magazine publisher once noted that 70 percent of a magazine is advertise-ments. If you want to save an article, rip it out, recommends Aslett. Then, in-stead of having messy piles of magazines that all need dusting and cleaning, you'll have a neat file of articles that you can store in a file drawer or folder.

Get organized.

Take a few minutes to look over the clutter that you have to keep and decide on an efficient arrangement. Use shelves, file cabinets and drawer dividers to organize things so that you'll waste less energy looking for what you need. "There's no exactly right way to organize," says Kramer. "It's a personal choice."

Organizing is an ongoing process, and often the ideal system is learned through trial and error, she says.

Tool Up for Energy Savings

Trying to houseclean without the right tools and without knowing how to use them efficiently will cost you plenty in both time and energy. Often, the job won't even be done right. Here's what the experts advise to speed you along.

Put out (and in) a welcome mat.

Most homes have welcome mats outside the front door and maybe the back, too, but what about inside the entrances to your home? By doubling the mats, which are cheap to buy, you'll keep a lot of dirt and grime from being tracked through your house.

"Proper matting alone could save the average household 200 hours of work a year, slow down structure depreciation 7 percent and save $160 in direct cleaning supply costs," notes Aslett. In terms of your energy, proper matting ultimately saves you 30 minutes of chore time a day.

Wipe away your work.

It takes only minutes to clean a bathroom if you wipe the fixtures and shower walls every day. It's especially efficient if you live in an area that has highly mineralized (hard) water, because that can leave unsightly whitish gray stains after the water dries. If you wipe up the water immediately, no stain.

After a shower, take 10 to 15 seconds to clean and dry the walls and fixtures. In fact, store a squeegee in the shower as a reminder and to make the job easier, Aslett advises.

Make every move count.

When you're cleaning any room, work around it once, always going from top to bottom, suggests Jeff Campbell, owner of The Clean Team, a San Francisco–based housing cleaning company, and author of *Speed Cleaning*. "It actually takes less energy to go around the room once doing everything you need to do as you come to it," he says.

Outfit yourself properly.

Carry your equipment and supplies with you as you work the room so that you don't make unnecessary trips back and forth, advises Campbell. He suggests wearing a work apron with about seven pockets that contain your tools and supplies. In the pockets you should have a toothbrush, a razor blade, a scraper, cleaning cloths, a feather duster and squirt bottles that contain the appropriate cleaners. Also, tote along a carryall tray, which doubles as permanent storage for your cleaning supplies.

Bag it.
Take along a gallon-size plastic storage bag so that you can easily pick up trash as you go, suggests Campbell. That way you just make one trip to the trash can.

Use two solutions.
You don't need specialized cleaners for each task, says Campbell. "Because we're Americans, we're bombarded with advertising about products that work wonders on a particular cleaning problem," he says. "It's almost a form of wishful thinking." You really need only two cleaning solutions: a light-duty cleaner such as Windex and a heavy-duty cleaner such as Formula 409 or Fantastik.

"It's much smarter to get one cleaner that will do ten things than ten different cleaners that will do one thing," he says. You will also save yourself the energy of hauling around all those unnecessary supplies.

Whistle While You Work

Don't look now, but your attitude about housecleaning could be depleting your energy before you even start. Here are a few tips from the experts on tackling your tasks with energy and enthusiasm.

Get in a project frame of mind.
If you're mentally ready to tackle the job, performing it will energize you. "Have fun with it," says Linda Mason Hunter, author of *The Healthy Home*. "I put on the radio or some music. I can work faster to certain music. It's more positive and uplifting."

Do it in small doses.
Take a few minutes to clean up whenever you can rather than putting it off until later, Aslett advises. "Later takes more time, more hot water, more scrubbing and more equipment." People often wait until the chores seem overwhelming, he notes, but if you wait too long, the chores are overwhelming and your energy level will be no match for them. "You wouldn't pay your bills once a year," observes Aslett, and you shouldn't put off housecleaning.

Let there be light.
Besides making it easier to see what you're cleaning, light is a great mood lifter. And if your mood is cheery, you'll have more energy, says Hunter.

Take a break.

There's nothing wrong with taking a pleasurable break from your task and doing something healthy for yourself. "If you're feeling lethargic and apathetic or your energy level is running on low, try taking a walk," says Hunter.

Enjoy your accomplishments.

There's nothing like finishing a job and feeling good about it. "Once you've moved a mountain, or even a molehill or two, you'll find yourself clicking your heels and ready to start on the next," notes Aslett. "One accomplishment just provides the fuel for more."

Low Self-Esteem

*Y*ou're worthless. You're incompetent. You're stupid, foolish and ugly to boot."

If anyone talked to you that way, you would punch him in the nose—or at least have a few choice words to give in return. But when it's your own brain dishing out the slurs, there's nowhere to run and no one to punish—except yourself.

The price, of course, is a whopping loss of energy. "Mind, body and spirit constitute an ecosystem," says Layne Longfellow, Ph.D., a psychologist in private practice in Prescott, Arizona. "If you damage one part, the energy flow in other parts can be blocked. If you constantly worry about your worth, that much less energy is available for other uses."

Even when you try to ignore or suppress those infernal internal messages, the result is a net loss of energy. "If there are aspects of yourself that are hard to accept, you need to invest energy in keeping them out of your awareness," says Stan Taubman, a doctor of social work, an instructor at the University of California, Berkeley, and author of *Ending the Struggle against Yourself*.

Fortunately, the cloud that's raining epithets on your parade is not a permanent part of the horizon. You helped create it, say the experts, and you can make it go away.

Onward and Upward

"The only way to improve self-esteem is to do things that give you a real reason to feel good about yourself," says Michael W. Mercer, Ph.D., an industrial psychologist with Mercer Group in Barrington, Illinois, and author of *How Winners Do It*. Here's what experts advise.

Do something well.
It doesn't matter what it is. Doing anything to the best of your ability will cause your self-esteem to rise and help quiet the energy-draining, self-criticizing back

talk, says Perry W. Buffington, Ph.D., a psychologist, lecturer and radio talk-show host on Amelia Island, Florida.

"Find a niche and master it," says Dr. Buffington. It doesn't have to be anything big. Consider the satisfaction that you get from completing a challenging crossword puzzle or working out a brainteaser. Something as simple as improving your vocabulary can have large benefits. "Once you find worth from behaviors, you can start finding worth on your own," he says.

Move your career forward.

There's nothing like making progress on a career path to help you feel good about yourself. You don't have to be sitting in the CEO's seat to feel as though you've made it. Small progress brings big rewards. Dr. Mercer recommends focusing on four key areas.

1. Set deadlines. Then meet them. This will impress your bosses, and you'll prove to yourself that you mean what you say.

2. Improve your skills. Anything that makes you more valuable at work will pay off in energizing self-esteem. Enroll in training programs. Take a business class at the community college. Read upbeat books and articles about succeeding in business.

3. Make a good impression. The best achievements won't counteract bad posture or sloppy work habits. Always doing a good job and acting like a pro can make a huge impression on those who affect your future—and this in turn will help you feel better about yourself.

4. Demonstrate your bottom-line impact. Let your employer know how you are improving profits or decreasing costs. Anything you do that benefits the company is going to benefit you—and your enthusiasm for the job as well.

Get moving.

When you're feeling tired, depressed and unappreciated, probably the last thing you want to do is work out. Do it anyway, advises Thomas R. Collingwood, Ph.D., president of Fitness Intervention Technologies in Richardson, Texas, and author of *A Piece of the Puzzle.*

"Getting active physically is the single best thing you can do," he says. "You get immediate feedback so you know if it's working or not; the outcomes are clear and you can see fairly quick results."

In addition, fitness makes you more resilient and better equipped to deal with stress, he says, which may explain why people who get regular exercise tend to be more motivated and energetic than those who don't. How you go about getting exercise is important, he notes. Here are his guidelines.

1. Find an activity you can easily do. If it's not enjoyable and convenient, you aren't going to stick with it. Walking is great exercise since you can do it anywhere and it doesn't require any start-up fees. If you decide to sign up at a

A Blueprint for Change

When you think about everything that goes into your personality—how old you are, who you went to school with, what your parents were like—making even small changes can seem all but overwhelming.

Yet even the most intricate structure is made up of smaller—and more manageable—parts. According to Nathaniel Branden, Ph.D., a Los Angeles psychologist and author of *The Six Pillars of Self-Esteem*, there are six key strategies that you can use to improve self-esteem.

1. Live consciously. "As with a muscle, you make the mind strong by using it," he says. "Think through the consequences of your actions. Pursue goals and seek the information that you need to achieve them and the feedback to correct yourself if you fall off course." Most important, of course, is to think about those things that bring you down—and those that make you stronger. "Pay attention to what energizes you and what drains you," says Dr. Branden.

2. Practice self-acceptance. "If you're busy disowning certain of your thoughts, emotions and actions, you're denying aspects of yourself, and it takes energy to sustain that denial," says Dr. Branden.

---

health club, choose one that's nearby. If you have to drive a half-hour to get there, you'll soon be making excuses for staying home.

2. Set incremental goals. Don't hold yourself to unrealistic standards. You aren't going to look like Arnold Schwarzenegger by the end of the month. What you can do, however, is get a little better—that is, stronger, more flexible and more energetic—each time you go. Every time you work out, try to improve your performance by pushing yourself a little further, says Dr. Collingwood. "Do an extra sit-up, beat your time by five seconds, do one more repetition—this will enable you to stretch your effort and give you more confidence every time you work out."

3. Don't get competitive. There are a lot of taut, well-muscled people out there, and you're going to want to match them pound for pound, step for step. Don't do it. "Your initial competition should be with yourself," Dr. Collingwood says.

Dress the part.
"People feel good when they look good," says Dr. Mercer. It's the little touches like getting regular haircuts, for example, or wearing a sharp suit that can change your overall appearance and make you feel better about who you are.

3. Practice self-responsibility. "Take responsibility for your own life and well-being, for your own choices and actions, for the attainment of your own desires and goals," urges Dr. Branden. "Nothing is more exhausting than waiting for someone else to do something, and nothing is more empowering than realizing that no one is coming."

4. Practice self-assertiveness. "Treat your thoughts and feelings with respect in your encounters with others," says Dr. Branden. "Stand up for what you believe and feel, as opposed to concealing who you are to get someone else to like you."

5. Practice living purposefully. Goals and purposes provide a grid for organizing your time and energy, Dr. Branden explains. "Monitor your behavior to see if it's in alignment with your action plan," he says. "This gives you control over your life and a sense of empowerment."

6. Practice personal integrity. Tell the truth, keep your promises and honor your commitments, says Dr. Branden. When you don't, it demoralizes you and undercuts your sense of efficacy, he observes.

Watch your finances.

In modern society it's almost impossible not to equate self-worth with dollars. Seeing your balance increase is a great way to boost your self-esteem. "Save at least 10 percent of your paycheck," advises Dr. Mercer. "You'll feel better knowing that you're building a nest egg."

Stick a wad in your pocket.

Speaking of money, here's a trick Dr. Buffington recommends: "Keep a money clip with a bunch of dollar bills in your pocket and put your hand on it from time to time. You'll feel better just knowing there's a little extra cash in your pocket."

List your achievements.

Making a list of all your accomplishments and carrying it with you is a great way to remind yourself that you matter. "Peek at it when you need to feel more enthusiastic about yourself," says Dr. Mercer.

Find a purpose.

"It's difficult to have a sense of worth if you feel that your life is without consequence," says Dr. Longfellow. "Find something or someone to care about. Do something for people who are less fortunate than you or get involved with a cause in your community. Altruism is caring directed outward, but it produces self-caring as well."

Family and Friends

Spouses, lovers, parents, co-workers, bosses and friends—they all affect how you feel about yourself. Good relationships can make you feel strong and energized. But when the relationships are negative, self-esteem and energy plummet.

To get the most from your relationships, here's what experts advise.

Don't take it personally.
Nothing drains energy and motivation like feeling put down. In most cases, however, even when someone is critical about your choice of suits, for example, or the quality of a report at work, they're not talking about *you*. "Taking things personally means assuming that a particular remark or action was intended to hurt you," says Mark Goulston, M.D., assistant clinical professor of psychiatry at the University of California, Los Angeles, and author of *Get Out of Your Own Way*.

Try to understand the other person's true intention, advises Dr. Goulston. Assuming they're really friends, what they're usually trying to do is criticize an action and not you personally. Once you feel comfortable enough to accept criticism, you'll feel less compelled to burn tons of energy mounting a defense.

Listen to yourself.
People with low self-esteem are always listening to what others have to say. "You spend much of your life trying to prove things to others, show them you're worthy, hide unpleasant truths from them and please them, all in an effort to feel worthy yourself," says Dr. Goulston. When you spend all your energy trying to make others feel better, you can't feel very good about yourself. "Try to seek out relationships in which you feel valued for doing nothing—for who you are, not what you do," he says.

Disconnect from harmful people.
In the real world, of course, this isn't always easy to do. But when you find yourself spending time with "friends" who are constantly critical, your energy is sure to suffer. "Stay away from those who put you down," advises Dr. Mercer. "Hang around with people who are positive and upbeat about your accomplishments."

Hand out compliments.
"When you show appreciation to others, people appreciate *you* more," Dr. Mercer says. And when you get positive feedback, you feel better about yourself— and more prepared to take on even more challenges.

Major Life Changes

Major life changes can make you want to sleep as long as Rip Van Winkle. Things like getting divorced, losing your job, starting a new job, getting married, retiring or having your children leave home are all considered major life changes. Note: Even positive changes—things that should be pleasant—fall into the category of major life changes that can produce unpleasant, energy-depleting symptoms related to stress.

Luckily, there are many steps that you can take to put the bounce back in your step and a grin back on your face, no matter what you're going through. Read on for tips on how to maintain your energy levels throughout some of the most common major life changes.

Boosting Energy during Crisis

When our habits, patterns and relationships get shaken up, most of us feel edgy, anxious or even depressed. To find the energy to go on despite such feelings, here are some suggestions from the experts.

Sob—on a budget.
You have just lost a loved one or a career, or your children have moved away. Of course you feel sad.

Ignore advice to snap out of it immediately, says Coralie Scherer, Ph.D., a psychologist at the San Jose Marital and Sexuality Center in California.

"Take the time to grieve," she says. If you fear that once you start to cry you'll never stop, sob on a budget. Give yourself the freedom to feel sad, even to sob uncontrollably, for 15 minutes a day until you begin to feel better, Dr. Scherer suggests.

Temporarily decrease your expectations.
"Make a list of all the tasks that you think you need to accomplish and then do a quarter of them," suggests Maria Mancusi, Ph.D., a clinical psychologist in pri-

vate practice in Fairfax Station, Virginia. "Looking after your mental health is much more important. And you'll be a good role model for your family—they'll see you taking the time to slow down and plan out your life."

Talk it out.
"You might not want to overload one friend with everything that's wrong, but you may be able to confide in a few different friends about a few of things that are ailing you," Dr. Scherer suggests.

Write about it.
Take 10 to 15 minutes a day to write about how you're feeling, suggests Dr. Scherer. Expressing your emotions can help you recover more quickly and give you a sense of how to move on.

List the nice things.
When terrible things happen—you have been fired from your job or your spouse has walked out—you're likely to feel like a failure for a while. Just try to keep reminding yourself that it's not true. You may be going through a difficult time, but you have had life-affirming experiences in the not-too-distant past.

To remind yourself of those experiences, "make a folder of the nice things that people have given you, including birthday and congratulations cards and even photographs of happy events," suggests Dr. Scherer. Then write a description of several pleasant memories. When you're feeling down, take out your folder and your notes and consciously focus on the good things that have happened to you. This practice can help pick you back up and energize you.

Look on the bright side.
"Chances are, this isn't the first life change you have made or crisis you have experienced," says Renee Magid, Ph.D., president of Initiatives, Center for the Advancement of Work and Family Life in Fort Washington, Pennsylvania. Remember that you lived through those earlier changes and came out smiling. It'll happen again. Just remembering that you're a survivor may put some pep back in your step, she says.

Cut yourself some slack.
When you go through a crisis, something's got to give. Accept that you may not do an A+ job in all the aspects of your life.

"Let your boss know that you're going through a difficult time and that she may need to lower her expectations of you," says Constance Ahrons, Ph.D., professor of sociology at the University of Southern California in Los Angeles and author of *The Good Divorce*. Chances are that you'll not only get her support but also lighten some energy-sapping pressure.

Relax.
"Sometimes the best way to replenish your energy is to take a break—and get quiet," says Myrna Hartley, Ph.D., a psychologist in private practice in West Los Angeles, California. Even if you can only spare a few minutes from your hectic day, relax whatever way works best for you. Some suggestions: Take several deep breaths, meditate or, if you have more time, try a yoga class.

Remember to have fun.
Paradoxically, when we're depressed or stressed out, we often resist or forget about pleasing activities that may lighten our moods and rejuvenate us so that we're better able to go on.

"If nothing tempts you, make a list of what you used to enjoy," recommends Dr. Scherer. Then choose an item a day, whether it's buying flowers, taking a bubble bath, gardening or listening to the Rolling Stones belt out "(I Can't Get No) Satisfaction."

Act like a kid.
"If you really can't think of anything that you want to do, think back to what you liked to do as a kid, whether it was bicycling, drawing cartoons or even playing with your dolls, and then go out and do it," says Frederick Flach, M.D., adjunct associate professor of psychiatry at Cornell University Medical College in New York City and author of *The Secret Strength of Depression*. Going back to a favorite childhood activity will give your spirits a lift.

Remembering Your Health

It's all too easy to neglect the basics of good health when you're feeling fatigued and anxious because of a major life change. Here are a few things to remember.

Eat right.
"Overeating saps your energy and ultimately makes you feel more depressed," Dr. Flach says. It's especially important when you're going through a major life change to stick to a healthy diet, he says. The best choice is a low-fat, high-carbohydrate diet.

It's also a good idea to eat slowly, enjoying each morsel. There's a practical reason for that. "Your brain sends a message to your stomach to stop eating when you have had enough, but when you eat too quickly, the brain can't deliver that message fast enough," says Dr. Flach.

Ban the bottle.

You may feel more relaxed after a drink, but alcohol is a depressant—which means it'll sap your energy, says Dr. Flach. If you don't drink, don't start. If you do, watch your intake. The latest guidelines from the National Institute on Alcohol Abuse and Alcoholism are for men to consume no more than two glasses of wine or beer daily, while women should stop at one glass.

Move that body.

"Exercise not only is good for you but also has been shown to improve people's moods," says Dr. Flach. Even just a couple of hours of aerobic exercise—walking or swimming or any activity that gets your heart pumping a few days a week—will literally lift your spirits and give you more energy, he says.

Medication

When it comes to sapping energy, sometimes the cure seems worse than the disease.

If you read drug labels, you know that common side effects of medications are drowsiness and fatigue. But even if you're taking a medication with those warnings on the label, it doesn't necessarily mean that the medicine will make you feel as though someone pulled the plug. On the other hand, after you take your medicine, you may just feel as though your own legs are the heavy machinery that the label says you're not supposed to operate.

But whatever your reaction, sometimes you just have to take your medicine. When the benefits clearly outweigh the costs and there are no alternative cures at hand, the best that you can do is reduce the risk and inconvenience of the side effects. (If the drug causes drowsiness, for instance, you better join a car pool or take public transportation instead of driving.) Experts recommend being well-informed before you put any drug in your body. Owning or referring to a library copy of *USP DI, Volume II, Advice for the Patient*, also known in bookstores as the *Complete Drug Reference*, or another source of drug information for consumers is a good idea, says Arthur Brownstein, M.D., medical director of the Princeville Medical Clinic in Kauai, Hawaii, and staff physician for the Preventive Medicine Research Institute in Sausalito, California. Here are some other tips for being an informed customer.

Get the whole story.

Before you leave a doctor's office with a prescription, be sure to ask about possible side effects, advises Dr. Brownstein. If your doctor is too busy to go into detail, ask for written material about the drug, perhaps a photocopy of the relevant pages from a reference book.

Talk to your pharmacist.

Whether it's a prescription drug or an over-the-counter remedy, ask your pharmacist about it. "Counseling patients is one of the most rewarding parts of being

(continued on page 360)

What Are the Med Effects?

A wide variety of prescription and over-the-counter drugs can dull your system and make you feel as lethargic as a rag doll. Some, like sleeping pills, are meant to do just that. Others, like appetite suppressants or decongestants, have a stimulating effect at first but can lead to fatigue as a rebound effect. Antidepressants, to cite another example, are meant to help depression, but many people wind up feeling sedated when they first start taking them.

With most drugs that drain your energy, tiredness is an unfortunate by-product. Here's a rundown of drugs that can leave you feeling run-down. If you find a drug that you're taking on this list and you feel that it's having a negative impact on your energy level, discuss your options with your doctor.

Antidepressants
Desyrel (trazodone)
Elavil (amitriptyline)
Pamelor (nortriptyline)
Sinequan (doxepin)

Antidiarrhea
Lomotil (diphenoxylate and atropine)

Antihistamines
Benadryl (diphenhydramine)
Chlor-Trimeton (chlorpheniramine)
Compoz (diphenhydramine)
Dimetapp (brompheniramine)
Nytol with DPH (diphenhydramine)
Sominex Formula (diphenhydramine)

Appetite suppressants
Adipex-P (phentermine)
Pondimin (fenfluramine)
   Note: Pondimin is for short-term treatment of obesity and can cause sedation and drowsiness initially.
Tenuate (diethylpropion)

Beta-blockers
Inderal (propranolol)
Lopressor (metoprolol tartrate)
Tenormin (atenolol)

Other blood pressure–lowering drugs
Aldomet (methyldopa)
Ser-Ap-Es (reserpine, hydralazine, hydrochlorothiazide)
Note: Ser-Ap-Es may cause unusual tiredness when you begin taking it.

Cough and cold preparation
DayQuil (pseudoephedrine, dextromethorphan, acetaminophen)
NyQuil (doxylamine, dextromethorphan, acetaminophen, pseudoephedrine)

Decongestants
Dimetapp (phenylpropanolamine, phenylephrine, brompheniramine)
Sudafed (pseudoephendrine)

Minor tranquilizers
Valium (diazepam)
Xanax (alprazolam)

Motion sickness medications
Bonine (meclizine)
Dramamine (dimenhydrinate)

Muscle relaxants
For trauma to your muscles such as whiplash injuries:
Flexeril (cyclobenzaprine)
Norflex (orphenadrine)
To relieve muscle spasm caused by conditions such as multiple sclerosis or injury to the spine:
Dantrium (dantrolene)
Lioresal (baclofen)

Neuroleptics (major tranquilizers)
Haldol (haloperidol)
Thorazine (chlorpromazine)

Painkillers containing narcotic analgesics
Darvocet-N (acetaminophen and propoxyphene)
Tylenol with codeine (acetaminophen and codeine)
Vicodin (acetaminophen with hydrocodone)

a pharmacist," says pharmacist Donald Sullivan, Ph.D., a drug information consultant and the author of two books on pharmacy. "They like it when people take the time to ask questions."

You should ask the following five questions, says Arthur I. Jacknowitz, Pharm.D., professor and chairman of the Department of Clinical Pharmacy at West Virginia University in Morgantown.

1. What is the name of the drug and what is it supposed to do?
2. How and when do I take the drug and for how long?
3. What foods, drinks, other medicines or activities should I avoid while taking this drug?
4. Are there any side effects, and what do I do if they occur?
5. Is there any written information available on the drug or drugs I am taking?

In some states prescriptions must be accompanied by counseling, whether in verbal form or as a written insert. If you ask for patient information about a particular medication, pharmacists can provide a printout.

The best time to reach a pharmacist, says Dr. Sullivan, is late in the evening and on weekends, when most doctors' offices are closed. (They're busiest when doctors' offices are open.) No matter which pharmacist filled the prescription, call any pharmacy when you have a question, he says.

And regardless of the time of day, pharmacists should make the time to answer your drug therapy–related questions, says Dr. Jacknowitz.

Read the label.

Over-the-counter labels have been made more user-friendly. When you purchase something over the counter, make sure that you examine the list of ingredients. Many products are made up of combinations of drugs, and it's not advisable to take anything that you don't really need, says registered pharmacist Ron Finley, a lecturer and assistant clinical professor at the School of Pharmacy at the University of California, San Francisco.

Antihistamines, for example, don't do much for the common cold. So why expose your body to their sedating side effects when you can substitute antihistamine-free drugs to alleviate the symptoms that you do have? Multisymptom medications may not help the common cold, either. Pick and choose the right drug for your specific symptoms, says Dr. Jacknowitz.

Beware of combinations.

Mixing drugs can make side effects even worse, because the chemicals can interact to magnify the drowsiness or fatigue caused by any single one. Let your doctor and pharmacist know what you're already taking before you add a new medicine.

Watch out for alcohol.

Some over-the-counter liquid products contain a fair amount of alcohol (NyQuil Adult Nighttime, for example, is 25 percent alcohol), says Finley. "This can compound side effects, like fatigue and lethargy, and interact with some prescription drugs." So be sure that you read labels to avoid the high-alcohol medications. If you have questions, ask your pharmacist, says Finley.

Make Some Changes

With many prescription drugs side effects like fatigue and drowsiness begin to wear off after you have been taking them for a while. "There is a tendency to become tolerant to those side effects," says Charles Lacy, Pharm.D., director of Drug Information Services at Cedars-Sinai Medical Center in Los Angeles. "If you give the therapy an adequate trial, you may get rid of the energy-sapping effects and still retain its therapeutic benefits."

You may want to stick it out and give your system a chance to adapt to the drug, he says. With beta-blockers, for example, two to four weeks is considered a fair trial. In the meantime, here are some ways you can minimize the impact of energy-sapping side effects.

Adjust the dose.

"Consult with your doctor or pharmacist about changing the dosage," advises Kenneth Lem, Pharm.D., associate dean for educational affairs and lecturer in clinical pharmacy at the University of California, San Francisco. Because of differences in metabolism, individuals vary in their response to medication. Also, your metabolism may change as you age. It may be necessary to reduce the dosage and still obtain the benefits of the drug.

Take a test run.

The first few times you take a drug that is known to cause drowsiness (antihistamines, for example), take it in the evening, when you won't suffer any major mishaps by nodding off. "In that way, you can see how it affects you personally," says David Tatro, Pharm.D., a drug information consultant in San Carlos, California.

Adjust the time you take it.

If the drug has to be taken only once a day, ask your doctor if you can take it in the evening, says Dr. Tatro. The therapeutic effect of long-lasting drugs won't be diminished by such a schedule, and you won't have to feel drowsy all day long, he says. If it's a twice-daily drug, take it for the first time as late in the day as possible to see how it affects you.

Try a different format.

If the drug has to be taken frequently because the duration of its action is short, find out if a similar medication has the same therapeutic effect but is longer-acting than your current drug, suggests Dr. Jacknowitz.

Or find out if the drug comes in a sustained-release formulation or perhaps as a transdermal patch. Taking it in those ways may reduce the side effects, says Dr. Lacy.

Switching Medications

Since the effects of medication vary with individual chemistry, you may be able to find an alternative that works without causing side effects. Here are some suggestions.

Go from day to night.

A lot of manufacturers of cold and flu remedies have come out with day and night formulations, Dr. Sullivan points out. "Day products usually have just a decongestant, while the night products have a decongestant and an antihistamine," he says. You may want to see if you can get by with just a decongestant during the day and save the antihistamine for night, when drowsiness does not present as much of a problem.

Try nonsedating antihistamines.

If, because of allergies for example, you need to take an antihistamine during the day, try those that are least sedating.

"The antihistamine that probably causes the most tiredness is diphenhydramine found, for example, in Benadryl," says Dr. Sullivan. "Next in line would be products with brompheniramine in them, like Dimetapp." The least sedating over-the-counter antihistamine is chlorpheniramine, the active ingredient in Chlor-Trimeton.

Manufacturers of some antihistamines, most notably loratadine (Claritin), terfenadine (Seldane) and astemizole (Hismanal), claim that these medications do not cause drowsiness at all. They are, however, much more expensive and available by prescription only, although experts expect that they will be available over the counter soon, says Dr. Jacknowitz. Ask your doctor if this form of antihistamine is appropriate for you.

Lower your pressure another way.

If you're taking beta-blockers to lower your blood pressure and you find that they cause intolerable tiredness, ask your doctor about ACE inhibitors and calcium channel blockers, says Dr. Sullivan. ACE inhibitors lower blood pressure

Take the Natural Route

If energy-depleting side effects from medications are sidelining you, you may want to investigate natural alternatives to drugs.

The popularity of alternative medicine is due largely to the relative absence of side effects, says Oscar Janiger, M.D., associate clinical professor at the University of California, Irvine, and author of *A Different Kind of Healing*. "Your condition might respond to herbs or homeopathy or chiropractic or body work or psychological therapy or some combination of things," he says. "It's worth investigating, as long as you don't make things worse by rejecting good conventional care."

Some drugs that cause drowsiness are used to treat conditions such as insomnia, anxiety and depression, Dr. Janiger points out. These can often be treated with psychotherapy, stress-reduction techniques, nutritional supplements and herbs. Also, high blood pressure and cardiac conditions can often be managed without the draining effects of certain heavy-duty medications—such as ACE inhibitors.

"I prefer to use conventional Western medicines for high blood pressure only when necessary. I try to get people off them as soon as they have learned alternative approaches," says Arthur Brownstein, M.D., medical director of the Princeville Medical Clinic in Kauai, Hawaii, and staff physician for the Preventive Medicine Research Institute in Sausalito, California. He tries to accomplish that by recommending a variety of procedures—biofeedback, breathing techniques, meditation, guided imagery, yoga—along with a low-fat diet, herbs, an exercise program and group support.

When looking for an alternative practitioner, advises Dr. Janiger, get recommendations from people you trust, and make sure that the person you choose is properly licensed or certified. "Ideally, your point of entry should be an M.D.," he says. "Don't be afraid to ask your doctor for a recommendation. It helps assure that you'll have a proper diagnosis and a responsible referral."

by inhibiting an enzyme produced in the kidney that causes blood vessels to constrict. Calcium channel blockers lower blood pressure by decreasing blood vessel resistance to blood flow throughout the body. Neither causes as much fatigue as beta-blockers, he says. Other medications have other side effects, however, so discuss these choices with your physician.

If you and your doctor conclude that a beta-blocker is your best option, you may want to try one with reduced fat solubility, suggests Dr. Lacy. They don't penetrate as much into the central nervous system and may not cause as much fatigue. Your pharmacist or physician will be able to tell you which beta-blockers have reduced fat solubility, he says.

Get stimulated.

A lot of drugs that cause sedation or fatigue come packaged in a form that combines them with a stimulant such as caffeine. Some examples of prescription drugs with stimulants are Cafergot, Empirin with Codeine, Darvon-N Compound and Fiorinal. Some examples of these over-the-counter drugs are Midol Maximum Strength and Vanquish. "If you can tolerate them, these products may be a reasonable way to counteract the sedating effects of the medicine," says Dr. Lacy.

Meetings

*A*round the table, 15 corporate employees alternately stare at the yellow tablets in front of them or look out a conference room window. A few watch the guy at the head of the table who's talking about wingnuts, bafflebarts and ring dings.

Occasionally, someone shifts in a seat or writes something on a pad. But for the most part, no one moves, no one talks and no one blinks. Some don't even seem to breathe.

We have all been trapped in meetings during which our heartbeats slow, our eyes glaze over and our breathing becomes shallow. We have felt the ebb of attention turn into a desperate battle to keep our eyes open, our heads up— and to take a few notes. But there's something in the very structure of meetings that seems to push our pummeled senses over the edge of exhaustion.

Depleting Meetings

Whether a meeting is part of your job or a mandatory part of community service, you're sure to wonder—perhaps often—whether the meeting is necessary at all.

Why do you feel so exhausted when you're trapped in one?

"In looking at thousands of pet peeves from employees in the Pittsburgh area, we found that the reasons for exhaustion cluster into three categories," says Sharon M. Lippincott, a staff development coach with TeamWorks PLUS in Monroeville, Pennsylvania, and author of *Meetings: Do's, Don'ts and Donuts.* "One, the meeting lacks a clearly defined purpose; two, the meeting is unfocused; and three, 'everybody' knows that nothing ever happens as a result of them."

If a meeting has these flaws, everybody who attends is likely to feel drained and exhausted from just sitting there trying to figure out what's going on. Or they all may be worrying whether things that need to get done will, in fact, even be addressed. But fortunately, there are ways to avoid the exhaustion of meeting stupor. Here's what to do.

Rock the boat when you can.

Some meetings you can change—others, you can't. But how do you tell the difference?

"The two types of meetings are formal and informal," explains Bernie DeKoven, head of the Institute for Better Meetings in Palo Alto, California, and author of *Connected Executives*. "The formal meeting is usually ritualistic." That's the annual marketing meeting or the weekly sales review, which are primarily designed for organizational approval. Since these meetings are very orchestrated, he says, there's really nothing you can do to change them.

What you can change are the more informal meetings, which are set up to get work done, says DeKoven. "You're supposed to come up with something like a new plan, product idea or design." To get one of these meetings back on track, just ask, "What are we hoping to accomplish here?" and "How are we going to do it?" Once those questions are asked, you're likely to find that the meeting gets much more focused—and far more energetic—fast!

Know when to fold 'em.

"Most people attend far more meetings than they need to," says Lippincott. To figure out whether you should be there in the first place, "ask yourself two questions before every meeting," Lippincott suggests, " 'Do I have a significant contribution to make to this meeting?' and 'Is there something that will happen in this meeting in which I need to be involved?' "

If the answers are no, says Lippincott, ask the person who's called the meeting if you can attend just part of it or be excused.

Insist on an agenda.

Be clear about the purpose of the meeting that you're going to attend, says Lippincott. If necessary, call the person who scheduled the meeting and say, "Let me make sure I understand what the meeting's for and what I need to do." Then follow up by asking him to send you a copy of the meeting's agenda.

If there's no agenda, make one.

To prevent the aimless meandering that wears everyone out, the agenda should clearly present the meeting's purpose. If you haven't received an agenda before the meeting starts, ask the meeting facilitator to run through the list of topics to be covered, suggests Lippincott. "That list can act as an agenda, which in turn will act like a road map to keep the meeting focused."

Plan for conflict.

Conflict can be draining—especially when people have to take sides—so avoid head-on confrontations by preparing in advance. "If you know there's going to be some controversy during the meeting, talk to people ahead of time, particularly those whom you know will disagree with your position," says Lippincott. "You can find out what their objections are and address them before the meeting."

Rethink the meeting.
Visualize the meeting as part of a series of communications rather than a single event where all available information needs to be on the table at once. A lot of the information that you need to share with your co-workers can be presented in other ways, says DeKoven.

Use e-mail or a typed memo before a meeting to lay out your ideas or to provide necessary information, says DeKoven. It will cut down on the amount of time that the meeting takes. That way, people won't nod off during long talks that just present facts and figures.

Skip the doughnuts.
If you sit down to a meeting where food is served, skip the food and stick to the coffee, urges Lippincott. Otherwise, she says, the warm fuzzy feeling that you get from eating will zap your energy and prevent you from staying focused.

Steer toward the topic.
"If you're being held hostage in an unfocused meeting, you might try to hijack it," says Lippincott. "If, for example, everybody's jumping around from one topic to another and people are looking at their watches, you can wait for a pause, then jump in and ask, 'Can we save that thought for later? Let's get back to the topic.' Or you can say something like, 'Gee, Tom, that sounds interesting, but what does it have to do with which software package to buy?' "

Risk a heroic act.
"Don't worry about how you'll be perceived if you do take the reins and guide the meeting back to the task. If you have been sitting there nervous and upset because the meeting is wandering around and things aren't getting done, so are a lot of other people," observes Lippincott. "And if you're the one with the guts to do something about it, everybody will think you're a hero."

You not only will have made their jobs easier but also will have reduced the exhaustion that results from trying to follow disjointed discussions.

Mononucleosis

It has been dubbed the kissing disease, but mononucleosis isn't spread by bussing alone. Caused by a virus, this contagious condition, like the common cold, can be passed by sharing utensils, drinking from the same glass or being on the receiving end of a cough or sneeze.

Despite its affectionate nickname, mono is anything but romantic. Symptoms range from fever, swollen glands, sore throat and poor appetite to headaches and nearly overwhelming fatigue. While most of the flulike symptoms disappear within a week or two, the fatigue may feel as though it's never going to end. In some cases people have felt under the weather for up to two years after being infected.

For some college students mono almost seems like a rite of passage. Studies show that between 1 and 3 percent of college students are infected with mono each school year. But you don't have to be in college to be susceptible. If you have ongoing fatigue and those telltale flulike symptoms, be sure to see your doctor, who can quickly determine whether mono is the problem.

If it is mono, following the doctor's orders is step number one. But here are some things that you can do to harbor your energy and speed your recovery while the kissing disease is nipping at your heels.

Take a daily nap.
It sounds obvious, but people with mono need lots of sleep, says James F. Jones, M.D., senior staff physician at the National Jewish Center for Immunology and Respiratory Medicine in Boulder, Colorado. Taking even a short nap will help keep you rested and your energy levels up.

Come back slowly.
A virus doesn't care if the bills are late, your Christmas presents need wrapping or that big project is due next week. Its only job is to replicate itself, and if that happens to make you tired, well, that's just too bad. Don't try to push too hard in the face of obvious illness, advises Dr. Jones. "If you make yourself ill or just more tired, you've done too much."

Avoid liftoff.

Here's another reason to take it easy: When you have mono, the spleen enlarges and becomes brittle, meaning that it can rupture. Be sure to avoid heavy lifting, vigorous sports or anything else that can create large amounts of pressure in the abdominal cavity. This is particularly true in the early stages of the illness, three weeks to about three months after being infected, says Luther Rhodes III, M.D., chief of infectious diseases at Lehigh Valley Hospital in Allentown, Pennsylvania. It's also important to avoid alcohol, since that puts extra strain on a liver that may already be weakened by illness, he adds.

Don't neglect exercise.

Too much bed rest can backfire as badly as too little, says Dr. Rhodes. "A person normally loses about 10 percent of his body strength for each week of bed rest. And studies show that total bed rest can undermine your health even after recovery."

He recommends doing some regular, light activity as soon as you're feeling up to it. Jogging is probably too vigorous, but walking will help keep you fit and energized—so will pedaling a stationary bike or working in the yard. Dr. Rhodes advises doing mild workouts of 10 to 15 minutes, three times a week, until you feel stronger. You'll have energy highs and lows each day, so take advantage of the highs—and don't fight the lows.

Take a supplement.

Blood tests show that mono patients tend to have low folic acid levels, which can make infection-fighting white blood cells work less efficiently. Plus, it's hard to eat when you're feeling run-down, which is why people with mono often are low in a number of key nutrients. Dr. Rhodes advises taking a multivitamin that contains folic acid.

Get gut-level relief.

The evidence isn't all in, but preliminary research suggests that cimetidine (Tagamet), a drug used for treating ulcers, can help get people with mono back on their feet. (Tagamet is available in both prescription and over-the-counter forms.) According to Jay A. Goldstein, M.D., director of the Chronic Fatigue Syndrome Institute in Anaheim Hills, California, cimetidine can help ease symptoms of mono in as little as one to two days.

While many experts feel that it's too early to say for sure if this treatment is effective, Dr. Goldstein says that the underlying principles are sound. In people with mono the immune system churns out an increasing number of specialized cells (T-cells) that help battle infection. While T-cells help keep you healthy, they also secrete chemicals called cytokines, which are in part responsible for the blahs caused by mono. Cimetidine decreases the production of cytokines, which in turn can help relieve fatigue, Dr. Goldstein says. He suggests asking your doctor if this treatment may be right for you.

Don't suffer too long.

If it has been a month and you're still feeling exhausted, Dr. Jones says it's definitely time for another checkup. Occasionally, people with mono develop a secondary condition in which the body's normal sleep patterns are severely disturbed. You may feel sleepy all the time but still be unable to get the kind of deep sleep that helps restore your energy. So if the exhaustion never seems to end, don't assume it's only the mono. Ask your doctor if an underlying (and undiagnosed) sleep disturbance may be involved.

Moving

New home. New friends. New schools. New life. New worries. A big move may be exciting and challenging, but that doesn't mean it's energizing. In fact, it's often just the opposite.

Don't let those smiling real estate agents and welcome wagon ladies fool you. Relocating is one of the biggest energy robbers out there. "Moving is very stressful for most people, usually ranking among the top five stressful situations we face—just behind the death of a loved one and divorce," says Thomas Olkowski, Ph.D., a psychotherapist in Denver who specializes in counseling families that are relocating and the author of *Moving with Children*. "There is always a sense of a loss because you're saying good-bye to familiar people, places and comfortable situations, so a portion of your identity is lost. That kind of overwhelming stress typically causes you to feel depressed, out of control, overwhelmed, inefficient—feelings that rob you of your energy."

Anxieties Abound

The fatiguing effects of relocating typically last six months after the move but start well before the "For Sale" sign is posted, says Fred Medway, Ph.D., professor of psychology at the University of South Carolina in Columbia who specializes in the psychological effects of moving. "A lot of the stress associated with moving begins as soon as the expected move is announced, which can be months before the actual physical move.

"And since the majority of moves these days are for corporate relocations, it's usually hardest on those who have less say—the spouse of the jobholder and the children. The spouse can be the husband, but still is usually the wife. And whether she's working or not, she usually feels lonely and has a fear of the unknown and not meeting friends or of not being accepted . . . all of these definitely impact energy levels negatively."

Just talk to Sylvia Kidd, wife of a career military man, who has moved about every 3 years during their 27 years of marriage. The energy-draining challenges of moving are all too familiar to her. "I'm one of those people who never likes to leave where I am because I put down roots quite easily," she says. "No matter where we were going, I was prone to fight against leaving."

Unexpected Stress

Children's energy can also be zapped by moving, but usually not as much as parents fear. "Like spouses, children tend to be affected by the anticipatory stress of moving; there's a lot of anxiety about how bad it will be," says Dr. Medway. "But more schools these days are aware of this and have programs to help children adjust better. There are now good data that it's more of a myth that it's hardest on high school–aged children.

"Actually, I'd say that it's toughest on those in early adolescence, seventh and eighth graders, because they're dealing with all sorts of self-esteem issues. And it's harder on boys than girls, because girls are more likely to actively take part in social and extracurricular activities at school. But research shows that children as young as three and four can also be affected by the stress of moving."

And the one who initiates the move—typically the breadwinner—has his own set of additional stressors. "Besides the stress of the actual relocation, there are issues about the new job, how he will fit in," adds Dr. Medway. "And because corporate relocations often involve a promotion, it usually means working longer hours and spending more time away from home."

Moving with Motivation

Here's what the experts recommend for making a move less stressful and fatiguing.

Delegate.
The less stress you face, the less draining a move will be, so experts recommend avoiding as much stress before the actual move as possible by delegating many relocating responsibilities. "That means having a moving company handle the move, having a real estate agent handle the sale of your house and basically delegating as much as possible to professionals," advises Dr. Medway. "In most major corporations there tends to be a relocation expert who can provide you with a list of doctors, churches and the like in your new town as well as give you information about schools and stores in different neighborhoods."

Look where other transfers live.

"One of the better ways to make the adjustment easier is to look for your new home in a part of town where there are other people who have moved from elsewhere," advises Dr. Medway. "If you move to an area where families have lived for generation after generation, they probably won't be as welcoming because they don't have as much of a need to make new friends. You'll likely make friends easier in a part of town where there are other new people who have relocated."

He suggests telling real estate agents that you're interested in living in a part of town where there are other transferees or, for corporate moves, having the relocated-employee network at work help you meet other recent transfers.

Divide and conquer.

"As soon as I knew we were going to move, I started going through closets and decided what to take and what to leave behind," says Kidd. Besides making the actual move easier, cleaning out is therapeutic and can energize by giving you a fresh-start feeling, she discovered.

Talk about it.

One way to help family members deal with the move is to sit them down and discuss their feelings, suggests Dr. Olkowski. "Stress the positives of the move—how it will be tough but how you'll deal with it as best you can as a family unit."

"It's also important to have a united front, especially if you have children," adds Dr. Medway. "If one spouse is for the move and one is against it, that adds to the stress and fatiguing effects—especially to children. You really need to talk up the new town and all the opportunities that await you there."

Mingle to meet.

Once you arrive, it's important to get involved as quickly as possible in organizations. "This helps make the transition go so much smoother," says Dr. Medway. "One of the most de-energizing aspects of moving is not knowing anyone, and mingling helps you meet new people."

Let repairs wait.

A surefire way to lose energy is to immediately tackle home repairs and renovations at the new house. "It's natural to want to get the new house in the best possible shape as quickly as possible, but there is so much else on your mind and taking your time that you may be biting off more than you can chew," says Dr. Medway. "My advice is to give yourself a few months before tackling any big jobs."

Overweight

Carrying weight takes energy. Whether you're trying to haul a sack of potatoes up the stairs or toting a backpack on an afternoon hike, you're drawing on your energy supply. And when you're carrying extra pounds on your body in the form of fat, the energy drain never lets up. Put bluntly, it's exhausting to be overweight.

"That's not at all surprising," says nutritionist Carla Wolper, a registered dietitian at the Obesity Research Center at St. Luke's–Roosevelt Hospital Center in New York City. "Imagine having to lug 50 pounds of groceries but having to carry them all day without respite. That kind of physical activity would consume a great deal of energy by the end of the day, just as it does for anyone who is 50 pounds overweight."

Doctors who specialize in treating people who are overweight frequently hear complaints of low energy and fatigue from their patients.

"Fatigue is almost invariably the reason why patients come to see me for the first time," says Steven B. Heymsfield, M.D., director of the Obesity Research Center at St. Luke's–Roosevelt Hospital Center in New York City.

Heavy Losses, Major Gains

Doctors are aware of plenty of other reasons, besides hauling around too much poundage, why the less-than-svelte may feel sluggish. The most common causes are poor nutrition and eating habits, sedentary lifestyle, diseases such as diabetes and conditions such as sleep apnea. (Sleep apnea develops when airways become blocked by excess tissue, making breathing so erratic that it disrupts sleep.)

The good news is that whether you're very overweight or struggling to take off just a few pounds, there are things that you can do to recoup your energy. In fact, people who lose weight often report a boost in their energy levels when they have lost as little as five to ten pounds.

Here are some strategies from weight-loss experts to ensure more bounce to the ounce as you shed excess weight.

Start with a checkup.

If you are overweight and exhausted, let your doctor make sure that there are no other problems underlying your low energy levels, says Dr. Heymsfield.

"Fatigue is a cardinal symptom of disease," he explains. "As a physician, my first approach is to rule out disease. I check for any kind of metabolic disturbance, like hypothyroidism (a sluggish thyroid)."

Once every two weeks, says Dr. Heymsfield, he discovers a case of diabetes among the overweight people who come in for their first checkups. Unmanaged diabetes is more than extremely exhausting; it can also be life-threatening.

Fight fat with food.

Nutrition experts agree that smart eating habits are the key to losing weight.

"To keep your diet low in fat, make sure it's well-rounded," says assistant professor Wayne C. Miller, Ph.D., of the Exercise Science Programs at George Washington University School of Medicine and Health Sciences in Washington, D.C. "Our studies over the last several years have found that overweight people eat significantly more fat and refined sugars and less dietary fiber than normal weight people."

He recommends skewing your diet away from processed foods, which tend to be high in sugar and fats and low in fiber, toward wholesome low-fat foods, like fruits, vegetables, whole grains, beans and legumes.

Follow the 75 percent rule.

Eating a lot of fat at one sitting may make you feel sluggish, says Wahida Karmally, R.D., director of nutrition at the Irving Center for Clinical Research at Columbia–Presbyterian Medical Center in New York City. On the other hand, eating complex carbohydrates—like fruits, vegetables, grains and beans—provides the most enduring energy charge, she says.

"Complex carbohydrates consist of long chains of sugars that need to be broken down, so the energy gets released slowly," says Karmally. "I recommend using the U.S. Department of Agriculture Food Pyramid as a model and filling your plate with 75 percent complex carbohydrates."

Don't forget the protein.

Make sure that low-fat protein foods make up the remaining 25 percent on your plate, suggests Karmally. Good protein choices include lean beef, chicken, fish, low-fat dairy products and low-fat tofu.

Try grazing.

Eating smaller portions more frequently throughout the day can help you lose weight and keep your energy levels up. "A small number of people are fatigued or hungry after eating large meals," says Wolper. "This may be the result of low blood sugar, a result of large amounts of insulin released to the blood to absorb a meal. If blood sugar is too efficiently dispatched, fatigue can be the result. Grazing is definitely an appropriate tactic for these people."

Power up with breakfast.

Researchers at the University of Nevada School of Medicine in Reno and at Baylor College of Medicine in Houston studied the breakfast eating habits of nearly 500 normal weight and overweight men and women.

They found that the overweight people who ate breakfast took in significantly more fat than their slimmer counterparts, but the slim set tended to eat more calories.

They also found that some overweight people skipped breakfast entirely. Skipping meals often produces overeating or bingeing instead of having the intended result, says Wolper.

Eating a nutritious, low-fat breakfast can help short-circuit this behavior cycle and keep your appetite—and energy—on a more even keel, she says. So, what's the ideal breakfast? "Starting your day with cereal, fruit and skim milk will energize you and improve your alertness, too," says Karmally.

Keep on moving.

"Resting is rusting," says Harvey B. Simon, M.D., assistant professor of medicine at Harvard Medical School. "One of the most common reasons for fatigue that we see is underuse of the body."

Experts view exercise as important for maintaining your energy levels no matter what your weight. "Fit people have a greater capacity to expend energy over a greater length of time," says Dr. Heymsfield. "It's like having a bigger engine that doesn't lose power so easily. Like pulling a load down the highway with a V-8 instead of a four-cylinder."

If you're overweight, it's a good idea to take a slow, steady approach to upping your activity, says James O. Hill, Ph.D., associate professor of pediatrics and medicine and associate director of the Center for Human Nutrition at University of Colorado Health Sciences Center in Denver. In fact, it's hard to lose and maintain weight by changing what you eat alone, he says.

"Spend less time being sedentary," he advises. "Work on staying active for half of each day. Look for opportunities to be more active as part of your routine—take the stairs instead of the elevator, walk instead of driving. You'll get the best results if you don't worry about what's best for burning fat and just do what's fun."

Get help if you snore.

If your sleeping partner complains that you snore, or if you find yourself waking up again and again during the night, discuss it with your doctor. Both snoring and frequent wakings are possible symptoms of sleep apnea—a problem that is more common among overweight people.

While the problem may disappear as you lose weight, it is important to get treatment in the meantime, says Dr. Heymsfield. He treats some of his patients with a procedure know as CPAP (an acronym for continuous positive airway pressure), which involves wearing a masklike device to bed at night. "CPAP is like a reverse vacuum cleaner that blows air through your nasal passages to keep the airways open," he explains.

It may sound cumbersome, but CPAP does help people with apnea get a good night's sleep. The result is higher levels of energy during the day, says Dr. Heymsfield.

Lift the weight of depression.

"Depression is tightly related to gaining weight," says Dr. Heymsfield. "It's depressing to be overweight, to be out of control. Weight gain is also a sign of depression."

If you can't seem to shake off feelings of depression, you should discuss it with your doctor, who may want to treat you for depression even as you're losing weight, he adds.

Poor Posture

What comes first, bad posture or low energy? It's a vicious circle: Reduced energy levels make you slump and slouch, but slumping and slouching drains your energy, forcing your back and neck muscles to work overtime to support your torso.

The downside of poor posture doesn't stop with strained muscles. When you spend a lot of time in chairs, your chest can compress downward. Instead of filling to 100 percent capacity, your lungs are constricted, their capacity reduced up to 30 percent. "When oxygen flow is compromised, the body runs on a compromised energy source," says Arthur Brownstein, M.D., medical director of the Princeville Medical Clinic on Kauai, Hawaii, and author of *Back to Life*. "It's like choking off the air-intake valve on your carburetor. You lose combustion."

Also, if you sit with your head bent forward—a head position that often goes along with poor posture—you can impede the blood flow to your brain, sinking your moods and sapping your mental energy. Poor posture also dramatically increases the workload on your cardiovascular system and can interfere with normal digestion and elimination. Add to all of this the possible impingement of nerves in the spinal column, which can affect every organ in the body, plus the effort it takes to compensate for aches and pains caused by improper alignment, and you end up with what can amount to an energy crisis.

Unfortunately, at this point, good intentions might not be enough. "In my 20 years of clinical practice, I have yet to see anyone improve his posture by reminding himself to sit erect," reports Lucien Martin, D.C., a specialist in rehabilitation and maximum performance who is in private practice in Santa Monica, California. If you've been sitting, standing and moving the wrong way, straightening out takes practice and re-education. Here's how to do it.

Sit Right, Feel Right

When you slouch or hunch in your chair, you place one to two times as much pressure on your back as when you sit up straight. And your poor neck muscles have to support a bowling-ball-weight head that's drooping under the pressure of gravity. So a good sitting technique—along with the right kind of chair—is the first step toward better posture and more energy. Here's how to take a better seat.

Choose the right chair.

"Sitting is most comfortable when the body's weight is taken primarily by the feet and the bony haunches at the base of the pelvis," says Rob Krakovitz, M.D., a medical doctor in private practice in Aspen, who specializes in alternative medicine, and the author of *High Energy*. To achieve this, your chair should enable you to sit with your feet on the floor and your thighs parallel to it, and you should be able to contact the back of the chair without slumping.

Seek support.

Good support for your lower back helps prevent slumping and lessens the strain on your spinal muscles, according to Dr. Krakovitz. "The support should start about five inches above the seat, so there is a hollow space for the buttocks," he advises.

Get a little laid back.

"Unless you're reclining in your chair, your back muscles are under constant exertion," says Chris Grant, Ph.D., an ergonomist with F-One Ergonomics in Ann Arbor, Michigan. "Research suggests that the optimum position is at least a ten-degree recline." That's only about as much as the average folding chair. (Ergonomics, or human engineering, involves designing environments that are comfortable, healthy and efficient.)

Get the right angle.

"You shouldn't have to hunch your shoulders to get your arms on your desk," says Scott D. Minor, P.T., Ph.D., assistant professor of physical therapy at Washington University School of Medicine in St. Louis. "When you type, your forearms should extend 90 to 95 degrees from your upper arms, sloping a bit downward so that your elbows are slightly higher than your wrists."

Raise your reading level.

"The top of what you're reading should be at eye level," says Dr. Minor. If you're at your desk, prop up your reading material and position your computer equipment so that the top of the screen is at eye level.

Avoid the neck swivel.

Sit so that you don't have to bend your neck. If you read in bed, prop yourself up with pillows so that your back and neck are supported in line, says Dr. Minor. Avoid using pillows only under your head, because that will bend your neck forward, he says. Hold up your reading material. If that's too tiring on your arms, Dr. Minor recommends getting a book stand or something like a hospital tray table that tilts.

Switch positions.
That may not be good advice for politicians, but for someone who sits a lot it's golden. "There are good postures and bad postures, but there is no posture that anyone should be in all the time," says Dr. Grant. "When you're moving, you have better blood flow and oxygenation, which means more energy." So lean forward, lean back, lean to the side, look up, look down, stand up.

"Make it a habit to get up and move," stresses Dr. Grant. For example, when the phone rings, stand up to answer it. If you refer to something regularly, store it where you have to walk a few steps to get to it.

Customize your posture.
Adopt the posture that's most balanced and comfortable at any given moment, advises Harold H. Bloomfield, M.D., a psychiatrist in Del Mar, California, and co-author of *The Power of 5: Hundreds of 5-Second to 5-Minute Scientific Shortcuts to Ignite Your Energy, Burn Fat, Stop Aging and Revitalize Your Love Life.* "To find your own best sitting position, first balance your neck. Close your eyes and gently tilt your head to the left, then the right, then return it to center. Then lean your head slightly forward, then back, and return to the spot that you sense is the exact center." You can then balance the rest of your torso by bending at the hips instead of the neck.

Walk Like a Man—Or Woman

"Efficient walking consumes minimal energy," observes Howard J. Dananberg, D.P.M., medical director of the Walking Clinic and a podiatrist in Bedford, New Hampshire. When you use your body inefficiently, your muscles have to work harder and you increase energy expenditure sixfold, he says. Here's how to save energy as you glide about the Earth.

Walk tall.
Walk with your head high, your neck and shoulders relaxed and your lower back flat, says Dr. Bloomfield. "Touch your heel down first, roll your weight forward across the sole of your foot and gently push off with your toes." Your feet should point straight ahead, he adds, and your legs should not be hyperextended.

Be a swinger.
Not only does posture influence the way you walk, how you walk affects your posture. "Studies show that if you don't allow your arms to swing, energy con-

sumption increases," notes Dr. Dananberg. "The power in walking comes when the left arm swings as the right leg kicks, and vice versa." Relax your hips and shoulders, allowing them to move naturally, he adds.

Try wearing orthotics.
If you're not walking properly due to an anatomical problem such as a rigid big toe joint, flat feet or a discrepancy in leg length, you may benefit from wearing an orthotic device in your shoes. Over time, compensating for such conditions can cause postural changes and energy drain, says Dr. Dananberg, and an orthotic device can make the compensation for you. A chiropractor, osteopath or podiatrist can determine whether you would benefit from an orthotic.

Posture-Enhancing Exercises

"Good posture is a position in which the least amount of energy is expended to hold you there," says Joanna R. Shaw, P.T., coordinator of clinical education at Affinity, an outpatient rehabilitation service in Allentown, Pennsylvania. "It boils down to adequate balance between opposing sets of muscles." If that balance has been thrown off by bad habits, some muscles need to be strengthened and others need to be stretched. These exercises will help get you balanced.

Get your back up.
For most of us, men in particular, the muscles of the chest and front of the shoulders are tighter and stronger than the muscles of the rear shoulders and back. Wayne Westcott, Ph.D., fitness research director at the South Shore YMCA in Quincy, Massachusetts, recommends the following exercises to correct that imbalance.
   • *Neck and upper back.* Holding a dumbbell in each hand, arms at your sides, bring your shoulders upward toward the ears in a shrugging movement. Slowly lower your shoulders and repeat 8 to 12 times.
   • *Rear of shoulders.* Lie facedown on a bench. Hold a light dumbbell straight down in each hand, with your palms facing inward. Now move your arms up and back, while bending your elbows and squeezing your shoulder blades together. Lift until your upper arms are parallel to the floor. Lower slowly and repeat 8 to 12 times.
   • *Middle back.* Place your right knee and hand on a bench so that your back is horizontal. Hang your left arm straight down, holding a dumbbell with your palm facing your body. Pull the dumbbell up to your armpit area. Lower slowly and repeat 8 to 12 times. Switch sides and do the same.

Move into Good Posture

These three practices have helped countless people improve their postures and move with greater energy efficiency, according to the experts.

Alexander Technique. With this technique, the goal is to learn to use your body efficiently while using the least amount of tension, allowing you to sit, stand and move with ease and grace. "In a series of private lessons, you learn about habits that may cause misuse of your body," says Pamela Blanc, executive director of the Alexander Training Institute of Los Angeles. "These old patterns cause tension and bad posture." For information and a list of certified teachers in your area, call the North American Society for the Alexander Technique (NASTAT) at 1-800-473-0620 or write to NASTAT, P.O. Box 517, Urbana, IL 61801.

Tai chi. A Chinese martial art, it's usually taught as a gentle exercise form to men and women of all ages. "It's practiced mainly for its health-enhancing and stress-reducing benefits," says Lana Spraker, a dance therapist and tai chi master in Los Angeles. Consisting of slow, energizing movements, tai chi teaches you to move through space in good alignment.

The result is natural improvement in posture and more effortless movement, says Spraker. She recommends finding an experienced teacher and observing a class to see if you would feel comfortable with the instruction. Your local YMCA or university may have an instructor.

Yoga. This ancient system from India links awareness, breath and movement, says Bija Bennett, a yoga therapist in Aspen and author of *Breathing into Life*. "Yoga positions are designed to create a healthy spine, which enhances the health and energy of the entire body." If you practice yoga correctly, she says, you will naturally start to have better posture.

There are numerous classes in every major city. Check your yellow pages or ask at your local Y to find classes near you. Make sure that you get some individual attention at first, says Bennett, so that a teacher can address your personal needs.

Stretch out your front.

To further correct the front-to-back imbalance, stretch the front shoulder and midsection muscles. Here are Dr. Westcott's suggestions.

• *Do the cobra.* Lie facedown on a mat. Keeping your hips on the floor and using your hands to push off, slowly raise your head, then chest, then stomach. Hold for five seconds, then slowly lower yourself—stomach, chest and finally your head. Don't strain yourself, only lift your body as far as you are able. Repeat three times.

• *Use the door.* Stand with your back to a doorway, an arm's length away. Reach back with your right hand and grab the doorjamb. Turn gently to the left. Hold the stretch for 30 seconds. Then do the same with your other hand and stretch to the right.

Strengthen the mid-back.

For the all-important muscles on either side of the spine, try these exercises recommended by Shaw. Lie facedown with your head resting on the floor, face to one side and stretch your arms over your head on the floor. Raise your arms up an inch or two and hold that position for a few seconds. Then, place your arms out to the side, raise them a few inches and hold. Repeat the routine 10 to 20 times, twice a day.

Hang around.

The best way to improve the energy capacity of your posture, says Dr. Martin, is to regularly stretch downward and backward. This is most simply achieved, he says, by hanging from a bar with your feet on the floor supporting most of your weight and by breathing deeply to unlock your ribs and spine. Then place one foot forward while tilting your head backward and thrusting your chest forward. Dr. Martin advises installing a secure bar in a doorway of your home so that you can stretch your spine and ribs regularly. "It releases hindrances to the natural flow of energies." In addition to hanging out, he recommends these exercises.

• *Lengthen your spine.* Lie on your back, arms at your sides, legs fully extended. Keeping your legs relaxed, rotate your pelvis upward by pulling in your abdominal muscles. You should feel your lower back flatten against the floor. Hold for a few seconds, and then relax the abdominal contraction. Repeat this process until you're comfortable doing it. Then extend your arms as far as you can above your head. Take a deep breath as you rotate your pelvis upward and flatten your lower back against the floor. You should feel your chest opening up and your spine elongating. Then exhale and let your pelvis relax. Repeat the procedure at least ten times.

• *Do the shoulder squeeze.* Sit no more than halfway back into a firm chair and slide one foot under the chair. This will make your pelvis roll forward. Rest your hands on a nearby table or desk. Straighten your spine and neck. Take a deep breath and lift your chest up, forcing your breastbone forward and squeezing your shoulder blades inward and downward. Then lean slightly forward as you keep squeezing for three or four seconds. Then exhale and relax. Repeat at least three times.

Tuck in your chin.

To strengthen the neck muscles, Shaw recommends this exercise: Rest your upper back and the back of your head against a wall. Slide your chin in toward your neck, flattening out the arch in the back of the neck. Hold for 10 to 15 seconds and repeat ten times. She advises doing the exercise twice a day.

Straighten up and breathe right.

"Your posture and your breath are intimately linked," says Bija Bennett, a yoga therapist in Aspen and author of *Breathing into Life*. "The inhale creates a stretching and expanding of your spine. The exhale creates a rounding of the lower back, strengthening your base of support." She recommends the following exercise.

Sit quietly for a few moments with your eyes closed. Begin to deepen your breath as you notice the natural relationship between your breathing and the movement of your spine. Then stand with your feet hip-width apart. Slightly drop your chin to release and free the back of your neck. Allow your spine to lengthen and your back to widen. Inhale and exhale through your nose, creating a soft, whispering sound from the back of your throat—it's the sound you would hear if you whispered the word "ha," but with your mouth closed. As you inhale, bring both arms up over your head. You will feel your spine lengthen and your head move up slightly. When your breath is full, hold for a few seconds, then exhale slowly while bringing your arms down. Do 10 to 12 slow repetitions, coordinating your movements and breath.

Pregnancy

*I*s there any event in a woman's life as turbulent and emotionally intense as pregnancy? Those nine months between conception and giving birth are a veritable roller coaster of emotions, with vibrant highs often followed by prolonged, energy-draining lows. Add to this all of the physical changes in a woman's body, and it's inevitable that her energy is going to suffer.

Although every woman (and every pregnancy) is different, there are a few things that every woman can do to stay strong and keep her energy level high. Indeed, medical experts attest that the positive changes you make during your pregnancy will help keep you energized even after the baby arrives. "You have the opportunity to change your life forever when you're pregnant," states Pamela Fenton, M.D., an obstetrician at Cedars-Sinai Medical Center in Los Angeles.

Interior Body Building

The nine months of pregnancy consist of some of the hardest work you'll ever do. After all, you're building a brand-new human from scratch. To help ensure that your pregnancy goes smoothly while at the same time you're staying energized and alert, here are a few tips to try.

Eat a little—more often.
Rather than eating three meals a day and letting your tank run empty in between, try eating smaller meals more often, says Jennifer Niebyl, M.D., professor and head of obstetrics and gynecology at the University of Iowa Hospitals and Clinics in Iowa City. This can help reduce the energy-draining nausea that sometimes occurs during pregnancy.

Pregnant women were traditionally advised to keep crackers at the bedside for a quick, healthy snack. It's still good advice today, says Dr. Niebyl. Also, be sure to have a small breakfast in the morning, followed by a midmorning snack.

Follow a light lunch with a midafternoon snack. Eat a small dinner and save your dessert for bedtime. "The idea is to keep your stomach full, so eating small portions is a good idea," she says.

Take your B₆.

Although taking vitamins during pregnancy won't eliminate fatigue, a large dose of vitamin B_6 can help alleviate energy-draining nausea. "B_6 is the only vitamin that's effective against nausea. I usually tell patients to take a 50-milligram pill and break it in half. Take a half, two to three times a day as needed," says Dr. Niebyl. Check with your doctor before taking B_6 supplements.

Iron out anemia.

In some cases fatigue during pregnancy is caused by iron-deficiency anemia. If that's the case with you, your doctor may recommend that you take iron supplements, which can help restore energy, says Carolyn Hadley, M.D., a perinatologist at Medical College of Pennsylvania and Hahnemann University in Philadelphia. Just as with B_6—or any other supplement—you should always get your doctor's okay. Taking supplements on your own is not a good idea during pregnancy, doctors say.

Take it easy.

"You can be physically active and maintain a normal schedule during your pregnancy, but don't do things that you don't need to do," says Dr. Niebyl.

"In the old days people who were pregnant were treated with kid gloves," she says, "but today the pendulum has swung in the other direction. Yet, pregnant women still need family support to help with the children so they can get rest. And mothers need to nap instead of cleaning or doing the dishes."

Get more sleep.

Your body needs more rest while you're pregnant, so don't resist the urge to sleep, says Dr. Niebyl. Adjust your life so that you can catch those extra winks by going to bed earlier in the evening and by napping during the day if you get a chance.

Look for outside help.

Especially if you already have young ones at home, parenting groups can be helpful when you're expecting. "It gives you a chance to talk about what it's like to raise a baby in the first year," says Marion McCartney, a certified nurse-midwife at The Maternity Center in Bethesda, Maryland. "Sometimes it's lonely out there." To find groups in your area, ask a midwife or nurse at your hospital birth center or look through the phone book blue pages for organizations that specialize in children and youth services.

Many of these organizations hold parenting classes. They can help you feel more comfortable about what you're doing. "If you're feeling okay about yourself, you'll feel better," says McCartney. These groups also serve as a great referral source for babysitters.

Consider a maternity massage.
A special maternity massage can help a woman relax and lessen some of the discomforts of pregnancy, according to Connie Cox, author of *Maternity Massage* and owner of massage centers in New York City and Scottsdale, Arizona. "A maternity massage is lighter than a regular massage and does not disturb the baby," she says. "A massage reduces tension and headaches, and it improves blood flow." Ask your obstetrician or a midwife for a referral to someone who does maternity massage in your area.

Sign up for childbirth education classes.
"These classes are a must," says McCartney. "You'll learn to let go and find the strength that's inside of you. It's there. You just have to learn how to tap into it."

Energy from Exercise

Pregnancy is no reason to give up exercise. "Childbirth is a physical event," says McCartney. "The more in shape you are, the more stamina you'll have at the end. Women who are runners and dancers do well in labor."

Even if you're not a hard-core athlete, you'll most likely benefit from walking or swimming during pregnancy if you already indulge in these activities, says Dr. Hadley. You won't want to overdo it, however. After the 25th week of pregnancy, your heart rate during exercise should not exceed 120 beats a minute.

Dr. Fenton put this tip into practice herself. She made daily exercise part of her routine when she became pregnant. Today, years later, she still exercises for a half-hour as soon as she gets home from work. "It gives me the energy to deal with what is often a difficult transition for the working mom—that of changing from the professional to the mommy role. At the same time I get to take time to take care of *me* without incurring any guilt," she explains.

Mental Boosters

While pregnancy can be a stressful time, it's also exciting. Keeping things in perspective will help you feel more energized throughout your pregnancy. Here's what experts recommend.

Keep a positive attitude.

Stress is one of the biggest energy drains there is. The more you know about pregnancy, the less anxious you'll be about the future. "Read books about pregnancy and what's going on in your body," says Dr. Hadley. "Take classes given by nurses about pregnancy so that you know what to expect. It takes away a fear of the unknown."

Know when to tune out.

Everyone likes to talk about her own experiences. Sometimes, however, the stories are less than positive. Every pregnant woman has had the experience of having well-intentioned, but misguided people alarm her by telling horror stories about pregnancy. In the next nine months you'll hear—often from total strangers: You're too big. You're not big enough. You're too active. Or not active enough.

"Shore yourself up against such talk," says Dr. Hadley. "Turn a deaf ear to such comments or say, 'Stop. This is not what I need to hear.' "

Ask before worrying.

Pregnancy is a time of unknowns, and it's almost impossible not to worry about every detail. Don't suffer alone. Call your doctor, advises Dr. Hadley. "I'd rather talk to patients and put their minds at ease than have them worrying at home," she says. If you don't feel comfortable calling your doctor, or if your doctor is always too busy to take your calls (or at least return them), Dr. Hadley has a simple piece of advice: Find another doctor.

Visualize your baby.

A good way to chase away worry and fatigue when you're pregnant is to lie in bed and meditate about your baby, says Diane Ross Glazer, Ph.D., a psychologist at Encino-Tarzana Regional Medical Center in Tarzana, California. "Lie in bed, close your eyes and massage your tummy. Try to picture your baby as whole and comfortable," suggests Dr. Glazer. "Talk to the baby. Tell the baby, 'I'm here and eager to meet you.' Try to think of positive things you can say to your baby."

Put your world in order.

"Make sure your surroundings are as wonderful as they can be because that helps your emotional state," says Dr. Glazer. "Put your house in order. Make a baby's room. Clean your files. If your external world is in order, you can feel more in order internally and then you'll have more energy."

Join together.

Before the baby is born, talk to your older children about the baby. "It's a really good thing for older children to be empathetic, to take care of you a little bit," says Dr. Glazer.

Older children are naturally curious about pregnancy. "There are wonderful books available for children that explain the baby's growth inside of you," she says. "Read the pregnancy books with them. It's a way to relax while educating and entertaining your older children."

Be kind to yourself.

Some new parents want the birth of their babies to match something they read in a magazine or see on TV. They may insist, for instance, that they want to give birth in a Jacuzzi. Don't waste energy fretting about birthing the trendy way. Instead, get all the information you can and then relax. You're about to take part in the oldest ritual of life. "The birth of your child is not a designer experience," says Dr. Fenton.

Premenstrual Syndrome

We often think of the menstrual cycle as being a veritable clock, ticking away at a regular monthly rhythm. But for many women, it's anything but. Periods can be surprisingly light one month and disturbingly heavy the next. Or they may come earlier than expected for three months in a row, then come late for the next six. Sometimes it seems that the only predictable thing about menstrual periods is that they're unpredictable.

Yet one aspect of the monthly cycle is nearly universal: Virtually all women, between the time of puberty and menopause, will experience at least some monthly discomfort—not during the period itself, necessarily, but for days (or even weeks) before it arrives.

Experts estimate that as many as nine out of ten women suffer from lethargy, mood changes or other forms of premenstrual discomfort. Not last on this long list of possible discomforts is fatigue. And the fatigue can be profound, sometimes dragging on for days or weeks at a time. All of these energy-sapping premenstrual discomforts are also unpredictable. For some women, they begin at mid-cycle. For others, they hit just before the period.

Putting Symptoms behind You

Fortunately, there often are ways to keep premenstrual fatigue and other premenstrual syndrome (PMS) discomforts under control. "Lifestyle changes offer the most help to women," says Annette MacKay Rossignol, Sc.D., professor in the public health department at Oregon State University in Corvallis.

But by planning ahead, you can help ensure that you're in a position of strength when the downtimes hit. Here's what experts advise.

Start with a diary.

One of the most difficult aspects of battling premenstrual-related fatigue is being sure that what's happening is related to your period—that there isn't some other problem that's wearing you down. "You should appreciate that your symptoms are real and that there is not something psychologically wrong with you," says Dr. Rossignol.

Premenstrual discomfort, when it occurs, always just precedes your menstrual cycle. Keeping a diary will help you understand whether your discomfort is, in fact, related to your periods. Look for a pattern. In most women premenstrual discomfort peaks 24 to 48 hours before menstruation begins, says Dr. Rossignol. Once you have the symptoms charted, you'll know when to expect the letdown—and you can plan your schedule accordingly.

Plan ahead.

Many women make it a point to avoid scheduling stressful or unnecessary events during the time they expect their energy to be low, says Jean Endicott, Ph.D., chief of the Department of Research, Assessment and Training at Columbia–Presbyterian Medical Center in New York City.

Staying in Charge

For women suffering the premenstrual blues, even the simplest things such as going to a movie, calling a friend or taking a walk around the block can become uncomfortable, energy-draining burdens. But withdrawing from life isn't even a short-term solution; it makes the blues worse.

At every opportunity, particularly when you're feeling down, "follow those things in life that make you blissful and go do them," advises Terry Oleson, Ph.D., director of the Department of Behavioral Medicine at California Graduate Institute in Los Angeles. "Anything that gives you pleasure can give you energy."

Pick up the telephone.

No one feels friendly and sociable when they're feeling down, but sometimes hearing the voice of a good friend will make you feel better and more energetic, says Dr. Oleson. So don't suffer alone. Call your friends. Make plans to meet. Or just chat for a while. The human contact can go a long way toward making you feel energized again.

Stay active.

"Sometimes it seems like a catch-22 to exercise when you're not feeling energetic, but it's one thing I do recommend," says Marcia Szewczyk, M.D., director of the PMS Clinic at Bowman Gray School of Medicine of Wake Forest University in Winston-Salem, North Carolina.

Getting energized doesn't require hard-core workouts, either. Brisk walking for about 20 minutes, even if it's around the block or around the house, can provide as much (or more) of a pick-me-up as napping, says Dr. Endicott.

Stay regular.
Don't wait until you're exhausted before getting started with activities, say medical experts. It's important to exercise regularly, not just during the days or weeks preceding your period.

Motivate with companionship.
To help yourself stay motivated, Dr. Szewczyk recommends inviting a friend to share your workouts. Exercise is more fun when you have company. In addition, you'll be less likely to backslide when someone is depending on you. "You're more likely to stick to the exercise routine if you feel as though you're committed to somebody else," she says.

Get plenty of rest.
It sounds obvious, but one of the keys to not feeling run-down before or during menstruation is to get enough rest. In today's high-stress world many women simply neglect to take the necessary downtime. Sleep eight hours at night and, if possible, take a nap at some point during the day, recommends Dr. Endicott.

Recharge with meditation.
Simply taking a half-hour to completely and utterly relax is a great way to get more energy. "Focus your mind on something very basic, like your breathing. Breathe slowly in and out. Envision the air going in and out of your abdomen like a balloon. Encourage your mind to release distressing or bothersome thoughts," Dr. Oleson says.

Get visual.
Another meditative technique that you may want to try is called visualization. "You imagine something like sunlight flowing into you. Imagine that light filters through your body as it does through the trees in the forest and brings the energy into your body. Having a mental picture of being energized by light can make it real for people," says Dr. Oleson.

Try acupuncture.
Some women say that a great way to escape premenstrual energy drain is with acupuncture. They may be onto something. "Acupuncture activates invisible energy in your body," says Dr. Oleson. You can ask your doctor or gynecologist to recommend a reputable acupuncturist in your area.

Energizing Diets

No doubt about it, what we eat affects our energy levels. Here's what experts recommend that you should do—and what you should avoid—to beat premenstrual energy drain.

Eat regularly.
This is good advice for everyone, but particularly for women with premenstrual fatigue. "Women who skip meals have less energy," says Dr. Szewczyk. "Even when you're not feeling hungry, be sure to eat a small amount of something to keep your energy up."

Go easy on caffeine.
"I recommend reducing caffeine intake for a couple of months and seeing if that helps," says Dr. Rossignol.

Cut back on sugar.
"It aggravates every symptom of PMS," says Guy E. Abraham, M.D., a researcher in premenstrual syndrome and owner of Optimox Corporation, a Torrance, California–based company involved in the manufacture and distribution of vitamin and mineral supplements. He recommends eating 60 percent of calories as complex carbohydrates, which are found in large amounts in whole grains and cereals.

Try apples and oranges.
When your sweet tooth strikes, reach for a piece of fruit. Fruit contains fructose, a form of sugar that can help satisfy those cravings without contributing to PMS problems, say medical experts.

Target your nutrients.
Women who increase their intake of foods rich in magnesium—such as tofu and leafy vegetables—often report feeling dramatically better, according to Dr. Abraham. "Within a month of switching to this program, their skin looks better, they look younger, their minds are sharper and they are more energetic," he says.

Be wary of dairy.
Large amounts of calcium may block the body's ability to absorb energy-releasing magnesium, says Dr. Abraham. Use dairy wisely and increase your consumption of vegetables to get magnesium. By eating a well-balanced diet that includes plenty of vegetables, you'll get plenty of calcium along with the magnesium, he adds.

Get an added boost from B₆.

Women who increase their intake of vitamin B_6 may experience less fatigue and other types of premenstrual discomfort, says Dr. Abraham. Some good food sources of vitamin B_6 include fish, chicken, turkey, potatoes and bananas. You can also take vitamin B_6 supplements under a doctor's supervision. For many women, taking 50 to 100 milligrams of supplemental B_6 daily may make a big difference. Or balance your B vitamins by taking a B-complex supplement, advises Dr. Abraham.

Think C.

While you're thinking about nutrients, don't forget vitamin C, which may help relieve energy-draining stress, says Susan M. Lark, M.D., medical director of the PMS and Menopause Self-Help Center in Los Altos, California. The vitamin is plentiful in broccoli, brussels sprouts and raw peppers. Fruit and fruit juices are also excellent sources of vitamin C.

Consider herbal remedies.

Although there is little scientific evidence that herbal remedies can relieve premenstrual fatigue, many women say that they help. Herbs that may offer a gentle stimulant effect include oat straw, ginger, ginkgo, dandelion root and Siberian ginseng, says Dr. Lark in her book *The Woman's Health Companion*.

Situational Insomnia

"O sleep! O gentle sleep!
Nature's soft nurse, how have I frighted thee,
That thou no more wilt weigh my eyelids down
And steep my senses in forgetfulness?"

Unlike the troubles of Shakespeare's Henry IV, what's keeping you awake will not affect the fate of a nation. Nevertheless, all that tossing and turning makes you want to scream—and not in Shakespearean verse, either.

Falling asleep is not supposed to be difficult. Most of the time, the hard thing is to stay awake.

But if you have the problem that doctors call situational insomnia, you start seeing a very different pattern. Now, the harder you try to catch some Zzzs, the more elusive they become.

Perhaps you're staying in a hotel on business or visiting your daughter in another state. Maybe you're in the middle of doing your taxes and you have a lot of financial concerns swirling around inside your head. Anything that robs you of sleep when you normally have no trouble nodding off is situational insomnia. The good news is that you don't have to let this fleeting nighttime problem rob you of your daytime energy.

Trying to Nod Off

What can you do about it? To begin with, don't panic. Worrying about insomnia is sure to keep you awake at night. It may even drive you to desperate measures, like trying to drink yourself to sleep or doubling your daytime coffee intake to boost your energy. Such tactics will only make things worse, says Joyce Walsleben, Ph.D., director of the New York University Sleep-Wake Center in New York City.

Sleep deprivation can diminish energy, and not only that, it can reduce your motivation and attentiveness. You may find yourself becoming irritable, listless and depressed in the bargain. But despite these considerable setbacks, a tempo-rary sleep deficit is probably not as bad as you think.

"People have been kept up as many as ten nights, and they could still func-tion," reports Peter Hauri, Ph.D., co-director of the Sleep Disorders Center and di-rector of its insomnia program at the Mayo Clinic in Rochester, Minnesota, and author of *No More Sleepless Nights*. "It might feel as though you're not functioning adequately and that you have no energy, but you can be sure that if an emer-gency arises, you'll still be able to function. The adrenaline will wake you up."

Although you may want to let someone else drive, for the most part you should go about your life as if you had slept like a baby, says Dr. Hauri.

Boosting Your Snoozing

Insomnia is not an illness, it's a symptom. Something has disrupted the nor-mal functioning of your nervous system. If it persists for more than three to four weeks, see a doctor who's familiar with sleep disorders. But if you know for sure that it's temporary, you can try to identify the cause and deal with it, says Michael Stevenson, Ph.D., clinical director of the North Valley Sleep Disorders Center in Mission Hills, California.

Your body will bounce back. All it needs is, well, a good night's sleep. Here's how to summon slumber to your bedside.

Get to the bottom of it.
In most cases, insomnia is a perfectly reasonable response to a stressful situa-tion—an emotional or financial crisis, a deadline, an illness—and will pass once the circumstances change. The cause, however, is not always obvious. To zero in on it, look to these four areas, says Dr. Stevenson.

1. *Stress.* Not just the heavy, negative stressors like losing a job or a spouse, but minor annoyances like a traffic ticket can affect you. Even the anticipation of positive events can keep you awake.

2. *Environment.* "Some people are very sensitive to their sleep environ-ments," says Dr. Stevenson. New bed? New pillow? New sleep partner (or the old one is absent)? Has it become noisy? Too much light? Too hot or too cold?

3. *Sleep schedule.* Have you altered your sleep patterns? Flown to a new time zone? Started working a new shift? Stayed up later than normal?

4. *Medications.* "Any drug that acts as a stimulant can cause insomnia," says Dr. Stevenson. Common sleep robbers include beta-blockers, blood pressure medications, prescription drugs containing amphetamines and, of course, caf-feine. Going *off* drugs can also be a problem. "If you abruptly discontinue a sleep medication or any drug that makes you feel drowsy, you can get what's

called rebound insomnia," explains Dr. Stevenson.

Just knowing what's causing your sleep problem should set your mind at rest and help you put it behind you.

Lose time.

Set an alarm so that you don't lose sleep because you're afraid to oversleep. Then shove it in a drawer. Put your watch away. If you can see the time on your VCR, cover it up. "Seeing the time can make you nervous," explains Dr. Hauri. "It's always the wrong time in the middle of the night."

Don't try to sleep.

The harder you try, the less likely you are to succeed. "Keep your mind on something else," advises Dr. Hauri. "Read, listen to music or watch a videotape." Don't just watch TV, he adds, since it will make you aware of the time. If these activities disturb your spouse, take a blanket and pillow to a guest room or to the living room sofa.

Try to stay awake.

Go ahead, see if you can. "Keep your eyes open and focus on your breathing," recommends Dr. Stevenson. "This is very difficult to do. It reassures you that you're a lot sleepier than you think and that you're going to fall asleep eventually."

Have a big white out.

You may also want to try a white-noise generator. "It creates sounds like rain or wind to mask the intermittent noises that tend to wake you up," says Dr. Stevenson. These are available at electronics stores.

Relax your body.

Anything that helps you settle down will hasten sleep. There are dozens of audiotapes that provide instruction in meditation or visualization. Some of them are designed specifically as sleep aids. If your local library carries them, you can sample the tapes before you go out and buy them. You can purchase audiotapes at some bookstores. Let personal taste be your guide in selection. The tapes that Dr. Stevenson uses with his own patients are put out by Inner Health and can be purchased only through your physician or sleep disorders center. If you are interested, have your doctor write to Inner Health, P.O. Box 1609, Idyllwild, CA 92549.

Progress into rest.

With or without an audiotape, you can ease yourself toward sleep with a technique called progressive muscle relaxation, recommended by Harold H. Bloomfield, M.D., a psychiatrist in Del Mar, California, and co-author of *The Power of 5: Hundreds of 5-Second to 5-Minute Scientific Shortcuts to Ignite Your Energy,*

Summoning the Sandman

You can't sleep. You want to sleep. You know that all it takes is one little pill. But should you do it?

Sleep specialists are uniformly opposed to the long-term use of medications to induce sleep and are reluctant to prescribe sleeping pills for chronic insomnia. That's because these drugs are habit-forming and disrupt natural sleep cycles. During a temporary sleep-robbing situation, however, experts say that sleeping pills are not likely to do any damage and may be useful.

"Depending on your overall health, judicious use of medication may be sensible," says Joyce Walsleben, Ph.D., director of the New York University Sleep-Wake Center in New York City. "It will get you to sleep so that you can deal with the situation more effectively the next day." Just don't rely on drugs every night.

While sleeping pills are available over the counter, it's advisable to consult with your doctor before taking them, says Dr. Walsleben. The choice of medication is best made in light of your physical condition, other drugs you may be taking, your work schedule and other factors.

Burn Fat, Stop Aging and Revitalize Your Love Life. "People can relax a muscle to a much greater degree after first tensing it," he says. "The method systematically tightens and releases every major muscle group in the body."

To perform this technique, begin with your right leg, foot and toes. Become fully aware of those areas and any sensations you may feel in them. Then tighten those muscles, taking a few seconds to feel the tension. Take a deep breath and hold for a moment. When you exhale, relax and let go, fully releasing all the tension in those areas.

Then repeat the same procedure with the rest of your muscle groups in this order: left leg, foot and toes; hips and buttocks; abdomen; chest; back; shoulders; right arm, hand and fingers; left arm, hand and fingers; neck; jaw; tongue; eyelids; face and scalp.

Breathe your way to slumber.
An exercise called the calming breath is recommended as a sleep inducer by Bija Bennett, a yoga therapist in Aspen and author of *Breathing into Life*. "It can calm your mind, stabilize your entire system and help you sleep better," she says. Here's how to do it.

1. Lying in your most comfortable sleeping position or sitting in a relaxing posture, breathe through your nose, making a soft whispering sound from the

When you take sleeping pills, be aware that you may experience side effects such as daytime drowsiness. And when you stop taking the medication, be prepared to sleep poorly for two or three nights. To minimize this effect, which is called rebound insomnia, Dr. Walsleben recommends taking medicine for no more than two weeks, then giving yourself a week to gradually taper off.

If you're reluctant to use sleeping pills, you may want to try some natural remedies. Medical research has shown that several traditional sleep-inducing herbs are both safe and effective, says Melvyn Werbach, M.D., a Los Angeles physician and author of *Healing with Food*. Valerian reduces the time it takes to fall asleep. The calming properties of chamomile are so popular that major companies market it in tea-bag form. Hops, catnip, skullcap and other herbs have also earned reputations as sleep aids. All can be found in health food stores. They come in a variety of forms. Valerian, for example, may be sold as a dried root, tincture, fluid extract or solid extract, says Dr. Werbach. A large-size health food store should carry several choices for many of these herbs.

back of your throat. (It's the sound you would hear if you whispered "ha," but with your mouth closed.)

2. Inhale deeply, but naturally, without straining.

3. Pause for a moment, then exhale slowly and easily using the whispering sound. Pause before inhaling again.

4. As you continue, gradually increase the duration of the out-breath. Let it be long and slow.

5. Lengthen the pause after each out-breath. When it feels comfortable, pause for three to five seconds, feeling the silence before inhaling again.

6. After about five minutes, allow your breath to come back to normal and feel the silence. Let your attention be effortlessly in your body.

7. If you don't fall asleep in a while, repeat the routine.

Courting Sleep during the Day

If your situational insomnia persists for several days, don't wait until bedtime to deal with it. You can start fixing the problem from the minute you wake up in the morning.

Rise and shine.

Get out of bed at your usual time, no matter what happened during the night. "Maintaining a normal wake-up time helps you keep a regular rhythm of sleeping and wakening," says Dr. Walsleben.

"Don't stay in bed longer thinking that you'll catch up on your sleep," adds Dr. Hauri. "The longer you stay in bed, the more shallow your sleep gets. It's like water being spread over a large area; it thins out. Whereas if you confine it to a small space, it gets deeper. If anything, get up earlier; you'll be that much more tired when you hit the hay that night."

See the light.

Get out in the morning and spend some time in the sun. If you can't, turn up the lights indoors. Your body rhythms are regulated, in part, by light—and getting enough in the daytime helps you fall asleep when you should at night by resetting your biological clock, explains Dr. Stevenson.

Nip your naps.

It's best to maintain one major sleep cycle during every 24-hour period. "Don't snatch an hour of sleep here and there," says Dr. Walsleben, who observes that these catnaps can interfere with nighttime sleep. If napping represents all the sleep you're going to get and you need it to function, by all means take some time out. But try to limit it to a half-hour or so, she advises.

Nix the coffee.

"If you use caffeine to compensate for feeling tired, it can keep you from sleeping the next night," says Dr. Hauri. The research is clear: Caffeine reduces sleep time and increases the number of awakenings. Ideally, you should cut it out altogether, especially after lunchtime.

Get some exercise.

Research shows that vigorous exercise during the day increases the deepest stages of sleep. A good workout several hours before sleep may deepen sleep because it increases body temperature, explains Dr. Walsleben. "One of the functions of sleep is to cool the brain down, so you sleep deeper when you go to bed with a higher temperature."

But don't do your workout too late in the evening since that can interfere with your falling asleep. The best time, experts agree, is in the late afternoon, about six hours before bedtime.

Take a hot bath.

A nice, long, warm soak can be a boon to sleep, says Dr. Walsleben. "A 40-minute bath will raise body temperature a degree or two." Bathing about three hours before you go to sleep seems to produce the best results.

Wind down before bed.

Leave your work at the office and keep your evening stress-free. "Give yourself a quiet period before your projected bedtime," says Dr. Walsleben. She recommends setting this aside as "a block of time in which you can relax and cool out."

Eat right, sleep tight.

You know what happens when you overeat or wolf down fatty or spicy meals: Your stomach punishes you by keeping you awake. Eat moderately in the evening hours.

"Ideally, lunch should be the larger meal and supper the lighter meal," says Brian Rees, M.D., medical director of the Maharishi Ayurveda Medical Center in Pacific Palisades, California. "Supper should not be eaten too late." He also recommends chewing thoroughly, taking a moment of silence before eating and, when you're done, sitting quietly for five minutes or so.

Have a snack.

While eating too much too close to bedtime can keep you awake, so can having an empty stomach. Dr. Stevenson suggests a light snack of complex carbohydrates if you're hungry: "Foods like cereal, rice, pasta or bread tend to make you a little drowsy."

Try some tryptophan.

An essential amino acid, tryptophan helps the body produce serotonin, a neurotransmitter that plays an important role in the brain's regulation of sleep. Eating some foods rich in tryptophan an hour or two before bedtime may be helpful, says Dr. Walsleben. Good sources are dairy products, meats, soy products and fish.

Pass on dessert.

Skip the after-dinner treats not because of the calories, but because of the sugar. "When your body metabolizes it, you may have a sudden drop in blood sugar, and that can act as an arousal mechanism," says Dr. Walsleben.

Make a list, check it twice.

"One of the things that makes it hard to fall asleep is anticipatory anxiety," says Mark Goulston, M.D., assistant clinical professor of psychiatry at the University of California, Los Angeles, and author of *Get Out of Your Own Way*. If worry about tomorrow keeps you aroused, he suggests relieving your anxiety by making a list of things to do, in order of priority. "Knowing how you're going to approach the next day can put your mind at ease," he says.

Smoking

You really need another reason to quit smoking, right?

Well, here it is anyway: It's robbing you of energy. Oh, sure, it doesn't feel that way. In fact, it feels as though it gives you energy. That's because nicotine is a stimulant. It ignites the nervous system and jacks up the heart rate, blood pressure and respiratory rate. But medical experts have found that these effects translate into just a temporary buzz, and it's ultimately depleting.

"The body needs more oxygen to handle this heightened activity, but it can't get it," explains Garland DeNelsky, Ph.D., a psychologist and head of the psychology section and director of the Smoking Cessation Program at the Cleveland Clinic in Ohio. That's because the carbon monoxide in smoke lowers the oxygen level in your blood, so your cells and tissues can't produce energy.

Less Breath

Heard enough? Sorry, there's more. Smoking also reduces your lung capacity, so you can't get the oxygen that you need to support high-energy activity. Plus, with all the nicotine and other poisons in your blood, your body needs more sleep to function effectively, but nicotine interferes with sleep. So while you need more, you actually get less.

Smoking retards your body's response to exercise, making it harder to get in shape and less likely that you'll even try. People who are addicted to nicotine are more likely to get depressed, and you know what that does to your energy.

Smoking does all these things . . . plus boosts the risk of energy-depleting illness, from colds to cancer.

Is it any wonder that the military bans smoking in basic training? They're not doing it to be politically correct but to be battle-ready. Studies show that smoking reduces readiness by impairing physical fitness and increasing illness. If that's what smoking does to 18-year-old recruits, what is it doing to you?

If you're a smoker, maybe a voice in your head is saying, "At my age, why bother? The damage is done." Well, studies show that people who already have health problems from smoking benefit from quitting regardless of age. Most damage is reversible, and it's never too late. If you're ready to reclaim the energy that's gone up in smoke, here's some expert advice.

Take the Middle Path

There are basically two ways to quit: cold turkey or tapering off gradually. Many experts favor a middle path, which Dr. DeNelsky calls prepared cold turkey. Here's how it works.

Choose a Quit Day.
Choose a day within the next month, mark it on your calendar and make a firm commitment that you will stop smoking that day. You may want to pick a weekend, when you're likely to have more control over your time and circumstances.

Make a list and check it twice.
Write down all the reasons why you want to be an ex-smoker—everything from living longer to protecting your loved ones from secondhand smoke to smelling better. Referring to the list will help keep you motivated.

Tell your friends and family.
Announce your intention to quit and specify the quit date. This has two advantages: You'll be more motivated knowing that others may hold you accountable, and you'll have people to turn to for support if you waver.

Get out of your rut.
During the preparation period, shake up your smoking rituals. Throw away your lighter and start using matches. Carry your cigarettes in a different place. At home keep them in drawers or coat pockets instead of on tabletops—make them somewhat harder to get to. Change your brand. Breaking simple habits will make it easier to break the big one.

Cut down a bit.
There's no advantage to trying to cut down by one or two cigarettes a day, says Dr. DeNelsky. "You look forward to those so much that their reward value skyrockets." But, if you're a heavy smoker, it may be wise to cut down to a pack or so a day.

Skip some crucial smokes.
For every smoker, certain occasions provide special satisfaction: a cigarette after a meal, for example, with coffee or after sex. Those are the times that you'll

Facing Down Fat

There are good reasons why many people gain weight when they stop smoking. Once you quit, your metabolic rate goes down, more fat gets stored because nicotine isn't there to burn it up and cravings for sweets increase. Unfortunately, fear of fat leads many ex-smokers back to the weed.

The best approach to this dilemma, says Martin Katahn, Ph.D., professor emeritus of psychology at Vanderbilt University in Nashville and author of *How to Quit Smoking without Gaining Weight*, is to take preventive steps before you quit. Cut down on fat in your diet and get more exercise, he advises. Most people have to compensate for about 200 calories a day (which smoking burns up). This approach will help you cope with the stress of quitting, boost your confidence and maybe even eliminate a few pounds so that you have a cushion in case you gain weight later on.

If you do put on pounds after you stop smoking, don't go on a severe calorie-restricted diet until you're sure that you have quit for good. This type of dieting will only increase the tension, and that might intensify the cigarette cravings, notes Dr. Katahn. "It's far more dangerous to smoke than to gain ten pounds," he adds. The final solution to weight management is not dieting, it is usually healthful eating and increased activity.

miss it the most, and the times that you'll be most tempted. Identify your high-risk situations and prepare for Quit Day by regularly not lighting up after some of these situations.

Rehearse.

Write down things that you can do instead of smoking: Take a walk, drink water, sing, do stretching exercises, go to a library and so forth. You may want to spend some time with your eyes closed, imagining difficult situations and seeing yourself cope with them without smoking. What will you do, for example, when you're in a bar and a friend offers you a cigarette?

Say good-bye to smoking.

You're giving up something that's been a significant part of your life and has given you pleasure. Don't pretend that you won't miss it or that it won't feel like a loss. As often as necessary, remind yourself that on Quit Day you're going to say good-bye with no intention of inviting it back. Think up some kind of farewell ceremony, if it suits you.

Make plans for Quit Day.
Why make it worse by being ill-prepared? Arrange to spend time with friends who support your desire to quit, preferably ex-smokers who can empathize with what you're going through. Plan to go places where smoking is prohibited and to avoid social situations that may attract smokers.

What to Do When the Day Comes

Think of Quit Day as the day you start getting back your health and energy. The benefits of quitting begin with the first cigarette you don't smoke, says Terry Pechacek, Ph.D., an epidemiologist at the Office on Smoking and Health at the Centers for Disease Control and Prevention in Atlanta. Here's how to handle this important day.

Throw out your cigarettes.
Flush them down the toilet or soak them in water so that you're not tempted to pull them out of the trash. And while you're at it, wash your ashtrays and put them out of sight.

Change your morning routine.
If you're used to eating breakfast at home, go to a restaurant where smoking is prohibited. If you eat at the usual place, sit someplace else. Skip the coffee and drink orange juice instead. Go for a walk instead of reading the Sunday paper.

Pick up some snacks.
Nibbling will help you combat the smoking urge. Low-fat items are advisable, as are foods that are crunchy and chewy (you may need some oral gratification). So stock up on gum, sugarless candy, celery, carrots and apples. And don't forget to take some with you when you leave the house.

Use the four Ds.
Over the first few days, you will have the urge to smoke, immediately and repeatedly. To reduce the discomfort, remember the four Ds of the American Lung Association.
1. Drink. Keep lots of liquids on hand, preferably water or fruit juice. It will help flush the nicotine out of your system and alleviate the discomfort of a sore throat or dry mouth.
2. Delay. Wait out the urge. It will fade in a few moments and ultimately disappear. "People think that the craving won't go away unless they smoke," says Dr. DeNelsky. "They think, 'I can't live the rest of my life like this.' Of course they can't, but they can live the next 30 seconds like that." The urge will go away whether you smoke or not, he says.

3. Deep-breathe. Breathing deeply can help you cope with the tension of cigarette cravings. One way is with the "sipping breath," recommended by Bija Bennett, a yoga therapist in Aspen and author of *Breathing into Life*. "One of the things that smoking gives people is a relaxing inhalation," she says. "This exercise gives you the same sensation." It increases circulation, blood flow and energy, she adds. Here are her instructions.

- Sit comfortably, with your eyes closed.
- Allow your spine to lengthen, your head to lift and your back to widen as you free the back of your neck.
- As you begin to inhale, pretend that you are sipping through a straw. Make sure you hear a sound like a hiss as you sip.
- When you have inhaled fully, close your mouth, lower your chin toward your chest and exhale from the back of your throat. Use the "whispering breath" and create a soft sound from the back of your throat without vocalizing. The sound is created from your breath alone.
- Continue breathing for a few minutes—"sipping" on inhale, holding for a second or two and then exhaling through your nose using the whispering breath. After 10 to 12 breaths, allow your breath to come back to normal, keeping your eyes closed for about a minute. Feel the silence and be aware of the sensations in your body.

  Use the sipping breath whenever you crave a cigarette or as a short break a few times a day.

4. Do something else. In general, it's wise to keep busy on Quit Day. When the urge to smoke comes over you, do something. Call a friend, take a walk, brush your teeth, hop in the shower, go dancing, read your list of reasons to quit smoking—do anything but sit around fighting the urge or feeling sorry for yourself.

Reward yourself.

Before you call it a day, congratulate yourself on getting past the first hurdle. You may want to buy yourself a little treat with the money you would have spent on cigarettes.

Getting over the Humps

If you have been addicted to nicotine, you can expect to experience withdrawal symptoms. They usually peak in the first few days, then taper off until they disappear. But cravings continue to crop up months and even years after you thought you had seen the last of them, says Dr. DeNelsky. Keep using the four Ds and keep in mind these additional tips.

Know what to expect.

It helps to know that what you're experiencing is, in fact, withdrawal. The most common symptoms are anxiety, irritability, headaches, difficulty concentrating, poor sleep, changes in appetite, craving for sweets, lightheadedness and fatigue.

Exercise.

Working out is not just a great way to keep busy—it's hard to smoke while swimming or riding a bicycle. It also reduces tension and burns up calories, which may ease your concern about weight gain. Working out has one more plus—it stimulates pleasure-giving brain chemicals, which help take the sting out of missing tobacco. It's also a good way to reinforce your commitment, notes Dr. DeNelsky. Wait until you see how much more energy you have for workouts as an ex-smoker.

Learn to deal with stress.

The urge to smoke is likely to strike at anxious, pressurized moments. Anything that helps you relax and cope is useful, whether it's meditation, yoga, massage, biofeedback, psychotherapy, visualization or a course in stress management.

Keep your eye on the prize.

"Doing *with* takes the sting out of doing without," says Mark Goulston, M.D., assistant clinical professor of psychiatry at the University of California, Los Angeles, and author of *Get Out of Your Own Way.* "Try to focus on what you're gaining, not what you're losing." Place the benefits of not smoking at the center of your attention. "One of those benefits," he notes, "is the pride that comes from breaking a self-defeating behavior."

Reach out and touch someone.

Knowing that you're not alone will strengthen your confidence and determination, says Dr. Goulston. You can get support from friends and family members, or join a support group for ex-smokers.

Patch it up.

If you find that you need a little medical assistance to quit, nicotine replacement therapy provides transition doses of nicotine until the nicotine dependency is broken.

This therapy comes in two forms—a chewing gum that contains nicotine and a skin patch that delivers a steady supply of nicotine. Of the two available methods, most experts prefer the transdermal patch to nicotine gum, which is unpleasant to the taste and is less well-accepted among smokers trying to quit. When used in conjunction with proper educational information, the patch is of positive benefit in helping you quit, says Dr. Pechacek. He stresses that the patch is not a magical cure. It should be part of a larger program that also addresses behavioral change and psychological dependency.

Don't kid yourself.

"You have to completely quit and stay quit," says Dr. DeNelsky. "Many smokers think that they can have a cigarette now and then. They're wrong." One puff and you may be hooked again.

Don't give up.

If you do backslide, don't get down on yourself and don't think it's hopeless. "Stay in a positive frame of mind," urges Dr. Pechacek.

"Most people who successfully quit have made at least one previous attempt at quitting." Learn from your slip and stay with it until you get it right, adds Dr. DeNelsky.

Taxes

*L*ife, we're told, has only two definites: death and taxes. Neither, you'll notice, is particularly energizing.

The former speaks for itself. But Uncle Sam takes a different approach to extracting vitality from your mind and body—not to mention money from your wallet. The great American energy drain usually starts in January, when tax forms are sent out.

"Most people don't even think of taxes until they get their W-2s and Federal tax forms," says Cheryl Fellows, Ph.D., a Dallas psychologist who specializes in counseling people about financial matters and the author of *Dollars and Sense: The Psychology of Money.* "Then they simply stash them away: good ol' fashioned denial."

But as the April 15 deadline approaches and Uncle Sam still hasn't been paid, the stress kicks in and continues to build while your energy wanes. "Anything stressful hurts your energy levels and can fatigue you," says Dr. Fellows. "And for a lot of people that definitely includes preparing and paying their income tax."

A Lack of Control

Why are taxes so stressful?

"For some people it's not just having to pay the money that causes stress," explains Dr. Fellows. The problem is that they have no control over paying taxes, she says.

"Having to make car or house payments may be a financial burden and stressful in their own regard, but getting that house or car is our choice. With taxes, we're told we have to give up our money. It's basic human nature," says Dr. Fellows. "We don't like being told what to do."

Here's what she and other experts suggest for making tax time a little less taxing.

Take it slow.

"If you break up doing your taxes into manageable tasks, it'll probably be a lot less stressful," says Elliott Gale, Ph.D., a psychologist at the University of Buffalo in New York who specializes in stress management. "Most people try to tackle the entire job all at once. But my advice is to do one form each week or so. Maybe start by adding up your income and then put everything away for a while. Then come back and do your deductions later, and so on."

Don't wait.

Many people, according to Internal Revenue Service spokeswoman Jody Patterson, wait until the last minute to do their taxes. "We encourage our employees to file early," she says. "Let's face it, it's less stressful if you do your taxes early and get it over with."

She suggests starting on your taxes shortly after receiving your tax forms so that you have a full three months to prepare them.

Prepare all year long.

"Many people get stressed over their taxes because they're not well-prepared," says Dr. Fellows. "My advice is to take a more long-term approach to taxes and think of them all year long—not just in the weeks before the April deadline. For instance, you could keep all those monthly receipts in an envelope for that month and file it away at the end of each month. That can help keep you from getting fatigued in that mad dash for receipts at the last minute."

Get help.

Many people get fatigued by taxes because they don't understand their tax forms. "If that sounds like you, go to an accountant so that you won't be burdened with it," says Dr. Fellows. If you can't afford an accountant, the IRS has free tax-preparation clinics in local libraries or churches and a toll-free number offering answers to your questions. Call your local IRS office for more information on these programs. You can find the phone number in the blue pages of the phone book under the U.S. government office listings. If you are hooked up to the Internet, you have access to about 90 tax publications and other tax information.

Accept the "unfairness."

Some people may think that they'll feel better if they enclose an angry letter with their tax payments. Wrong!

"A lot of people get so stressed by taxes because they don't feel they are fair—that others don't pay their fair share while they do," says Dr. Fellows. "But it's probably not a good idea to voice these feelings in angry letters because you'll probably not get a response, and that might get you even more angry. Simply accept that life—and taxes—aren't always fair."

Teenagers

*I*t's two o'clock in the morning, and the hiss of whispered confidences—periodically punctuated by swiftly stifled giggles—has gone on now for hours.

Of course, your 14-year-old and several sleepover friends haven't done anything wrong. They're tucked in their sleeping bags, the lights are out and they're keeping the noise level low, just as you had asked. So there's nothing that will allow you to march down the hall and stifle the chitchat.

Not that you would want to anyway. After all, when you have worked from nine to five, then picked up your teen from basketball practice, picked up a pizza from the neighborhood pizzeria, gathered up the dirty clothes from your teen's bedroom floor and washed three loads of laundry—who has the energy?

Climbing toward Adulthood

Parenting a teen is an exhausting occupation. And it's not just dealing with sleepovers and picking up dirty clothes that can drain you. During the teen years parents are likely to experience lots of conflict with kids who want to remain dependent on their parents but also want to become independent. And all that conflict can lead straight to exhaustion.

"This independence versus dependence is a real tough number for parents to deal with," says Charles Wibbelsman, M.D., chief of the Teen Clinic at Kaiser Permanente Medical Center in San Francisco and author of *The New Teenage Body Book*.

"The adolescent wants the comfort of being a child—your bed is made, your laundry's done, the food is on the table—and the privileges of an adult— 'Well, I want to come home around midnight'—at the same time," explains Dr. Wibbelsman.

Making the situation even more draining is the fact that teens are unconsciously but actively looking for things to disagree about, says Judi Craig, Ph.D., a clinical psychologist who practices in San Antonio and the author of *You're*

Grounded 'til You're Thirty! "They have to," she adds. "If the nest is too cozy, they'll never leave. And their task is to tear themselves away from these parents who have protected them and to grow into a different relationship with them as adults."

Adolescent Adjustments

The key to reducing energy drain during the teen years is to reduce conflict, increase communication and make time for yourself, says Karen M. Zager, Ph.D., a psychologist with offices in both New York City and Hastings-on-Hudson, New York, who specializes in parenting and adolescence. Here's how to do it.

Honor yourself.
"We're all like a bag of chocolate chip cookies," says Dr. Craig. "If your bag is full and you have extra cookies spilling over the top, then you'll be nurturing, loving and packed with extra energy."

How can you see that your own bag stays full? "By nurturing yourself daily," she says. "Buy a fresh flower, play music, take time to play with your cat or read a novel."

Pick your battles.
"Probably a good 90 percent of the battles we fight with teens are hardly worth fighting," says Dr. Zager.

Forget about arguing with your teen about stuff like clothes dropped on the floor, advises Dr. Craig. This isn't an argument that you can possibly win anyway, since every teenager is likely to be sloppy about *something*. Certainly, remind your teenager about what you expect. But if you get angry or "lay down the law" every time your expectations are not met, you'll only exhaust yourself.

Know when to go along.
Often, parents want to take a firm stand in order to discipline their teens or draw a clear line. But that can lead to energy-depleting battles. Before you draw a line in the sand, ask, "Is this reversible?" suggests Dr. Zager. "As long as the choices that your teen is making are not harmful and they're reversible, there's very little you have to lose by going along with them."

You might not like having your teen dye her hair orange, but it's clearly reversible—so why pour your energy into fighting it? Allowing her to go out with a crowd that will be drinking and driving, on the other hand, could lead to a life-threatening accident; that's where the line should be drawn. Once you apply the reversibility test, you may be surprised at how many battles you don't have to fight.

Take a Meeting

If you're burning up energy during sporadic arguments with your feisty teen all week long, maybe you need a forum where cooler heads will prevail.

Every family should establish a family council that holds weekly meetings, suggests Raymond Corsini, Ph.D., a Honolulu psychologist and author of *The Practical Parent*. Make it a family rule that most disagreements (except, of course, life-threatening matters) are to be discussed only at the council meeting. Once you start having these meetings, you may be surprised at how many exhausting arguments can be avoided during the week, knowing that they'll be postponed until this get-together. You may have an agenda a mile long, says Dr. Corsini, but what you won't have is guerrilla warfare every night.

Here are some guidelines from Dr. Corsini for setting up these meetings and making sure that your teen participates.

- Open up the agenda. Start a list of things that need to be discussed—and let anyone add to it anytime.
- Change the chairperson. Let a different family member chair the meeting every week so that no one person is allowed to dominate.
- Bar interruptions. Make it a rule that no one can interrupt.
- Avoid criticism. Everyone should be allowed to have their say in the family meeting. Make sure Mom and Dad don't take this opportunity to catalog the teen's faults and demand compliance.
- Broaden the scope. In addition to resolving disagreements in this forum, use the time to make joint family decisions such as where to go on a family vacation or whether to buy a two- or four-door car.

Take a time-out.

Often, when teens ask for permission to have an ear pierced, buy a new compact disc player or take an overnight trip to the shore, we give an off-the-cuff "no." That's a word that can launch us straight into an emotion-draining argument, says Dr. Zager.

"To avoid these situations, I recommend a mutual time-out," she says. "A parent says, 'Okay, I'm not going to say no. But you think about it for a week, and I'll think about it for a week. And then after a week of thought, let me know if this is something that you really want to do.' A lot of the time, teenagers will come back and have changed their minds."

Recognize boundaries.

Most of us have enough to do managing our daily lives without trying to oversee someone else's as well. If you want to save more energy for your own "to do" list, keep your nose out of your teen's business if it doesn't affect you directly, says Raymond Corsini, Ph.D., a Honolulu psychologist and author of *The Practical Parent.*

Of course, some things affect you as well as your teenager, such as cars, allowance money, loud music in the house and crumbs in the computer. But there are plenty of things that do not affect you, such as who your teen likes and hates, who's calling and who's not and what rumors are feeding the high school's rumor mill. You can save yourself a lot of energy by letting your teen handle these issues alone.

Listen first, speak second.

Even when you disagree in a big way over key issues, you'll conserve energy if you avoid arguing, nagging or lecturing, says Dr. Craig. Any of these tactics can lead to a blowup, which is a big exhauster.

"Remain calm, matter-of-fact and open," she says. "Hear their views first before you air your own. Then try to acknowledge something in what they have said before you express your objections." Instead of saying, "Absolutely not. You're wrong," you might try: "That sounds like an interesting idea, but here's what I'm concerned about." Then go ahead and tell them what you think, suggests Dr. Craig. That simple change of approach may help you understand what your teen really wants—and why—and also gives you a far better chance of being heard.

Share the teen work.

Does your teen constantly resist must-do's like homework, meals and lights out? Often, you know you'll have to fight a few familiar little battles almost nightly. But if you're a two-parent household, you can divvy up the necessary nagging just as you do the chores, says Dr. Zager.

"It usually turns out that one parent bears the brunt of arguments," she observes. "It may be that one parent is simply more strict than the other." By teaming up on teen management, you allow one person a refreshing night off while the other keeps an eye on the teen. "If you argued on Monday," says Dr. Zager, "let your spouse take Tuesday."

Take your teen to breakfast.

A parent who has an open line of communication with his teen is a lot less likely to spend much time on the family battlefield, says Dr. Wibbelsman.

How do you open that line?

"What you really need to do is for Mom to take that 16-year-old girl shopping or to a movie, for Dad to take that 15-year-old boy to a basketball game or for Mom to take him to breakfast. Make it just you and your teen together," urges Dr. Wibbelsman. "Then it's just conversation about what's happening in your lives. And when issues or problems come up, you can be a friend."

Spending that extra time with your teen may seem like an extra obligation at first, but you get energy from sharing conversations and confidences, instead of spending energy in battles.

Negotiate limits.

All teens need a set of behavioral limits, says Dr. Wibbelsman. Otherwise, they feel unloved. But there's a way to set enforceable limits with a minimum of energy-draining nagging and arguments. Invite the teen into the limit-setting process, Dr. Wibbelsman suggests.

Instead of imposing a 10:00 P.M. bedtime, for example, raise the issue, say what time you feel is appropriate and explain why. Then ask your teen what time he thinks is appropriate. Your concept of a reasonable bedtime may differ from your child's, but the two of you can negotiate back and forth until you determine a third, mutually agreeable time. After that, it's harder for your teen to refuse to cooperate.

Let them talk.

Sometimes teens start family arguments to unload the stress they feel from hyper-busy lives, says Dr. Craig. But no matter why the argument starts, you get the brunt of it—at a cost to your energy. One way to reduce the need for confrontation is to let teens talk out problems with friends on the phone.

This usually does mean some awfully long conversations, says Dr. Craig. But if phone time gets excessive, negotiate some time limits. If you only have one phone at home, for example, everyone can say when they need to use it.

If you need the phone free from 7:00 to 8:00 P.M. to receive business calls, for example, let your needs be known. Let your teen discuss when he needs the phone, and the two of you can negotiate a telephone schedule that meets both your needs.

Television

Some things deplete your energy by placing excessive demands on your system. Television does it by demanding nothing.

Spacing out in front of the TV to unwind after a tough day is harmless enough. In small doses it may even be an effective stress reducer. Studies show that people who watch TV after a stressful day have fewer domestic arguments than those who interact with their spouses right away, says Daniel Anderson, Ph.D., professor of psychology at the University of Massachusetts at Amherst. And selective viewing that stimulates the mind can be as edifying and energizing as a good book.

It's when TV holds you captive three to four hours a day that it begins to earn the sobriquet "the boob tube." That's when you zone out instead of zooming in—and unless you take measures to free yourself, you could end up captive to that watched-everything, saw-nothing run-down reaction.

"It's a very seductive medium," says Robert Kubey, Ph.D., associate professor of communication at Rutgers University in New Brunswick, New Jersey, and co-author of *Television and the Quality of Life*. "You sit down and watch something you want to see and end up watching for hours. And the more you watch, the more likely it is that you'll feel enervated when you turn it off."

Switching Off the Siphon

Is the television set actually draining your energy like some kind of electronic vacuum cleaner? Of course not. It's what you're doing—and not doing—while watching that's the problem.

"From a commonsense perspective, the more time one spends sitting around not doing anything, the more tired one becomes," says Michael Morgan, Ph.D., a professor in the Department of Communication at the University of Massachusetts at Amherst.

Over-watching can also lead to overweight, which exacts another toll in lethargy. Since it gives you less time for exercise, the Vast Wasteland—as TV has been called—produces a vast waistline. So far, studies to prove this have only involved children and adolescents.

Would the same debilitated feelings show up if you spent that amount of time sitting around reading or chatting? Not necessarily. TV seems to be more insidious than other sedentary activities. Research indicates that when people watch TV, their metabolic rates slow down much more than when they sit and do nothing. What that means is that you burn about 10 to 15 percent fewer calories watching television than you do when you sit with the TV off. You're also more likely to be chomping on something—and not carrot sticks. TV viewing seems to go hand in hand with high-calorie, high-fat snacking, according to Dr. Morgan.

What TV Is Telling You

Heavy TV viewers tend to have complacent attitudes about health, at least in part because of what they see on TV, says George Gerbner, Ph.D., dean emeritus of the Annenberg School for Communication at the University of Pennsylvania in Philadelphia. The most common beverage consumed on TV during prime time is alcohol, for example, and you rarely see TV characters sit down to a wholesome meal. To some extent, viewers absorb these messages, Dr. Gerbner believes.

"TV is a powerful and pervasive teacher," says Larry A. Tucker, Ph.D., associate professor of health promotion at Brigham Young University in Provo, Utah. "You learn more from TV than you realize."

Fortunately, there's a lot you can do to balance out the equation. Here's some expert advice for enjoying TV while keeping your energy in prime time.

Turn Off, Tune Out

Chances are you already feel guilty about spending too much time in front of the tube. Studies show that most heavy viewers feel they ought to be using their time more constructively. But cutting down might not be as easy as it sounds.

Here are some ways to make it easier to hit the off button.

Do your own Nielsen rating.
Keep track of how much time you spend watching TV, suggests Dr. Kubey. Since we tend to underestimate how many hours we actually devote to it, the

shock of seeing the reality in black and white can be a strong motivator. Keep a notebook by the TV and make a habit of jotting down your start and stop times.

Keep a journal.

In addition to toting up the hours spent, note the names of the shows that you watch and what you think you got out of them. This increases self-awareness, says Dr. Kubey. You may realize you're investing a lot of time in something that depletes your energy while offering meager rewards.

Get the family involved.

It's hard to cut back on TV viewing if the people around you are glued to the set, says Dr. Kubey. If, like most families, yours has communal TV habits, try to get everyone to agree on a cutback plan.

Program yourself.

It's said that heavy viewers watch TV, not the programs *on* TV. They turn on the set and watch whatever pops up on the screen or channel-surf with their remotes.

To combat passive, automatic viewing, Dr. Tucker suggests looking through a program guide and selecting in advance the shows that you really want to see. Then stick to that schedule. Turn on the set when the show goes on and shut it off the minute the closing credits appear on screen. Don't get seduced into seeing what's on next.

Tape now, play later.

Make use of your VCR, advises Paul R. Thomas, R.D., Ed.D., assistant professor at the Center for Food and Nutrition Policy at Georgetown University in Washington, D.C.

"There are 12 to 15 minutes of advertising in every hour of programming," he points out. "If you watch two hours of TV and fast-forward through the commercials, you save a half-hour." You can use that block of time to get some exercise—and you'll make fewer trips to the refrigerator while watching your favorite shows on tape.

Make a list of alternatives.

Brainstorm on your own or with your family and come up with a list of activities that are fun, entertaining or challenging.

"At times when you may reflexively turn on the TV," says Dr. Kubey, "you can consult the list for constructive things you can do individually or together." If you need some help getting started, here are some suggestions from Harold

H. Bloomfield, M.D., a psychiatrist in Del Mar, California, and co-author of *The Power of 5: Hundreds of 5-Second to 5-Minute Scientific Shortcuts to Ignite Your Energy, Burn Fat, Stop Aging and Revitalize Your Love Life*:

- Listen to your favorite music.
- Play musical instruments, no matter how badly.
- Study the stars against the night sky.
- Write poetry or recite poems aloud.
- Read a good novel.
- Play cards or tackle some puzzles.
- Snuggle with your romantic partner.
- Play hide-and-seek with your kids or grandchildren.
- Take a walk, roller-skate or ride a bicycle.
- Go dancing.
- Look through a photo album and share stories.
- Do some gardening or arrange flowers.
- Write down your innermost thoughts in a journal.

"Choose activities that boost your heart and spirit," says Dr. Bloomfield. "You'll feel rejuvenated and give yourself a chance to engage more deeply in life."

Get support.

TV addiction has a lot in common with drug dependency, Dr. Kubey points out. "It's quickly rewarding; you tend to do it more than you intended; it interferes with other activities; and when you stop cold turkey, you go through a kind of psychological withdrawal." As with drug withdrawal, it can take awhile to adapt to less TV, and at times, you may be tempted to backslide.

If your trigger finger gets itchy on the remote control, call a friend, suggests Mark Goulston, M.D., assistant clinical professor of psychiatry at the University of California, Los Angeles, and author of *Get Out of Your Own Way*. "It's important to have someone to call when you're having trouble."

Get out of the house.

Remaining in the same environment in which you're accustomed to watching TV can be like going to a bar when you want to stop drinking, says Dr. Goulston. Try walking, going to the library or playing a game with a friend.

Accentuate the positive.

When breaking a habit, it's common to dwell on what you're giving up. When you find yourself focusing on the shows you're missing, think instead of what you're gaining, says Dr. Goulston. Focus on things like better health, intellectual stimulation, more vitality and closeness with your family.

Watch Something Else

It's not just how much you watch that can be a problem, but what you watch and how you watch it. Unlike reading, most TV fare requires very little skill and concentration.

People report feeling quite passive while watching, and there is evidence of what Dr. Kubey calls a spillover effect: "One or two hours after viewing TV, people report feeling more passive or tired than they do after more active pursuits, especially if they watch for a number of hours." Here are some tips for energizing your viewing habits.

Watch more challenging shows.
Changing your viewing habits may upset the networks, but it can boost your energy. "One could argue that most mainstream television acts as a kind of lullaby," says Dr. Morgan. "Intellectually stimulating shows—whatever that means for you—are probably more invigorating."

This doesn't necessarily mean a steady fare of public broadcasting. With the advent of cable it's easier for anyone to find programs that energize the mind rather than lull it to sleep.

Become an activist.
"You'll get a lot more out of watching TV if you watch actively instead of just vegging out," says Nicholas Roes, president of the Education Guild in Barryville, New York, and author of *Helping Children Watch TV*. Keep your mind engaged, he suggests, by using the shows you watch as a springboard for discussion.

"Look for things you can learn," he says. "Discuss the behavior of the characters and the issues raised. Use TV to make you think rather than as an excuse to stop thinking."

Don't use it to escape problems.
To a certain extent, TV is a healthy coping mechanism, says Dr. Anderson. There's nothing like a good comedy when life brings you down, and it sure beats getting drunk or taking your problems out on your family.

But, says Dr. Goulston, if you use TV as a way to avoid important issues, it can drain you in the long run. "It takes energy to numb your feelings or suppress unpleasant thoughts," he says. Suppression can also sap your energy by keeping you from solving the problems from which you're trying to escape.

Get up and move.
Sitting in one position for a long time can be enervating. "When you're moving, you have better blood flow and oxygenation," says Chris Grant, Ph.D., an er-

gonomist with F-One Ergonomics in Ann Arbor, Michigan. (Ergonomics is the science of designing environments for maximum health, efficiency and comfort.)

Moving while you're viewing means less fatigue and more energy. So make it a habit to move around while you watch TV, especially during commercial breaks.

Work out, don't space out.

While you're at it, why not exercise while you're watching TV? Place a stationary bike or a rowing machine in front of the screen. Or do some stretching exercises or isometrics, a form of exercise that requires stable resistance like pushing your palms against each other. It may take the boredom out of both TV and working out.

Watch What You Eat When Watching

One reason TV junkies tend to be overweight is the American way of snacking.

"When you're watching TV, you don't pay close attention to what you're consuming or how much you're consuming," says Dr. Thomas. As a result, you eat much more than you need and way too much junk. If you're overweight and lack the nutrients your body needs, you're going to feel tired. Here are some tips for munching while you're viewing.

Choose healthful snacks.

Obviously, some choices are better than others. You'll stay ahead in the energy game if your snacks are lower in calories, fat and sugar.

"Pretzels are better than potato chips," says Dr. Thomas. "Low-fat cookies are better than regular cookies. Diet soda is better than regular soda."

Popcorn is a good option, as long as you select a brand that's not buttered and has relatively little oil. And you can't go wrong by slicing up some fruits and vegetables, as long as you don't eat them with a rich, creamy dip.

Ration your snacks.

"Instead of bringing the whole bottle or can or bag into the living room, dish out a limited portion in a separate container," says Dr. Thomas. And don't go back for more.

Take your time.

You may eat less than you otherwise would if you nibble your snack slowly and make it last for the duration of your viewing, says Dr. Thomas.

Worry

The ability to foresee potential disasters is a powerful survival mechanism. It's one of the things that makes human beings special. Sometimes, however, rather than anticipating trouble, all we do is worry about it. Will I get the job? Will the water in the basement pipes freeze? Does my boss like my work? At the very least, worry can consume an enormous amount of time.

"It's not a passive pursuit," says Arthur Freeman, Ed.D., chairman of the Department of Psychology at Philadelphia College of Osteopathic Medicine and co-author of *The Ten Dumbest Mistakes Smart People Make, and How to Avoid Them*. "It requires energy. It burns calories."

Ultimately, of course, excessive worrying is self-defeating as well. "If you spend too much energy worrying about being successful," says Dr. Freeman, "you may not have the energy to be successful."

Habits Die Hard

To a certain extent worry is a natural part of our emotional lives, along with emotions such as love, anger or concern. On the other hand, chronic worrying is literally a self-destructive habit, like nail biting or smoking, says Dr. Freeman. Once you start letting your fears and anxieties wear you down, it can be difficult to get your energy back on track again. But worrying is a habit, and habits can be changed.

The problem is that many people value worry. They believe it makes them alert to potential problems. To some extent this is certainly true, says Dr. Freeman. But for most of us, frequent worrying is nothing less than an energy drain. It exhausts our strength without bringing us any closer to solving the issues that cause it.

Want to figure out what worrying has really done for you? Dr. Freeman recommends making a list with two columns. In one column write down all the things that you believe are helpful about worrying. In the other column list the disadvantages. "Does worrying actually help you be happier or more productive?" he asks. What you'll discover is that the costs of worrying are much higher than any potential benefits.

Don't confuse worry with concern, says Ken Druck, Ph.D., a clinical/consulting psychologist in Del Mar, California, and author of *The Secrets Men Keep*. "Concern activates us to think hard and anticipate what we need to do to be effective," he explains. Being concerned means that you're thinking about solutions. Worry, on the other hand, dwells on the problems, essentially becoming a rehearsal for failure.

Worry isn't even very helpful when it comes to identifying painful emotions. More often, it's a way of avoiding emotions, says Daniel M. Wegner, Ph.D., professor of psychology at the University of Virginia in Charlottesville and author of *White Bears and Other Unwanted Thoughts*.

Suppose, for example, that you spend the weekend worrying about a speech you have to give on Monday morning. Are you really worried about the presentation? Or are you dwelling on it because you'd rather not think about other, possibly more painful issues like lifelong insecurities or memories of childhood failures?

When we worry, says Dr. Wegner, "we think things through and talk to ourselves about our problems, and we don't really feel the emotions."

Working through Worry

Okay, so now you're worried about worrying and how it drains your precious energy reserves. (That's the thing about worriers; there's always something.) Don't be. There are a number of quick, effective ways to keep worry from getting you down. Here's what experts advise.

Let them out.
About the most exhausting thing you can do is to let worries run over and over in your head like a broken record. "Vent the things that worry you," advises Dr. Druck. Talk to a friend. Visit a support group. Try a few sessions with a therapist. "If you put it outside yourself where it can be mapped out, you get a reality check, a fresh perspective and new ideas," he says.

Give yourself a talking-to.
Having a sympathetic ear is nice, but it's not the only way to dispel worrisome—and wearisome—thoughts. "Get it down on paper or into a tape recorder," says Layne Longfellow, Ph.D., a psychologist in private practice in Prescott, Arizona. "The problem with worry is that you get caught up working the content over and over, around and around. Getting it out of your head breaks the cycle."

Planning Worry Time

Something's amiss. You start to worry about what might happen. Your mind starts racing, cooking up all sorts of awful scenarios. Pretty soon you're in a frenzy, you're losing sleep and you're driving your friends crazy. You realize you're worrying yourself sick, so you slam on the mental brakes. You promise yourself you won't think about it anymore.

Fat chance. "If you tell people to try not to think about a particular topic, soon they become obsessed with the very thing that they're trying to suppress," says Daniel M. Wegner, Ph.D., professor of psychology at the University of Virginia in Charlottesville and author of *White Bears and Other Unwanted Thoughts*.

Although you can't entirely suppress your worries, you can keep them under control. The trick, he says, is to put them on a schedule. In one study people who were big-time worriers were told to set aside time several nights a week just to worry. They were encouraged to use that time fully, to worry to the max. And they did, for several weeks. What the researchers found was that compared to people who worried at will, those who worried only at certain times wound up doing a lot less of it.

It sounds odd to encourage yourself to worry, but putting it on a schedule really does work, according to Dr. Wegner.

Another reason to get worry out in the open where you can see it, Dr. Longfellow adds, is that "expressing it exposes how exaggerated and illogical it is."

Think the worst.
It sounds contradictory, but giving your worry free rein, by imagining that whatever it is you're worrying about comes to pass, can be a great way to dispel the fear. Dr. Freeman calls this process de-catastrophizing.

"Sometimes, when you answer the question, 'What is the worst?' you immediately realize that it won't happen, or if it does, it won't be the end of everything," he says.

Think the best.
"There's a chatterbox inside our heads that drives us crazy with 'I should have done this' or 'What if that happens?' " says Susan Jeffers, Ph.D., author of *Feel the Fear and Do It Anyway*. Her advice: Replace negative thoughts with positive ones, what psychologists refer to as affirmations.

"When you start worrying, no matter what the what-ifs are, immediately interject, 'I'll handle it,' " she says. As you repeat these affirmations in your mind, the negative chattering will diminish and your body will relax and naturally become more energized.

Think your way to success.
When it comes to keeping worry in check, the mind can be a powerful friend—or foe. People who imagine positive outcomes, giving a great speech, for example, do better in the actual event than those who think the worst. "Research shows that we can practice behavior in our imagination and translate it into performance," says Dr. Freeman.

To keep worry from sapping your reserves, he recommends setting aside time every day for positive mental rehearsals. Replace images of failure and doom with images of success and happiness.

"But make sure the images are reasonable," he stresses. "If you're a man worried about rejection, for example, instead of seeing yourself at a bar besieged by gorgeous models, imagine talking to one attractive woman and getting a date."

Stay active.
"If you change your physiological state, your emotional and psychological states may also change," says Dr. Longfellow. Studies have shown that exercise burns off a stress chemical called adrenaline, while at the same time causing the release of "feel-good" chemicals called endorphins. Even a quick walk around the block will help boost your sense of well-being as you leave the worries behind.

Ask about biofeedback.
This is a technique in which you use the body's natural responses like muscle tension or body temperature to gain control over worry, stress or other negative emotions. "The techniques are simple and the devices are easy to obtain and use," says Dr. Druck. Ask your doctor if biofeedback would be a good approach for you.

Stay balanced.
If you're one of those people who gets deeply caught up in a single aspect of your life—it could be work, a relationship or even a hobby—chances are, you get more than a little worried when problems arise in that area, says Dr. Jeffers.

Even if you're passionate about what you do, never put all your eggs in one basket. There's nothing wrong with having one special relationship, as long as you maintain other friendships as well. It's good to take work seriously, but only if you also invest some time in play. "Create a life so rich that trouble in any one part of it doesn't wipe you out," she advises.

Make a difference.

"When you're self-involved, you're much more prone to worry," says Dr. Jeffers. "When you know that you're contributing to society in some meaningful way, the fear is greatly diminished."

No matter where you live, there are many opportunities for getting involved. Join a conservation group. Adopt a stretch of highway. Volunteer at the hospital. Join the Parent-Teacher Association. Be a mentor at the high school. Donate your talents at a senior citizen center. It doesn't matter what you ultimately choose. Just getting involved and helping others is one of the strongest motivators there is, experts say. You'll discover sources of energy that you never knew you had.

Index

Underscored page references indicate boxed text. **Boldfaced** references indicate primary discussion of topic.

ACE inhibitors, fatigue from, 362–63, <u>363</u>
Acetaminophen, for colds and flu, 300
Acupuncture, for managing
   pain with chronic disease, 285–86
   premenstrual syndrome, 392
   quitting alcohol habit, <u>258</u>
Adolescents, as energy demon, **411–15**, <u>413</u>
Aerobic exercise, 69–72
   approaches to, 70–72
   benefits of, 69–70
   bicycling as, 71
   for cardiovascular fitness, 72
   laughter as, 172
   for managing
      depression, 309
      headaches, 334
   runner's high from, 135
Affirmations, as energizers, **131–34**, 309–10
Aging, **247–53**, <u>250</u>
   attitude about, 247–48
   effects on
      brain cells, 250–51
      metabolism, 252
      muscles, 66, 247
      sex, <u>250</u>
      sleep patterns, 126–27
   managing
      diet, 252–53
      exercise, 251–52
      humor, 249
      mental activity, 249–51
      strength training, 252
      walking, 252
      weight lifting, 252
Air-conditioners, sleep and, 124
Air purification, plants for, 60–61
Alcohol, **254–58**, <u>256–57</u>
   addiction, 254, <u>256–57</u>
   colds and flu and, 303
   effects of
      dehydration, 243, 255–56
      energy level, decreased, 254, 356
      sex, decreased performance, 205
      sleep problems, 122–23

   managing intake of, 255–56
   medications and, 361
   quitting habit, 256–58, <u>258</u>
   water intake and, 243
Alcoholism, 254, <u>256–57</u>
Alexander Technique, for good posture, <u>382</u>
Allergens, types of, <u>260</u>
Allergies, as energy demons, **259–62**, <u>260–61</u>
Alpha brain waves
   concentration and, 190
   jasmine scent and increased, 59
   relaxation and, 96
   during sleep, 214
Alternative medicine, medications vs., <u>363</u>
Altruism, 95, **135–37**, 163–64, 310
Anemia, iron-deficiency, 23, 25–26, 386
Anger, managing, 158–60
Anorexia in elderly, 194
Antidepressants, 308–9
   sleep problems from, 122
Antihistamines
   with colds and flu, avoiding, 303
   fatigue caused by, 259, 362
   types of, 362
Anxiety
   anticipatory, 401
   stress induced, 156, 265, 332
Apples, 209, 393
Apple scent, sleep and, 119
Aromatherapy, **138–41**. *See also* Fragrances
Art, energizing colors in, 53
Asparagus, 26
Aspirin, for colds and flu, 300
Astemizole, 260, 362
Asthma, swimming and, 261
Autogenic relaxation, **98–100**
Avocados, 20, 26

Basil scent, 141
Bathing, **142–44**
   essential oils and, 140
   ginger and, 142

Bathing *(continued)*
　herbs for, 143–44
　insomnia and, 117–18, 400
　for relaxation, 142–44
Beans, 15, 20, 26
Beef, 16
Benadryl, 259, 362
Bergamot scent, 140
Beta agonists, sleep problems and, 122
Beta-blockers, fatigue from, 362
Beta brain waves, 59, 214
Beta-carotene, 209
Bible, reading for energy, 199
Bicycling, 71
BioDots, for mood evaluation, 104–5
Bioenergetics, 159, 164
Biofeedback, **101–6**, 104–5
　benefits of, 101–2
　equipment, 97, 101, 103–4
　for managing
　　allergies, 260, 262
　　stress, 101, 285
　　worry, 425
　for relaxation, 101–6, 104–5
Bird feeder, 196
Blood fat level, 194
Blood pressure
　increased, 90
　laughter and, 171–72
　pet ownership and, 194
　spikes in, 72
Blood sugar level
　glycemic index and, 6
　low, 20, 21
　pet ownership and, 194
　protein and, 13
　sugar and, 10–11, 253, 300
Blood tests, 18–19
Body clock
　energy peaks and, 69
　in scheduling for energy, 111
　sleep and, 126–27, 214–16
Boredom, **263–68**, 266, 268
Boring people, dealing with, 92
Boysenberries, 26
Brain cells, aging and, 250–51
Brain waves. *See* Alpha brain waves; Beta
　brain waves
Bran, 19
Breads, whole-wheat, 5, 23
Breakfast, energizing, 27, 376
Breakup of relationship, stress of, 79, 89
Breathing. *See* Calming breathing; Deep
　breathing
Brewer's yeast, 22
Broccoli, 22
Brompheniramine, drowsiness from, 362

Bronchodilators, sleep problems and, 122
Burnout, **269–75**
　managing, 271–75
　signs of, 270–71
B vitamins, **16–17**
　deficiencies in, 16, 25
　energy metabolism and, 4, 28
　for headaches, 335
　immune system and, 204–5
　sources of, 16–17, 205
　supplements, 17

Cafergot, stimulant in, 364
Caffeine. *See also specific sources*
　colds and flu and, 303
　effects of
　　dehydration, 152, 243
　　energy boost, 150–51
　　headaches, 333–34
　　heart rate, increased, 150–51
　　sleep problems, 122, 400
　hypoglycemia and, 11
　in medications, 122, 153, 364
　nicotine and, 152
　pregnancy and, 153
　premenstrual syndrome and, 393
　reducing intake of, 152
　smoking and, 152
　sources of, 150
"Caffeine buzz," 151
Calcium, premenstrual syndrome and,
　393
Calcium channel blockers, 363
Calming breathing, sleep and, 398–99
Calories
　burning, 3–4, 238
　from dietary fat, 10
　soldiers' amount of, 21
Candy, 13
Carbohydrates, **4–8**, 6–7
　complex, 4, 253, 300
　energy bursts from, 28
　exercise and, 66
　fat in, dietary, 8
　glycemic index and, 5, 6–7
　metabolism of, 5, 16
　simple, 253
　sources of, 4–5, 8, 209
Carbo loading, 8
Carpooling, 306
Celiac disease, gluten allergy and, 262
Cereals, 17
CFS. *See* Chronic fatigue syndrome
Chamomile scent, 141
Chi (positive energy), 62–63
Chicken, 15
Childbirth classes, 387

Child rearing, **276–82**. *See also* Teenagers
  communication in, 281–82
  decision making in, 281–82
  discipline in, 281–82
  fun in, 279–80
  shortcuts in, 276–79
Chlorpheniramine, drowsiness from, 362
Chlor Trimeton, drowsiness from, 362
Chocolate, 209
Cholesterol level, 16–17, 194
Chores
  bartering, 114
  housecleaning, 343–47
  meditation with, 180
  scheduling, 112
  sharing, 84, 278
Chromium, **20–23**
Chronic disease, **283–86**. *See also specific*
    types
Chronic fatigue syndrome (CFS), **287–97**,
    290, 292, 294–95. *See also* Fatigue
  diagnosing, 288–89, 291–93
  energy management with, 293
  fibromyalgia and, 288
  help hotline for, 292
  Lyme disease and, 288
  managing
    aromatherapy, 141
    exercise, 289, 291, 294–97
    individual cases of, 294–95
  memory loss with, 288, 291
  symptoms of, 287–88, 290
Cigarette smoking. *See* Nicotine; Smoking
Cimetidine, mononucleosis and, 369–70
Cinnamon, 22
Circadian rhythms, naps and, 191
Circulation, laughter and, 171–72
Citrus scents, 60, 140
Claritin, drowsiness from, 362
Classes, educational, 95
Clay bath, 143
Clothing
  energizing colors of, 56
  self-esteem and, 350
Cloves, 22
Clutter, cleaning as energizer, **114–15**
Codeine, stimulant in, 364
Coffee, **150–53**. *See also* Caffeine
  colds and flu and, 303
  controversy about, 150
  effects of
    dehydration, 243
    situational insomnia, 400
  energy from, 150–51
  iron absorption and, 25
  tannins in, 25
"Coffee nerves," 151

Cognitive problems, with chronic fatigue
    syndrome, 288, 291
Cognitive therapy, for boredom, 268
Colas
  caffeine in, 150–51
  dehydration from, 243
  headaches and, 333–34
Colds and flu, **298–304**, 301
  cautions about, 303–4
  energy loss from, 298
  managing, 299–303, 301
  remedies, 300–303, 301
Collaboration in relationships, 84
Colors, **52–56**, 54–55
  of clothing, 56
  for energizing environment, 52–56,
    54–55
  personality and, 53, 55–56
  psychological effects of, 52, 54–55
  of toys, 227
Commitment in relationships, 85
Communication
  art of, 81–84
  in child rearing, 281–82
  of chronic disease, 284
  in marriage, 85
  with teenagers, 414–15
Commuting, **305–7**
  exercising while, 306
  prayer during, 201
Contrast bath, 143
Cooking, when entertaining, 318–19
Cravings, food, 12
Crying, anger and, 159
Cultural differences in touching, 167, 221

Dairy products, premenstrual syndrome and,
    393
Darvon N Compound, 364
Daydreams, as energizer, **154–55**, 178–79
De-catastrophizing, worry and, 424
Decision makers, types of, 145–46
Decision making, **145–49**, 147
  in child rearing, 281–82
  energy needed for, 145–49, 147
Deep breathing, **156–57**
  benefits of, 156
  exhaling in, 157
  in-bed, 325
  inhaling in, 157
  for managing
    burnout, 273–74
    child rearing, 282
    depression, 309
  technique for, 157
Dehydration, 152, 242–43, 255–56
Delegating work, **113–14**, 372

Depressants, 254
Depression, **308–11**
  boredom and, 267–68
  overweight and, 377
  problem of, 308
Dessert, health benefits of, 12
Dessert scents, stress and, 59
Diabetes, 20, 22
Diaries. *See* Logs
Diet, **3–27**. *See also* Eating for energy;
    Recipes for energy
  for managing
    aging, 252–53
    allergies, 262
    burnout, 272
    colds and flu, 300
    life changes, 355–56
    premenstrual syndrome, 393–94
    situational insomnia, 401
  vegetarian, 17
Dieting, 4
Difficult people, as energy demons, **312–16**,
   313
Digestion, overeating and, 9
Dimetapp, drowsiness from, 362
Dimmers, psychological effects of, 57–58
Diphenhydramine
  for allergies, 259
  drowsiness from, 362
Dock weed, magnesium in, 20
Dress
  energizing colors of, 56
  self-esteem and, 350
Drinking problem, 254, 256–57
Driving. *See* Commuting
Drugs. *See* Medications; *specific types*

Earplugs, sleep and, 123
Eating for energy, **3–27**. *See also* Diet;
    Recipes for energy
  biochemistry changes and, 18
  B vitamins, 16–17
  carbohydrates, 4–8, 6–7
  chromium, 20–23
  energy bars, 21, 24
  energy metabolism and, 3–4
  glycemic index and, 5, 6–7
  insulin spikes, 11–13
  iron, 23–26
  light meals, 252
  magnesium, 17–20
  minimeals, 27, 252, 385–86
  overeating, avoiding, 8–10
  protein, 13–15, 14
  schedules in, 9, 27, 393
  soldiers' intake, 21
  sugar, 10–11

Echinacea, for colds and flu, 302
Eggs, 15–17, 26
Ejaculation, vitamins lost with, 204
Emotional loss, as energy demon, **326–30**,
  328
Empathy
  difficult people and, 316
  forgiveness and, 160
Empirin, stimulant in, 364
Endorphins, 174, 238–39
Energy bars, 21, 24
Energy metabolism, **3–4**, 11, 23, 28
Energy peaks, 69
Entertaining, **317–21**
Environments for energy, **51–65**
  color, 52–56, 54–55
  feng shui and, 62–63
  fragrances, 58–60
  lighting, 56–58
  manipulating, 51
  plants, 60–61, 61, 64
  temperature in house, 65
Essential fatty acids, 273
Essential oils, in aromatherapy, 139–41
Exercise, **66–78**. *See also* Aerobic exercise;
    Walking; Yoga
  while commuting, 306
  eating and, 27, 208
  effects on
    carbohydrate consumption, 66, 208
    immune system, 66
    sleep, 122, 127
  fat burning during, 151
  fatigue and, 69
  during holidays, 341
  ideal prescription for, 219
  in bed, 323–25
  logs, 77
  for managing
    aging, 251–52
    allergies, 261–62
    boredom, 265
    burnout, 272
    chronic fatigue syndrome, 289, 291,
      294–97
    colds and flu, 301
    grief, 330
    headaches, 334
    life changes, 356
    mononucleosis, 369
    overweight, 376
    pregnancy, 387
    premenstrual syndrome, 391–92
    quitting smoking, 407
    situational insomnia, 400
  medical evaluation before, 68
  with music, 184–88

for posture corrections, 381–84,
382
prayer during, 201
program for, starting, 67–68, 68
runner's high from, 135–36
strength training, 72–74, 252
stretching, 74–77, 76
swimming, 261, 294–96
trainer for, 67
warm up before, 70–71, 73, 75
water intake before, 243
weight lifting, 72–74, 252
yoga, 74–75

Family meetings, teenagers and, 413
Fans, sleep and, 124
Fantasy, as energizer, **154–55**, 178–79
Fat, body, as energy demon, **374–77**
Fat, dietary
burning, 151
calories from, 10
in carbohydrates, 8
insulin and, 11
reducing, 10, 253, 300, 375, 404
saturated, 14
Fatigue. See also Chronic fatigue syndrome
(CFS)
in afternoon, 76
biochemistry changes and, 18
causes of
anemia, iron-deficiency, 23
antihistamines, 259, 362
chronic disease, 283
gluten allergy, 262
medications, 259, 358–59, 362–64,
363
moving, 371–73
nutrient deficiencies, 3, 16–18
stress, 332
exercise and, 69
managing
caffeine, 150
delegating work, 113–14
foot massage, 223
looking out window, 177
napping, 126
visualization, 98
operant, 179
Feng shui, 62–63
Ferritin levels, 25
Feverfew, for headaches, 336
Fiber, 209. See also Carbohydrates
Fibromyalgia, chronic fatigue syndrome and,
288
Fiorinal, stimulant in, 364
Fish, 15, 17, 19
Flatulence, 15

Floor coverings
energizing colors of, 56
in feng shui, 63
Floral oils, in aromatherapy, 141
Flu. See Colds and flu
Fluorescent bulbs, psychological effects of,
57
Folate, sources of, 16, 26, 209
Folic acid
deficiencies, 25–26, 369
sources, 26
Food. See also Diet; Eating for energy;
Recipes for energy; specific types
acidic, iron absorption and, 25
allergies to, 262
fast, 8, 10
leftover, as snack, 209
low-fat, 10, 13
Forgiveness, as energizer, **158–61**
Fragrances, **58–60**, 119, 121. See also
Aromatherapy
Fructose, sources of, 255, 393
Fruits. See also specific types
alcohol burning and, 255
beta-carotene in, 209
carbohydrates in, 209
dried, 209
fiber in, 209
folate in, 26, 209
fructose in, 255, 393
magnesium in, 209
nutrients in, 12
sugar in, 12, 393
vitamin C in, 209
Fun. See also Humor
in child rearing, 279–80
life changes and, 355

Garlic, for colds and flu, 302–3
Gas, reducing digestive, 15
Gender differences in sex drive, 203
Geranium oil, 141
Getting up in morning, **322–25**
Ginger, 22, 142, 336
Glucose, 4–5, 6–7, 11
Glucose polymers, 21
Glucose tolerance factor (GTF), 22
Gluten, food allergies and, 262
Glycemic index, 5, 6–7
Glycogen, 8
Grains
B vitamins in, 5, 17
carbohydrates in, 4–5
chromium in, 23
cooking, 5
magnesium in, 19
refined, 5

Grains *(continued)*
    as snacks, 209
    whole, 4–5
Gratitude, as energizer, **162–64**
Grazing, for overweight people, 375–76
Grief, as energy demon, **326–30**, <u>328</u>
Groups of people. *See also* Support groups
    energy from, 174
    for managing
        aging, 248–50
        boredom, 267
    vacationing with, 230
Grudges, dropping, **158–61**
GTF, 22
Guided imagery, as energizer, 154–55

Haddock, 19
Halibut, 19
Ham, 23
Headaches, 153, **331–36**
Health clubs, 73, <u>232</u>
Heart rate
    effects on
        aerobic exercise, 70
        caffeine, 150–51
        drumbeat, 185
        laughter, 171–72
        music, 184
        target, 71
"Helper's high," from volunteering, 135
Hemoglobin, iron and, 23
Herbs
    for bathing, 143–44
    for energy, 141
    for managing
        colds, 302
        headaches, 335
        premenstrual syndrome, 394
Hismanal
    for allergies, 260
    drowsiness from, 362
Holidays, as energy demon, **337–42**
Home diffuser, for essential oils, 139
Honey, 255
Honeymoon, reliving for romance, 86
Hops bath oil, 143
Hormone changes, insomnia and, 117
Housecleaning, as energy demon, **343–47**
Houseplants, 60–61, <u>61</u>, 64
Hugging, as energizer, **165–67**
Humidity, plants in controlling, 61
Humor. *See also* Fun
    as energizer, **171–75**, <u>175</u>
    for managing
        aging, 249
        child rearing, 281
        difficult people, 314–15

Hydroxyzine, for allergies, 259
Hyperglycemia, 20
Hypoglycemia, 11, 20, <u>21</u>
Hypothermia in elderly, 194–95

Imagination, for relaxation, **97–98**, 100,
    188
Immune system
    effects on
        exercise, 66
        iron, 23
        laughter, 171
        sleep, 299
        vitamins, 204–5
    T-cells and, 369
Incandescent lights, psychological effects of,
    57
Indoor lights, sunlight vs., 212–13
Insomnia. *See also* Situational insomnia
    causes of, 117
    incidence of, 116–17
    managing
        bathing, 117–18, 400
        fragrances, 119, 121
        lighting, 123–24, 127, 400
        mind games, 119–20
        television, 119
        worry diary, 120
    performance anxiety, 121
Instincts, 148, 341
Insulin, **11–13**
    chromium and, 20, 22
    fat and, 11
    hypoglycemia and, <u>21</u>
    protein and, 13
    small meals and, 252
    spikes, 11–13
    sugar's effects on, 11
Intelligence (IQ), <u>147</u>
Internal clock. *See* Body clock
Intimacy, touching and, 223–24
Iron, **23–26**, 386

Jasmine scent, 59, 141
Jet lag, as energy demon, 216
Job. *See* Work
Jokes, <u>175</u>. *See also* Fun; Humor
Journal writing, **168–70**, 329, 354. *See also*
    Logs
Juice
    fluid loss and, 243
    grapefruit, 13, 243
    iron absorption and, <u>24</u>, 25
    orange, 13, <u>24</u>, 25, 243
    potassium in, 13, <u>24</u>
    sugar in, 12–13
    vegetable, 13

Labels
food, 5, 17, <u>24</u>, 140
medication, 122, 153, 360
Laughter, as energizer, **171–75**, <u>175</u>. *See also* Fun; Humor
Lavender bath oil, 143–44
Lavender scent, for managing
insomnia, 119, 121
stress, 141
L-dopa, for restless legs, 123
Lean body mass, protein and, 14
Leisure activities, 107, 164
Lemon bath oil, 143–44
Lemon scent, 60
Licorice, for colds and flu, 302
Life changes, major, **353–56**
Life expectancy, increasing, 95
Lighting, **56–58**
in feng shui, <u>63</u>
for managing
insomnia, 123–24, 127, 400
seasonal affective disorder, 214–15
personality and, 56–57
Listening, relationships and, 82–83
Lists
organizational, **109–10**
"to do," 109, 149, 278, 401
of wonderful things, 163
Logs
activity, 110
energy, 169–70
exercise, 77
health, 289
laughter, 172–73
pleasure, 341
premenstrual, 391
for prioritizing tasks, 149
worry, 120
Looking out window, as energizer, **176–79**
Loratadine, drowsiness from, 362
Love letters, for romance in relationships, 86
Low self esteem, as energy demon, **348–52**, <u>350</u>
Lunch, energizing, <u>18</u>
Lyme disease, chronic fatigue syndrome and, 288

Magnesium, **17–20**
deficiencies of, 18–19
energy metabolism and, 4
for headaches, 336
sources of, 19–20, 209
supplements, 336
Magnesium aspartate, 20
Magnesium gluconate, 20
Marriage, 84–85

Massage
essential oils for, 139
foot, <u>223</u>
at health spa, <u>232</u>
maternity, 387
in pleasuring, <u>83</u>
self, <u>222–23</u>
Meat, 16, 25–26. *See also* Fish
Medical evaluation
before exercising, <u>68</u>
for overweight people, 375
Medications, **357–64**, <u>358–59</u>. *See also* specific types
alcohol and, 361
alternative medicine vs., <u>363</u>
caffeine in, 122, 153, 364
fatigue from, <u>358–59</u>, 362–64, <u>363</u>
labels on, 122, 153, 360
for managing
allergies, 259–60
headaches, 332–33
sleep problems, 122, 396–97
mixing, avoiding, 361
natural, <u>363</u>
with stimulants, 364
switching, 362–64
Meditation, **180–83**
during chores, 180
for laughter, 174
for managing
burnout, 274
premenstrual syndrome, 392
tai chi, 218–19
transcendental, 180, 274
during walking, 182
Meetings, as energy demons, **365–67**
Melissa scent, 141
Memory
chronic fatigue syndrome and, 288, 291
fragrances and, 59–60
Menopause, iron supplements and, 23
Menstrual cycle, insomnia and, 117
Mental focus, 182–83. *See also* Meditation
Metabolism
aging and, 252
of carbohydrates, 5, 16
energy, 3–4, 11, 23, 28
Methylphenidate, sleep problems and, 122
Midol Maximum Strength, 364
Minerals. *See also* specific types
for energy metabolism, 4
soldiers' intake of, <u>21</u>
Mononucleosis, as energy demon, **368–70**
Mood
effects on
aerobic exercise, 70
fragrances, 59–60, 140

Mood *(continued)*
  effects on *(continued)*
    laughter, 174
    lighting, 56–57
    music, <u>186–87</u>
Mood cards, <u>105</u>
Mood rings, <u>104–5</u>
Morale, pet ownership and, 194
Morning, as energy demon, **322–25**
Moving, as energy demon, **371–73**
Muscles
  aging and, 66, 247
  energy and, 72
  strength training and, 72–74
Music, **184–90**, <u>186–87</u>
  for depression management, 309
  for energy, 189–90
  exercise with, 184–88
  heart rate and, 184
  mood, <u>186–87</u>
  for relaxation, 188–89
  with visualization, 188

Naps, **191–92**. *See also* Resting
  circadian rhythms and, 191
  for managing
    child rearing, 276–77
    fatigue, 126
    mononucleosis, 368
    situational insomnia, 400
  sleep inertia and, 192
  strategies for, 192
Nasal congestants, sleep and, 122
Negative thinking, <u>133</u>, 155, 284
Nicotine. *See also* Smoking
  caffeine and, 152
  chewing gum, 408
  smoking and, 402
  supplement therapy, 408
Nutrients. *See also specific types*
  energy levels and, 252
  for energy metabolism, 4
  in fruits, 12
  for managing
    anemia, 25–26
    mononucleosis, 369
    premenstrual syndrome, 393
Nutrition, **3–27**. *See also* Diet; Eating for energy; Recipes for energy
Nuts, 19

Obsessing, boredom and, 265
Odors, **58–60**, 119, 121. *See also* Aromatherapy
Odor therapy, **138–41**.
Oranges, 26, 209, 393

Organizing. *See* Scheduling and organizing for engery
Overcommitment, **110–13**
Overeating, **8–10**, 355–56
Overload, <u>268</u>
Overweight, as energy demon, **374–77**
Overwork. *See* Burnout
Oxygen
  for energy metabolism, 23
  for red blood cells, 23, 25

Pain management of chronic disease, 285–86
Pain relievers, caffeine in, 153. *See also specific types*
Papayas, 26
Parsley, 26
Pasta, 8
Peanut butter, 19
Peanuts, 19
Pepper, 22
Peppermint scent, 141
Performance anxiety, insomnia, 121
Personality, **80–81**, 108
  colors and, 53, <u>55–56</u>
  lighting and, 56–57
  relationships and, 80–81
  toys and, 226
  Type A, 53, 174
Pets, **193–96**
  as energizers, 193–96
  health benefits of, 193–95
  touching, 224
Physical examination
  before exercising, <u>68</u>
  for overweight people, 375
Plants, for energizing environment, 60–61, <u>61</u>, 64
Play, as energizer, **225–27**
Pleasuring, touch and, <u>82–83</u>
PMS, **390–94**
Pork, 16
Positions, sex, 204
Positive thinking, **131–34**
  affirmations, 131–34
  with daydreams, 155
  for managing
    chronic disease, 284
    colds and flu, 300
    life changes, major, 354
    getting up in morning, 325
    pregnancy, 388
    worry, 424–25
Posture
  correcting poor
    exercises for, 381–84, <u>382</u>

sitting, 378–80
walking, 380–81
effects of poor, 378
feelings evoked by, 159, 164
Potassium, 13, <u>24</u>, 243, 253
Poultry, 15
Prayer, as energizer, **197–201**
Pregnancy, **385–89**
caffeine and, 153
energy loss from, 385
essential oils and, 141
insomnia caused by, 117
managing
childbirth classes, 387
exercise, 387
mental boosters, 387–89
Premenstrual syndrome (PMS), **390–94**
Prescriptions. *See* Medications
Problem solving, laughter and, 171
Progressive muscle relaxation, sleep and,
397–98
Props, laughter and, 173
Protein, **13–15**, <u>14</u>
alcohol burning and, 255
benefits of, 13–14
blood sugar level and, 13
lean body mass and, 14
light lunch high in, <u>18</u>
low-fat foods with, 375
sources of, <u>14</u>, 15
Prozac, 308–9
Psychotherapy for managing
boredom, 268
depression, 308–9
Pudding, sleep and, 119
Purslane weed, 20

Recipes for energy, **28–50**
Apricot Cinna-Muffins, 45
Bistro Pepper Steak with Herbed Oven
Fries, 37
Couscous Vegetable Medley, 38
Dilled Halibut Skillet Dinner, 35
Fruit-Bowl Cake with Orange–Cream
Cheese Frosting, 46–47
Garden Patch Pasta, 29
Gingery Date-Nut Bars, 44
Lentil Tacos with the Trimmings, 36
Northern Italian Tuna-Bean Salad, 30
Southwestern Pumpkin and White Bean
Chili, 33
Spinach-Orange Salad with Sesame, 40
Sweet and Spicy Snack Mix, 50
Tabbouleh, 39
Top Secret Chocolate Pudding, 41
Tropical Fruit Smoothie, 28

Turkey-Vegetable Wedges, 32
Tuscan Beans and Pork with Rice, 34
Vegetable Miso Soup with Ramen
Noodles, 31
Wheat and Walnut Bread, 48–49
Whole-Wheat Buttermilk Pancakes with
Blueberry Cinnamon Sauce, 42–43
Red blood cells, oxygen for, 23, 25
Relationship inventory, <u>88</u>
Relationships for energy, **79–95**
boring people and, <u>92</u>
breakup and, 79, 87–89
communication and, 81–84
groups of people and, 93–95
marriage, 84–85
personality and, 80–81
pleasuring, <u>82–83</u>
protecting self and, 89–91
romance, 85–87
temper tantrums and, <u>94</u>
at work, 91–93
Relaxation, **96–106**
alpha brain waves and, 96
autogenic relaxation, 98–100
bathing for, 142–44
biofeedback for, 101–6, <u>104–5</u>
meditation for, 180–83
music for, 188–89
progressive muscle relaxation, 397–98
smiling for, 77
tai chi for, 218–19
vacations for, 228–34, <u>231</u>, <u>232</u>
visualization for, 97–98, 188, <u>260</u>, 262
yoga for, 96–97, 100–101, <u>102–3</u>
Repetitive work, 189–90
Resistance training, 72
Resting. *See also* Naps
as energizer, 192
for managing
burnout, 273
colds and flu, 299
life changes, 355
pregnancy, 386
premenstrual syndrome, 392
Restless legs
iron-deficiency anemia and, 23
sleep problems and, 123
Retreats, vacations at, <u>231</u>
Rhinovirus, <u>301</u>
Riboflavin, 335–36
Ritalin, 122
Rituals
gratitude and, 163
holiday, 339
Romance, **85–87**
Rosemary scent, 141

Rose oil, 141
Rosewood scent, 141
Routines
    child rearing and, 277
    morning, 322–23
    quitting smoking and, 405
Runner's high, 135–36

SAD, 211–15
Salt, 24, 253
Sandalwood scent, 141
Scents. *See* Aromatherapy; Fragrances; *spe-cific types*
Schedules
    aromatherapy, 139
    coffee breaks, 152
    daydream, 155
    for eating, 9, 27, 393
    exercise, 78
    prayer, 200
    sex, 203–4
    sleep, 121–22, 396
    snack, 208
    vacation, 229
    walking, 240
Scheduling and organizing for energy,
        107–15
    body clock and, 111
    chores, 112
    for cleaning, 114–15
    delegating work, 113–14
    lists, 109–10
    overcommitment and, 110–13
    suggestions for, 107–9
Scream therapy, anger and, 159
Seasonal affective disorder (SAD),
        211–15
Seaweed, 20
Seeds, 19
Seldane
    for allergies, 260
    drowsiness from, 362
Self-acceptance, 350
Self-defense, 218–19
Self-esteem
    delegating work and, 114
    effects on
        pet ownership, 194
        volunteering, 136
    low, 348–52, 350
Senses, in daydreaming, 155
Serotonin production, 119, 401
Serum level, 18–19
Sex, **202–5**
    effects on
        aging, 250
        alcohol, 204

smoking, 204
    vitamins, 204–5
endocrine system and, 202–3
fragrances and, 59
gender differences and, 203
positions, 204
schedules, 203–4
Sexual harassment, 166
Sexual innuendo, 175
Shellfish, B vitamins in, 17
Shoes, walking, 241
Shrines, visiting, 200
Sick building syndrome, plants and, 60–61
Situational insomnia, **395–401**, 398–99. *See also* Insomnia
    causes of, 396
    managing, 395–97, 398–99, 400–401
Sleep apnea, 116, 118
Sleep inertia, 192
Sleeping for energy, **116–27**
    aging and, 126–27
    insomnia and, 117
    positions for, 124
    snoring and, 118
    strategies for, 117–24
    yawning and, 125
Sleeping pills, 398
Sleep mask, 123
Smells, **58–60**, 119, 121. *See also* Aroma-therapy
Smiling, **206–7**
    laughter and, 174
    for relaxation, 77
Smoking, **402–8**. *See also* Nicotine
    caffeine and, 152
    effects of
        colds and flu, 304
        sex, decreased performance, 205
        sleep problems, 123
    quitting, 403–8, 404, 407
Snacks, **208–10**
    healthy, 10, 12, 27, 421
    quitting smoking and, 405
    situational insomnia and, 401
Snoring
    overweight and, 376–77
    sleep problems and, 118, 123–24
Sodas, 150–51. *See also* Colas
Sodium, 24, 253
Soldiers' intake, 21
Soup, 9, 209, 303
Soy, 15
Spices, 22
Spinach, 20
Spirituality, as energizer, **197–201**
Spiritual retreats, 231
Sports drinks, 10, 21, 24, 255

Sports energy bars, 24
Spruce scent, black, 141
Stair climbing, 71
Starch. *See* Carbohydrates
Stimulants, sedative medications and, 364
Strength training, **72–74**, 252
Stress
   blood cells and, 156
   blood sugar level and, 194
   causes of
      breakup of relationship, 79, 89
      moving, 372
   effects of
      anxiety, 156, 332
      colds and flu, 300
      fatigue, 332
      headaches, 332
      situational insomnia, 396
   managing
      aerobic exercise, 70
      aromatherapy, 59, 141
      biofeedback, 101, 285
      controlling personal life, 137
      laughter, 171
      lemon-lavender bath, 144
      looking out window, 177
      pet ownership, 194–95
      quitting smoking and, 407
      support groups, 93–95
      volunteering, 136
Stress cards, 105
Stress points, 104–5
Stretching, **74–77**, 76. *See also* Yoga
   boredom and, 265
   in-bed, 325
   in midafternoon, 76
   for relaxation and laughter, 174
Sugar, **10–11**, 253, 393, 401
Sunglasses, light energy and, 212
Sunlight, as energizer, **211–17**
Supplements
   B vitamins, 17
   chromium, 23
   folic acid, 369
   iron, 23, 25
   magnesium, 20
Support groups. *See also* Groups of people
   for managing
      burnout, 274
      chronic disease, 285
      grief, 328
      quitting smoking, 407
      stress, 93–95
Surprise, for romance, 86
Sweets, healthy, 12

Swimming, for managing
   asthma, 261
   chronic fatigue syndrome, 294–96
Swiss chard, 20

Tagamet, mononucleosis and, 369–70
Tai chi, **218–19**
   for good posture, 382
   for relaxation, 218–19
Tannins, in tea and coffee, 25
Taxes, as energy demon, **409–10**
T-cells, immune system and, 369
Tea
   caffeine in, 150–51
   dehydration from, 243
   iron absorption and, 25
   tannins in, 25
Teenagers, **411–15**, 413
Television, **416–21**
   child rearing and, 279
   eating while watching, 421–22
   laughter from watching, 173
   over-watching, 416–19
   therapeutic value of, 196
Temperature in house, 65, 123
Temper tantrums, managing, 94
Terfenadine
   for allergies, 260
   drowsiness from, 362
Testosterone level, sex and, 204
Therapeutic activities
   journal writing, 168–70
   pets, caring for, 193–96
Therapy, for boredom, 268
Thinking. *See also* Positive thinking
   clear, **145–49**, 147
   creative, 171
Thyroid replacement drugs, 122
TM, 180, 274
Tofu, 20
Touching, **220–24**, 222–23
   ethnic differences in, 167, 221
   feedback about, 224
   hugging and, 165–67
   intimacy and, 223–24
   motives behind, 221
   pets, 224
   pleasuring and, 82–83
   self-massage and, 222–23
Toys, as energizers, **225–27**
Trainer, professional, 67, 71, 73, 75
Transcendental meditation (TM), for relaxation, 180, 274
Treadmill stress test, 68
Triglyceride level, 194
Troublemakers, types of, 313

Tryptophan
  serotonin production and, 401
  sources of, 119
Type A personality, 53, 174

Vacations, **228–34**, 231, 232
  creative, 229–30
  for depression, 310
  group, 230
  health spas, 232
  schedules for, 229
  solo, 231
  spiritual retreats, 231
  virtual, 233
Valerian bath oil, 143
Values, in decision making, 148
Vanilla scent, 119
Vegetables. *See also specific types*
  folate in, 26
  with pasta, 8
  protein in, 15
Vegetarian diet, 17
Vistaril, for allergies, 259
Visualization, **97–98**
  for managing
    pregnancy, 388
    premenstrual syndrome, 392
    situational insomnia, 397
  music with, 188
  for relaxation, 97–98, 188, 260, 262
Vitamins. *See also specific types*
  for burnout, 273
  effects on
    immune system, 204–5
    sex, 204–5
  ejaculation and, 204
  for energy metabolism, 4
  for headaches, 335
  soldiers' intake of, 21
Vitamin B$_6$
  for managing
    headaches, 335–36
    nausea during pregnancy, 386
    premenstrual syndrome, 394
  supplements, 17
Vitamin B$_{12}$, 25–26
Vitamin C
  for colds and flu, 301–2
  in fruits, 209
  iron absorption and, 25
  premenstrual syndrome and, 394
Vitamin E
  for headaches, 336
  sources of, 205
  supplements, 336
Volunteering, as energizer, 95, **135–37**,
    163–64, 310

Walking, **235–41**, 236–39
  benefits of, 70, 238–39
  for managing
    aging, 252
    chronic fatigue syndrome, 296–97
  medical evaluation before, 68
  meditation during, 182
  posture, proper, 380–81
  programs, 236–39, 297
  in rain, 212
  schedules, 240
  shoes, 241
  in sunshine, 212
Warm up, before exercise, 70–71,
    73, 75
Water, positive effects of, 177
Water intake, **242–43**
  alcohol and, 243
  before exercise, 243
  for managing
    burnout, 273
    colds and flu, 299–300
    dehydration, 152, 243, 255–56
  toxins and, flushing out, 273
Weight gain, as energy demon, **374–77**
Weight lifting, **72–74**, 252
Weight-reduction drugs, 122
Wheat, food allergies and, 262
White noise generator, 123, 397
Windows, as energizers, **176–79**
Word games, laughter and, 175
Work
  boredom at, 267
  burnout from, 269–75
  commuting to, 305–7
  difficult people at, 312–16, 313
  naps at, 192
  relationships at, 91–93
  repetitive, 189–90
  self esteem and, 349
Workaholism, 269–75
Workouts. *See* Exercise
Worry, as energy demon, **422–26**, 424
Writing, journal, **168–70**, 329, 354. *See also*
    Logs

Yawning, 125
Yin/yang, 62
Yoga, **100–101**, 102–3
  for boredom, 265
  for correcting poor posture, 382
  for exercise, 74–75
  for relaxation, 96–97, 100–101, 102–3

Zen Buddhism, 181
Zinc, 4, 204–5, 302
Zoo, 196